Guidelines for Nurse Practitioners in Gynecologic Settings

Joellen W. Hawkins, RNC, PhD, FAAN, has been a women's health nurse practitioner since 1969 and currently practices at the Sidney Borum, Jr., Community Health Center in Boston. Since 1983, Dr. Hawkins has been the director of the women's health nurse practitioner program at the William F. Connell School of Nursing, Boston College, teaching clinical and theory courses for that program, as well as the advanced practice role course. She is the nursing editor of *Taber's Cyclopedic Medical Dictionary.* Her research includes abuse during pregnancy; coalition building to address violence in a community; and historical work on individual nurses, advanced practice nursing, and women's health nurse practitioners. She is the author or editor of 34 books and more than 100 articles in professional journals.

Diane M. Roberto-Nichols, BS, APRN-C, is an OB/GYN nurse practitioner. She has been employed at Ellington OB/GYN, a solo physician practice, for 16 years. Her focus has been women's health, starting as coordinator of the Women's Health Clinic at the University of Connecticut where she was instrumental in making contraception and confidential heath care available to female students. She also co-developed a protocol and implemented an assault crisis center for sexually and physically abused students at the University, as well as co-authored the protocols that served as the prototype for this book. She has continued to provide education and health care to women throughout the life span.

J. Lynn Stanley-Haney, MA, APRN-C, is an Adult Medicine nurse practitioner with special practice areas in Gynecology and Psychiatry. Since graduation and certification in 1980, she has been involved in a variety of practice settings where she has had an opportunity to pursue advocacy in women's health and access to care. As the Director of Nursing for the University of Connecticut Student Health Services she worked with their Women's Health Clinic in assuring quality of care and also provided direct care to students. Along with her long time colleague and co-author Diane Roberto-Nichols, she co-developed and implemented a 24-hour sexual assault crisis service for physically abused and sexually assaulted women students as well as co-authored the protocols that served as the prototype for this book. Since leaving the university, she has worked to implement and manage, as well as work clinically in state funded school-based health services. She has also maintained a clinical practice at Planned Parenthood of Connecticut as well as her current private practice setting. In addition, she maintains a private psychotherapy and medication management practice.

Guidelines for Nurse Practitioners in Gynecologic Settings

Ninth Edition

Joellen W. Hawkins, RNC, PhD, FAAN, FAANP

Diane M. Roberto-Nichols, BS, APRN-C

J. Lynn Stanley-Haney, MA, APRN-C

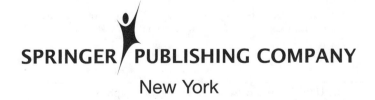

SPRINGER PUBLISHING COMPANY

New York

Springer Publishing Company, LLC.
11 West 42nd Street
New York, NY 10036
www.springerpub.com

Acquisitions Editor: Sally Barhydt
Production Editor: Carol Cain
Cover design by Joanne E. Honigman
Typeset by Apex Publishing, LLC

08   09   10/   5   4   3   2

Library of Congress Cataloging-in-Publication Data

Hawkins, Joellen Watson.

   Guidelines for nurse practitioners in gynecologic settings / Joellen W. Hawkins, Diane M. Roberto-Nichols, J. Lynn Stanley-Haney. — 9th ed.
       p. ; cm.
  Includes bibliographical references and index.
  ISBN-13: 978-0-8261-0300-0 (alk. paper)
  ISBN-10: 0-8261-0300-6 (alk. paper)
  1. Gynecologic nursing.   2. Nursing care plans.   I. Roberto-Nichols, Diane M.
II. Stanley-Haney, J. Lynn.   III. Title.
  [DNLM: 1. Genital Diseases, Female—nursing.   2. Nurse Practitioners.
3. Nursing Care—methods.   4. Patient Care Planning.   WY 156.7 H393g 2007]
  RG105.H368 2007
  618.1'0231—dc22   2007016187

Printed in the United States of America by Victor Graphics.

The authors dedicate this ninth edition to the memory of Dorothy Lewis, publisher and owner of Tiresias Press, New York City. Dorothy's belief in us made this project possible from its inception and through seven editions. Dorothy, you were an author's dream as a publisher.

Contents

PART II: APPENDIXES

Contents in Detail

Preface

This ninth edition of *Guidelines for Nurse Practitioners in Gynecologic Settings* has been revised extensively, using best evidence data from the literature, and is designed to guide the practice of nurse practitioners, nurse midwives, physician assistants, and other clinicians caring for women across the lifespan in ambulatory care settings. The concerns for which women may seek care include common gynecologic conditions, such as infections and sexually transmitted diseases, as well as managing life transitions such as menopause, fertility control, and preparing for pregnancy. Women also seek care and assistance when they encounter abuse; struggle with lifestyle issues such as weight management, smoking, stress and mental health; and face risks for heart disease and breast cancer.

The three authors of *Guidelines for Nurse Practitioners* are nurse practitioners in women's health care settings. All were actively involved in the development of the original guidelines and have continued to be responsible for updating these for each edition of the book. Several guidelines were developed by nurse practitioner colleagues with expertise in a particular specialty.

This ninth edition has several special features to assist you in your practice. In addition to a bibliography for each guideline, which are all new and reflect the latest literature and evidence-based practice, we have also included one or more Web site resources. Guidelines for sexually transmitted diseases, vaginitis, and vaginosis reflect the current CDC *Sexually Transmitted Diseases Treatment Guidelines 2006* and the recommendations of the American Society for Colposcopy and Cervical Pathology (ASCCP) Consensus Conference 2006 to revise the *2001 Guidelines for the Management of Cytological Abnormalities and Cervical Intraepithelial Neoplasia.* The information on hormone therapy, menopause, and osteoporosis reflects evidence-based practice generated through analysis of the emerging data from the Women's Health Initiative and other studies. Information on contraception is based on research articles and on the third edition of World Health Organization's *Medical Eligibility Criteria for Contraceptive Use* (2004). Information on natural family planning has changed significantly, and the revised guidelines have been prepared by an expert natural family planning (NFP) educator to reflect those changes.

New guidelines in the ninth edition cover vulvodynia, the contraceptive sponge, Implanon, Lea's Shield, FemCap, interstitial cystitis, as well as expanded information on polycystic ovary syndrome (PCOS), metabolic syndrome, and smoking cessation. All the patient education materials, which may be copied and given to patients, have been revised and updated, and several new ones have been created.

We hope that you, our colleagues in the care of women, will continue to find this ninth edition an invaluable source of current and reliable information in your clinical practice.

Joellen W. Hawkins
Diane M. Roberto-Nichols
J. Lynn Stanley-Haney

Acknowledgments

The authors wish to thank their colleagues whose contributions have enriched this ninth edition. The Breast Conditions guidelines were revised by Christine S. Edgerton, RNC, MS, Nurse Practitioner, Department of General Surgery, Breast Center, Lahey Clinic, Burlington, Massachusetts. The Medical Abortion guideline was created by Amy Kassirer, RNC, MS, MSW, Women's Health Nurse Practitioner at the Ob/Gyn Office of Dr. Marie Lemoier and at Four Women. Mary Finnigan, BA, MA, updated the Natural Family Planning guideline and appendix originally created by the late Eleanor S. Tabeek, RN, CNM, PhD, and revised in earlier editions by Nancy Keaveny, RN, BS. Linda Hansen Rodier, MS, RN, WHCNP, Dermatology Nurse Practitioner, Dartmouth-Hitchcock Dermatology Clinic, Manchester, New Hampshire, created the Vulvodynia guideline. Rosanna DeMarco, PhD, APRN BC, ACRN, Associate Professor, Community Health, William F. Connell SON, Boston College, updated the AIDS Risk Self-Assessment originally created by Richard S. Ferri, PhD, ANP, ACRN.

Introduction

Advanced practice nurses as well as other clinicians increasingly use clinical guidelines in their practice. Many states mandate that advanced practice nurses practice under written protocols or guidelines. Managed care systems often mandate the use of clinical guidelines by all their clinicians, particularly when the guidelines reflect best-practice standards and are generated from the literature on evidence-based practice. Such guidelines can also be linked to quality assurance programs.

There is empiric support for the fact that patient outcomes are at least 28 percent better when clinical care is based on rigorously designed studies (Fincout-Overholt, Melnyk, & Schultz, 2005). Having written this, we need to add that it often takes years for research to be incorporated into practice. Until the research–practice gap closes, clinical guidelines are one of the best ways for clinicians to stay up-to-date in practice and to apply the best available evidence to their care of patients.

REFERENCE

Fineout-Overholt, E., Melnyk, B. M., & Schultz, A. (2005). Transforming health care from the inside out: Advancing evidence-based practice in the 21st century. *Journal of Professional Nursing, 21,* 335–344.

PART I

Clinical Guidelines

CHAPTER ONE

Methods of Family Planning

HORMONAL CONTRACEPTION

I. Types of Hormonal Contraception

    A. Oral Contraceptives

      1. Definition:

Oral contraceptives (OC) (also known as birth control pills) are pills that when taken by mouth produce systemic changes that prevent conception.

        a. Types of Pills:

          1) A combination of synthetic estrogen and progestin

          2) Progestin only (also known as mini-pills)

      2. Directions for use (combination):

        a. The combination pill is taken for 21–24 days and an inert pill (or no pill) is taken for 7 days, during which time withdrawal bleed should occur; some packets have 21 oral contraceptive pills only, so the woman then takes no pills for 7 days.

        b. Consecutive use, 12 weeks or more, of a monophasic pill or Seasonal® (an 84 combination pill regime) may be considered in certain situations, or Lybrel® (ethinyl estradiol, levonorgestrel) (taken continuously) including:

          1) headaches regularly occurring during withdrawal weeks

          2) heavy withdrawal bleeds

          3) endometriosis after work-up

          4) patient's preference

3. Directions for use (progestin only):
   Progestin only pills are taken continuously.
   a. Indications for using progestin only pill:
      1) Is a good choice in situations when estrogen is contra-indicated:
         a) Smokers
         b) Lactation
         c) History/current deep vein thrombosis/pulmonary embolism
         d) Surgery with immobilization
         e) Valvular heart disease
         f) Severe headaches including migraine without focal neurological symptoms
         g) Gallbladder disease
         h) Seizure disorders
      2) Elevated blood pressure >/ = 140/90
   b. Other considerations for progestin only methods (advantages may outweigh risks):
      1) Undiagnosed breast cancer
      2) Gallbladder disease while on combination method
      3) Diabetes without vascular involvement (Type 1 or 2)
      4) Diabetes with nephropathy, retinopathy, or neuropathy
      5) History of current ischemic heart disease
      6) History of cerebrovascular accident
      7) Severe headaches, including migraines, with focal neurological symptoms
      8) Mild cirrhosis (uncompensated)
      9) Undiagnosed hypertension (not hypertension in pregnancy)
   c. Women who fit the above criteria after appropriate screening and physical exam may be candidates for progestin only, bearing in mind that irregular bleeding may present a major clinical problem. Since number of pills varies with manufacturer, carefully review instructions on use and pill pack.
4. Procedure for pill related bleeding problem, i.e., amenorrhea, scant menses, break-through bleeding:
   a. Rule out the following:
      1) Faulty OC taking (review packet)
      2) Pregnancy
      3) Uterine or cervical pathology—leiomyomata, polyp, cancer

    4) Pelvic or vaginal infection
    5) Drug interference
    6) Gastrointestinal problems
    7) Endometriosis
    8) Thyroid disorder
b. Based on information gained, treatment as follows:
    1) Amenorrhea or scant menses
        a) Reassure woman
        b) Consider method change
    2) Break-through bleeding
        a) During the first 3 months of hormone use, reassure only
        b) Consider method change
        c) Consider STD testing
        d) If treatment for a or b is unsuccessful and symptoms persist, consult with gynecologist.
    3) For hormonal amenorrhea:
        a) Pregnancy test
        b) If amenorrhea continues after 6 months and pill has not been changed, change pill; if no withdrawal bleed, discontinue pill and consider progestin challenge; if no withdrawal bleed, refer to amenorrhea protocol for work-up.
    4) If a woman is on any medications that decrease contraceptive effect, she should be offered the option of back-up contraception, such as condoms and/or spermicidal protection. Decisions about hormonal contraceptive use with medications should be individualized. If there is any question regarding drug interaction and interference of method with other drugs, consult with gynecologist or pharmacist.
5. Explanation of method:
  a. Ways in which oral contraceptives are taken:
    1) Start oral contraceptive on day 1 (first day of menses) OR Sunday start taking first pill on the first Sunday after the menstrual period begins OR Quick start taking the first pill at the time of the office or clinic visit regardless of cycle day (with the caveat that if this is after the 7th cycle day, patient could be pregnant at that time or become pregnant if a back-up method is not used for the first 7 days).
    2) Oral contraceptive must always be taken at the same time of day (within an hour either way).

3) Back-up contraception is necessary for 7 days (first cycle only) if OCs started later than the 5th cycle day.
4) In case of missed pills:
   a) One pill missed: woman to take pill when she remembers, and then take scheduled pill at regular time.
   b) Two pills missed in first 2 weeks: take 2 pills at regular time for 2 days. Use back-up contraception for the remainder of cycle.
   c) Two or more pills missed in third week, take 2 OCs daily until all OCs are taken; restart OC cycle with one pill daily within 7 days; use back-up contraception until OCs are restarted with new packet and for first 7 days of that packet.
   d) Three or more pills missed any time in cycle, restart OCs within 7 days with one pill daily. Use a back-up method for 7 days of that cycle.
   e) If one or more pills are missed, no back-up contraception is used, and no withdrawal bleed occurs, woman should be instructed to call to discuss possible pregnancy test.

B. Transdermal Contraceptive: Contraceptive Patch OrthoEvra®[1]
   1. Definition:
The contraceptive patch is a 3 layer transdermal polyethylene/polyester device about the size of a matchbook, with an adhesive on one side. It is impregnated with norelgestromin (NGMN), a synthetic progestin, and ethinyl estradiol (EE), a synthetic estrogen, and releases 150 micrograms of NGMN and 20 micrograms of EE every 24 hours.
   2. Directions for Use:
      a. Women weighing > 198 pounds (> 90 kg) are at an increased risk for pregnancy. An alternative method is recommended.
      b. Patch is changed weekly for 3 weeks then off for 1 week.
   3. Explanation of Method:
      a. Ways in which the patch is used:
         1) Apply the patch on first day of menses or on the first Sunday after bleeding begins; postpartum non-nursing 4 weeks or with resumption of menses.
         2) Apply to clean, dry, healthy skin on buttocks, abdomen, upper outer arm, or upper torso. Patch should not be applied to breasts.

3) Instruct woman not to use lotions, cosmetics, creams, powders, or other topical products in area of patch or area where patch will be applied.
4) Instruct the woman to press down firmly on patch for at least 10 seconds and then check that the edges adhere.
5) Instruct woman to check patch daily.
6) If patch detaches, instruct woman to immediately apply a new patch. Supplemental tapes or adhesives should not be used.
7) Apply a new patch the same day of the week 7 days after first patch. Repeat this in week 3.
8) No patch is applied in week 4.
9) Begin a new cycle on the same day of the week for week one and repeat cycle of 3 weeks on and 1 week off.
10) Withdrawal bleed will occur during 4th week.
11) If the woman forgets to apply a new patch and less than 48 hours have passed, she should apply a new patch as soon as she remembers and then apply that next patch on the usual renewal day.
12) If more than 48 hours have elapsed, the woman should stop the current cycle and immediately begin a new 4-week cycle by applying a new patch. The day for patch renewal will now change. Instruct her to use back up contraception for 1 week.
13) If missed change day occurs at the end of the 4-week cycle, instruct the woman to remove the patch and apply a new patch on the usual change day to begin a new cycle.

C. Intravaginal Contraceptive: Contraceptive Vaginal Ring Nuva-Ring®

   1. Definition:

The contraceptive vaginal ring is flexible, transparent, colorless, and about 2 inches in diameter. It is impregnated with etonogestrel, a synthetic progestin, and ethinyl estradiol (EE), a synthetic estrogen, and releases 120 micrograms of progestin and 15 micrograms of EE every 24 hours over a period of 3 weeks.

   2. Explanation of method and way in which ring is used:

     a. Insert ring into vagina between day 1 and day 5 of menstrual cycle.

     b. Keep ring in place for 3 weeks in a row.

     c. Remove ring for one week for withdrawal bleeding.

    d. If ring is removed and is out of the vagina for more than 3 hours, back up contraception is required for the next 7 days, except for hormone free week.
D. Intramuscular Contraceptive: Contraceptive Injectable (Depo-Provera®[3])
    1. Definition:

Synthetic hormonal substance in Depo-Provera (depot-medroxyprogesterone acetate or DMPA) that acts by blocking gonadotropin, thus preventing ovulation from occurring. This injectable decreases sperm penetration through cervical mucus and causes endometrial atrophy preventing implantation. Injected intramuscularly every 12 weeks into the muscle of the upper arm or buttocks.

    2. Explanation of use:

Depo-Provera is injected intramuscularly (in gluteal or deltoid muscle) or subcutaneously in the first 5 days of the menstrual cycle (after onset of menses), within 5 days postpartum, or, if breastfeeding, at 4–6 weeks postpartum.

The injection consists of one 150-milligram dose intramuscular or one subcutaneous injection of 104 milligrams of depot-medroxyprogesterone acetate every 12 weeks for as long as contraceptive effect is desired. If time between injections is greater than 13 weeks, do pregnancy test before administration. Inject IM with 1.5" up to 3" needle (depends upon size of woman since it needs to be deep intramuscular) or subcutaneously with a 1" needle, and do not rub the site as rubbing breaks up the microcrystals and increases absorption. Available in 150 mg/ml and 104 mg/0.65 ml prefilled syringes as well as single and multiple-dose vials.

Visit every 12 weeks for injection.
E. Contraceptive Implant: Implanon®
    1. Definition:

Single-rod implantable polymer contraceptive device impregnated with 68 mg of etonogestrel. It is effective for up to 3 years.

    2. Explanation of use:
        a. inserted subdermally on the inner side of the woman's upper arm the device releases a low, steady dose of progestin.

II. Physical Changes Occurring With Hormonal Contraception

    A. Ovulation is suppressed.
    B. The endometrium becomes deciduous making it unreceptive to implantation.
    C. The cervical mucus is altered, so it is hostile to sperm.
    D. Transport of the ovum may be altered.

E. Possible luteolysis.

F. Possible inhibition of capacitation of sperm.

III. Effectiveness

    A. 99.6% effectiveness rate for combination pill

    B. 97% effectiveness rate for progestin only pill

    C. 98–99% effectiveness rate for vaginal contraceptive ring

    D. 99% effectiveness for contraceptive patch

    E. 99%+ effectiveness for contraceptive injectable

    F. 99%+ effectiveness for contraceptive implant

IV. Contraindications

    A. Absolute contraindications to hormonal contraception (may vary with method)[2]:

        1. Thromboembolic disorder (or history thereof) including postpartum deep vein thrombosis, pulmonary embolism, or thromboembolism; stroke

        2. Thrombotic cerebrovascular accident (or history thereof)

        3. Coronary artery disease (or history thereof), or multiple risk factors for arterial cardiovascular disease; current angina pectoris; structural heart disease complicated by pulmonary hypertension; atrial fibrillation; valvular heart disease with complication

        4. Known or suspected carcinoma of the breast

        5. Major surgery with prolonged immobility or any surgery on the legs

        6. Known impaired liver function at present time; liver problems; hepatic adenoma; liver cancer, or history of active viral hepatitis; severe cirrhosis; benign or malignant liver tumor with prior OC use or other estrogen product

        7. Known or suspected estrogen dependent neoplasm (or history thereof) including endometrial carcinoma

        8. Over 35 and currently a smoker

        9. Triglyceride level greater than 350 mg/dl; hypercholesterolemia (type II hyperlipidemia)

      10. Known or suspected pregnancy

      11. Chronic hypertension and smoking or uncontrolled hypertension; vascular disease

      12. Weight > 198 lbs (> 90 kg); weight decreases efficacy

      13. Undiagnosed abnormal vaginal/uterine bleeding

      14. History of hormonal contraception-related cholestasis or cholestatic jaundice of pregnancy

15. Leiden factor V mutation
16. Allergic reaction to any components of the ring, patch, or Depo-Provera or any of its ingredients (check allergic reaction to local anesthetics for dental or other procedures—the carrier substance is the same for local anesthetics and Depo-Provera)
17. Migraines with aura at any age
18. Diabetics with nephropathy/retinopathy/neuropathy or diabetes of > 20 years duration
19. Breastfeeding < 6 weeks postpartum

B. Relative contraindications
1. Severe headaches or common migraines, which start or worsen with initiation of hormonal contraception use especially in women 35 or older
2. Hypertension with resting diastolic BP of 90 or more, or resting systolic BP of 140 or more on three or more separate visits, or an accurate measurement of 110 diastolic BP or more on a single visit
3. Impaired liver function (i.e., mononucleosis, acute phase, medication induced changes)
4. Hypertriglyceridemia; worrisome LDL : HDL ratio
5. Gallbladder disease: medically treated, current biliary tract disease

C. Other considerations (advantages of hormone contraception generally outweigh disadvantages):
1. Diabetes: without vascular disease
2. Congenital hyperbilirubinemia (Gilbert's disease)
3. Failure to have established regular menstrual cycle (without prior work-up) [See amenorrhea guideline]
4. Conditions likely to make it difficult for woman to use method correctly and consistently (learning disability, major psychiatric problems, alcoholism or other drug abuse, history of repeatedly taking oral contraceptives or other medications incorrectly)
5. Major surgery with no prolonged immobilization
6. Undiagnosed breast mass
7. Cervical cancer awaiting treatment; CIN
8. Use of drugs affecting liver enzymes (altering absorption of medication), eliphenytoin, carbamazapine, barbiturates, topiramate, primidone, rifampin, rifabutin, griseofulvin
9. Under 35 and heavy smoker (> 15/day)
10. Use in breastfeeding not yet approved for NuvaRing and OrthoEvra
11. Skin disorder that may predispose to application site reactions

V. Adverse Drug Interactions

A. All women prior to starting hormonal contraception and on a yearly follow-up basis should review and re-sign informed consent for method of choice—emphasizing drug interaction and knowledge of danger signs.

B. If a woman is on any medications that decrease contraceptive effect, she should be offered the option of back-up contraception such as condoms and/or spermicidal protection. Decisions about hormonal contraceptive use with medications should be individualized. If there is any question regarding drug interaction and interference of method with other drugs, consult with gynecologist or pharmacist.

C. Drug interactions with oral contraception. Some drugs can decrease the effectiveness of oral contraceptives by decreasing the available level of hormone. This can result in pregnancy. Drugs that may decrease the effectiveness of OCs include:

1. Antibiotics
   a. cephalosporins
   b. chloramphenicol
   c. macrolides
   d. penicillins
   e. tetracyclines
   f. sulfas
2. HIV protease inhibitors
   a. amprenavir
   b. nelfinavir mesylate
   c. ritonavir
   d. modafinil
3. Rifamycins
   a. rifampin
4. Anti-seizure medications
   a. barbiturates
   b. carbamazepine
   c. phenytoin
   d. primidone
   e. topiramate
5. St. John's Wart

VI. Laboratory

A. Lipid screen
   1. Lipid screen prior to using hormonal contraception
   Significant immediate family history

    a. Under age 50—stroke, coronary, or sudden death

Do lipid screen. If levels abnormal, consult with MD before starting hormonal contraception. If normal levels, start hormonal contraception and repeat test in 2 years.

    2. Lipid screen strongly advised if parents or siblings have hypertension, vascular disease, myocardial infarction, arteriosclerotic heart disease, and/or hyperlipidemia before age 50, or are on medication for hypertension.

  B. Monitor carefully any prediabetic and diabetic women using hormonal contraception. Consider screening with fasting blood sugar and/or 2-hour postprandial blood sugar if parents or siblings are diabetic or woman is otherwise at increased risk for developing diabetes.

  C. Liver profile if woman has had mononucleosis or mono-like illness within past year, or if patient has history of hepatitis or other liver disease or drug or alcohol history.

  D. In combination hormonal methods, Leiden factor V for women with personal or family history of venous thromboembolism.

VII. Follow Up

  A. For all methods of hormonal contraception:
    1. Blood pressure check as needed
    2. Smoking cessation counseling
    3. Review of side effects and danger signs
  B. For injectable:
    1. Depo-Provera
      a. Revisit every 12 weeks
      b. If greater than 13 weeks since last injection, use very sensitive pregnancy test prior to injection.[3]

See Appendix B for consent form and informational handout on oral contraceptives for patients. See other appendixes for informational handouts on other hormonal methods. See Bibliography. Web site: http://www.IMPLANON-USA.com.

INTRAUTERINE DEVICES (IUDS)

I. Definition/Mechanism of Action

  A. A sterile foreign body placed in the uterus to prevent pregnancy. This is accomplished through several mechanisms:
    1. A local sterile inflammatory response to the foreign body (i.e., the IUD) causes a change in the cellular makeup of the endometrium; with the copper devices there is an effect on

the endometrium of interfering with the enzyme systems, and with the progesterone device, an effect over time of a less well-developed endometrium.
2. A possible increase in the local production of prostaglandins that may increase endometrial activity.
3. Alteration in uterine and tubal transport.
4. IUDs probably exert an antifertility effect beyond the uterus and interfere with fertility before an ovum reaches the uterus.
5. Alteration of cervical mucus causing a barrier to sperm penetration (progesterone IUD).
6. Ovulation suppression first year with levonorgestrel intrauterine system (LNG IUS) Mirena®. Releases 20 mcg/day of levonorgestrel.

B. The exact mechanisms of action are not completely understood. One thing that has become clear is that the IUD does not act as an abortifacient.
C. Different types of IUDs use varying mechanisms of action to prevent pregnancy.

II. Effectiveness

A. Theoretically: 92.0–99.9% effectiveness rate
B. User: 92–99% effectiveness rate

The range is close, because the patient's participation is low, and therefore there is little possibility of patient error.

III. Contraindications

A. Absolute contraindications
1. Active pelvic infection (acute or subacute), including known or suspected gonorrhea or Chlamydia
2. Known or suspected pregnancy
3. Recent or recurrent pelvic infection; postpartum endometritis; postabortion infection (past 3 months)
4. Purulent cervicitis; untreated acute cervicitis or vaginitis
5. Undiagnosed genital bleeding
6. Distorted uterine cavity (bicornuate; severely flexed)
7. History of ectopic pregnancy
8. Allergy to copper (known or suspected) or diagnosed Wilson's Disease (ParaGard only); hypersensitivity to any part of Mirena®.
9. Abnormal Pap smear, cervical or uterine malignancy, or premalignancy (endometrial hyperplasia, cervical intraepithelial neoplasia, or cancer)

      10. Impaired responses to infection (diabetes, steroid treatment, immunocompromised patients)

      11. Presence of previously inserted IUD

      12. Genital actinomycosis

      13. Acute liver disease or liver tumor (Mirena®)

      14. Known or suspected breast cancer (Mirena®)

      15. Malignant gestational trophoblastic disease

      16. Known pelvic tuberculosis

B. Relative contraindications (benefits usually outweigh risks)

      1. Multiple sexual partners or partner has multiple partners

      2. Emergency treatment difficult to obtain should complications occur; this would primarily be a problem in very rural areas or developing countries

      3. Cervical stenosis

      4. Impaired coagulation response (ITP anticoagulant therapy, etc.)

      5. Uterus sounding less than 6 cm or more than 10 cm

      6. Endometriosis

      7. Leiomyomata

      8. Endometrial polyps

      9. Severe dysmenorrhea (Mirena® may be therapeutic)

      10. Heavy or prolonged menstrual bleeding without clinical anemia; consider oral iron or nutritional alterations to prevent with IUD (Mirena® may be therapeutic)

      11. Impaired ability to check for danger signals

      12. Inability to check for IUD string

      13. Concerns for future fertility

      14. History of PID; with subsequent intrauterine pregnancy, risk decreased

IV. Insertion Technique

    A. Procedure

      1. Woman is scheduled for appointment for insertion only during menses or within 7 days of onset of menses (Mirena®) and after

        a. Negative Papanicolaou smear (within 6 months)

        b. Negative gonorrhea/Chlamydia testing

        c. Appropriate medical and menstrual history is obtained

      2. Patient should be instructed to eat before coming to an appointment

      3. Take oral analgesic or nonsteroidal anti-inflammatory 30–60 minutes before procedure

4. IUD consent form (see Appendix B) and minor surgical consent form must be reviewed and signed at the time of an IUD consultation and evaluation, after discussion of
   a. Procedure
   b. Mechanism of the device
   c. Side effects and complications
   d. Relationship to woman's needs
5. Atropine 0.5 mg should be available at the time of insertion for severe vasovagal response.
6. Anxious woman, or woman for whom it is deemed necessary to perform a paracervical block and/or use IV atropine (to decrease likelihood of vasovagal reaction), should be referred to a gynecologist for insertion.
7. Insertion under sterile technique
   a. Bimanual examination to determine uterine position and size; insert warmed speculum
   b. Cleanse the vagina, cervix, and endocervical canal with iodine solution (unless allergic to iodine)
   c. Xylocaine gel or hurricane spray could be used to decrease discomfort of tenaculum
   d. Use tenaculum to straighten the uterine body and cervical canal
   e. Sound the uterus (depth less than 6 cm or more than 10 cm is contraindication)
   f. Insert specific IUD as instructed by manufacturer
   g. Spasm of the internal cervical os may occur; it is usually relieved by simply waiting. *Never* force entry of the sound or applicator.
   h. After insertion, observe the patient for weakness, pallor, diaphoresis, either bradycardia or tachycardia, hypotension, and syncope, which may occur (check blood pressure several times following insertion)
   i. If patient has mild cramping, the following may be used:
      1) Nonaspirin analgesic 650 mg every 4 hours, or
      2) A prostaglandin inhibitor (NSAID) such as Motrin® 400 mg orally 4 times a day.
   j. Explain to patient that the IUD is effective immediately. In some settings it is recommended that the patient abstain for 1 day due to disruption of cervical mucus barrier.
   k. Instruct patient to check for presence of IUD string post menstruation or after unusual cramping prior to relying on device for continued contraception effect.

l. Follow-up with appointment in 6 weeks to 3 months; at that time be sure the woman can feel the IUD strings.

V. Complications Following Insertion and What to Do About Them

A. Immediate, severe vasovagal response
   1. Notify physician
   2. Place patient in shock position
   3. Monitor pulse and blood pressure until stable
   4. Administer oxygen as needed
   5. Atropine 0.4 mg subcutaneously or intramuscularly may be administered if appropriate
B. Severe immediate cramping: remove IUD
C. Excessive pain or bleeding is often a sign of perforation (fundal); physician consult for management
D. Side effects or later complications
   1. Two or more missed periods: recommend a serum pregnancy test (e.g., Paragard®). With Mirena®, irregular, little or no bleeding is normal. Missed menses: 2 of 10 women have no menses after 1 year of Mirena®. Pregnancy is rare, but when this happens, there is a 50% chance of miscarriage. If IUD is removed, this drops to 25%.
   2. Pregnancy occurring while IUD is in place: it is now recommended that, due to risk of infection, the IUD should be removed at the time of diagnosis whether the pregnancy is continued or terminated. There should be consultation with a gynecologist prior to removal of the IUD by the gynecologist or nurse practitioner.
   3. Break-through bleeding related to IUD: use the following guidelines for removal:
      a. Bleeding is associated with endometritis
      b. Hematocrit falls 5 points
      c. There is a hematocrit of 30–32% or lower
      d. The IUD is partially expelled
      e. The patient wants the IUD removed
   4. Cramping and pelvic pain
      a. Rule out ectopic pregnancy
         1) Obtain a serum pregnancy test
         2) Consider ultrasound and surgical consult (physician consult)
      b. Pain or cramping caused by or associated with
         1) Partial expulsion of IUD
            a) Remove IUD

2) Pelvic inflammatory disease (a long-standing foul-smelling discharge in an IUD wearer is presumed to be PID until proven otherwise)
    a) Remove IUD
    b) Treat infection; culture, and sensitivity at time of removal and adjust treatment as indicated
    c) Consult a physician prior to inserting another IUD (some sources advise waiting a year)
3) Spontaneous abortion

5. Migraine headache
    1) First time or focal migraine with asymmetrical vision loss or other symptoms of transient cerebral ischemia, consult with a physician

6. Expulsion
    a. Objective findings when the cervix is visualized
        1) The IUD is seen at the cervical os or in the vagina
        2) The IUD string is lengthened (partial expulsion)
        3) The IUD string is absent (complete expulsion)
        4) The IUD cannot be located using various methods of probing (physician consult)
        5) The IUD is absent on ultrasound of abdomen
    b. Removal and reinsertion of IUD
        1) If partial expulsion occurs, IUD should be removed. IUD may be reinserted immediately if there is no infection or possibility of pregnancy, or with the next menses
        2) If completely expelled, a new IUD may be reinserted as outlined previously

7. Lost IUD strings
    a. Referrals for locating IUD include
        1) Exploration of canal with gentle probing; if not found, then,
        2) Ultrasound,
        3) Flat plate of abdomen, or
        4) Hysterosalpingogram

8. Difficulty in removing IUD
The following techniques may help in the removal of IUDs
    a. Remove only during menses
    b. Employ gentle, steady traction, remove IUD slowly. If IUD does not come out easily, physician consult is in order
    c. If IUD strings are not visible, nurse practitioner may probe for them in the cervical canal with narrow forceps

9. Uterine perforation (fundal or cervical), embedding of the IUD
   a. Objective findings include
      1) Absence of IUD string
      2) Inability to withdraw IUD if string is still present
      3) Demonstration of displaced IUD by ultrasound, hysteroscopy, or x-ray
   b. If perforation or embedding is suspected, referral to physician is in order
   c. Reinforcement of education that multiple partners increase the risk of infection, including HIV infection

VI. Follow-up

A. Yearly Papanicolaou test and pelvic examination with removal and reinsertion as the particular IUD requires (Mirena® 5 years; ParaGard T 380A® 10 years).
B. As needed for any of above-mentioned complications with physician consultation as necessary.

Appendix B may be photocopied for your patients as an informational handout as well as a consent form for using an IUD. See Bibliography. Web sites: http://www.paragardiud.com, http://www.Mirena.com/dtp.

BARRIER METHODS

Diaphragm

I. Definition/Mechanism of Action

A diaphragm is a shallow rubber or silicone cap with a flexible rim that is placed in the vagina so as to cover the cervix. It serves as both a mechanical barrier and a receptacle for (contraceptive) spermicidal cream or jelly, which must be used to insure effectiveness.

II. Effectiveness and Benefits

A. Method: 97% effectiveness rate
B. User: 80–85% effectiveness rate
C. May be inserted up to four hours prior to intercourse
D. May have some protective effect against transmission of certain sexually transmitted diseases
E. Effective form of contraception for women who have infrequent intercourse or in whom there are contraindications for other methods

III. Side Effects and Complications

  A. Allergic reaction of patient or her partner to rubber or to the spermicidal agent (a silicone diaphragm is available)
  B. Inability to achieve satisfactory fitting
  C. Inability of patient to learn correct insertion and/or removal technique
  D. Use may be associated with an increased incidence of urinary tract infection due to upward pressure of the rim of the diaphragm against the urethra
  E. Pelvic discomfort, cramps, pressure on the bladder or rectum can occur if:
    1. Diaphragm is too large
    2. Patient has chronic constipation
  F. Toxic shock syndrome: severe cases occurring immediately after use have been reported in diaphragm users during menses (although these appear to be related to damage to vaginal walls during scanty flow by tampon use rather than diaphragm use per se)
  G. Foul-smelling vaginal discharge may occur if the diaphragm is left in too long

IV. Types (Representative of Several Manufacturers)

  A. Arcing spring
    1. Sturdy rim with firm spring strength (spiral, coiled spring)
    2. Firm construction allows diaphragm to be kept in place despite rectocele, cystocele, mild pelvic relaxation, uterine retroversion
    3. Folds in an arc-shape
  B. Coil spring
    1. Spring in rim is spiral, coiled, and sturdy
    2. Best suited for women with good vaginal tone and no uterine displacement
    3. Folds flat for insertion
  C. Wide-seal
    1. Cuff inside rim
    2. Available in arcing and coil spring; also in silicone

V. Fitting

  A. Most diaphragms are available in sizes ranging from 50 or 55 millimeters to 95 or 100 millimeters (available sizes in 5 millimeter gradations)

B. Fit should be snug between the posterior fornix, pubic symphysis, and lateral vaginal walls, but should cause no pressure or discomfort

C. The patient may review and sign informed consent form (see Appendix B)

D. After a diaphragm has been fitted, instructions have been given, and the patient has demonstrated her ability to insert and remove it, she may be given an appointment for a follow-up visit in 1 week. During this week the patient is instructed to practice wearing the diaphragm for at least 8–hour intervals. (In many settings, 1-week follow-up may be unrealistic, so diaphragm fitting and use will be taught at one visit and the patient given the prescription or kit.) It is helpful for the patient to be given a phone number and times to call about any concerns or problems.

E. At optional follow-up appointment:
   1. Diaphragm is checked for fit and proper insertion
   2. Instructions are again reviewed and patient is given an opportunity to ask questions

F. If above criteria are met, patient is then given prescription for diaphragm

G. Yearly diaphragm check is recommended, but the patient should return for recheck sooner if:
   1. Diaphragm does not seem to fit well or can be displaced; this can occur with weight gain or loss of > 15 lbs
   2. She has any pelvic surgery
   3. She has a miscarriage, abortion, or wishes to resume using diaphragm after giving birth
   4. She is having problems with use

Appendix B may be photocopied and used as an informational handout on the diaphragm, as well as a consent form, for your patients. See Bibliography.

FemCap

I. Definition/Mechanism of Action

The contraceptive FemCap is a prescription-only contraceptive device that is used to hold spermicide and to provide a partial barrier to sperm when placed over the cervix.

II. Effectiveness and Benefits

   A. 96–98% effectiveness

B. May be inserted before intercourse and left in place for up to 48 hours
C. Latex free
D. Reusable for more than a year

III. Side Effects and Disadvantages

A. Vaginal irritation from the device
B. Vaginal irritation from the spermicide used with the device
C. Sensation of something in the vagina
D. Requires a prescription and pelvic examination

IV. Contraindications

A. Allergy to spermicide
B. Allergy to material device is made of
C. Partner allergy to device or spermicide
D. Device is expelled repeatedly during use
E. Cannot be used during menses
F. Known or suspected uterine or cervical cancer
G. History of toxic shock syndrome
H. Current infection of vagina or cervix, PID
I. Cannot be used during postpartum or after an abortion for 6 weeks
J. Adhesions between cervix and vaginal walls
K. Third-degree uterine prolapse
L. Cut or tear in vagina or cervix noted on pelvic examination

V. Types

A. Available in 3 sizes: 22 mm, 26 mm, and 30 mm

VI. Fitting

A. A pelvic examination is needed to rule out anatomical or pathological contraindications and to evaluate size and position of cervix.
B. Select size based on woman's history and examination findings: small for nulligravidas; medium with history of abortion or cesarean section; large for women with one or more vaginal deliveries.
C. Follow-up for any concerns or problems; annual examination. Web site for FemCap information: http://www.FemCap.com.

Lea's Shield

I. Definition/Mechanism of Action

Lea's Shield is a contraceptive device that is used to hold spermicide and to provide a partial barrier to sperm when placed over the cervix.

II. Effectiveness and Benefits

    A. 86% effectiveness—limited data
    B. May be inserted before intercourse and left in place for up to 48 hours
    C. Latex free
    D. Reusable for more than a year

III. Side Effects and Disadvantages

    A. Vaginal irritation from the device
    B. Vaginal irritation from the spermicide used with the device
    C. Sensation of something in the vagina
    D. Difficulty in removing
    E. Requires prescription

IV. Contraindications

    A. Allergy to spermicide
    B. Allergy to material device is made of
    C. Partner allergy to device or spermicide
    D. Device is expelled repeatedly during use
    E. Cannot be used during menses
    F. Known or suspected uterine or cervical cancer
    G. History of toxic shock syndrome
    H. Current infection of vagina or cervix, PID
    I. Cannot be used during postpartum or after an abortion for 6 weeks
    J. Adhesions between cervix and vaginal walls
    K. Third-degree uterine prolapse

V. Types

    A. Available in one size

VI. Fitting

    A. A pelvic examination is needed to rule out anatomical or pathological contraindications and to evaluate size and position of cervix.

B. Follow-up for any concerns or problems; annual examination. Web site: http://www.leasshield.com.

Vaginal Contraceptive Sponge

I. Definition/Mechanism of Action

The vaginal contraceptive sponge looks like a small doughnut with a hollow area in the center. The hollow area fits over the cervix. The sponge measures about 1 3/4 inches in diameter. Across the bottom is a string loop to provide for easy removal. The sponge is polyurethane and contains the spermicide Nonoxynol 9. It provides a barrier between sperm and the cervix, traps sperm within the sponge, and releases spermicide to inactivate sperm over 24 hours.

II. Effectiveness and Benefits

    A. 89–90.8% effectiveness
    B. May be inserted before intercourse and left in place for up to 24 hours
    C. Latex free
    D. Over the counter
    E. No need to add extra spermicide within 24 hours

III. Side Effects and Disadvantages

    A. Vaginal irritation from the sponge
    B. Vaginal irritation from the spermicide in the sponge
    C. Sensation of something in the vagina
    D. Difficulty in removing
    E. May have a relationship to development of toxic shock syndrome if not used as directed
    F. Frequent use of Nonoxynol 9 can cause genital irritation and increase the risk of HIV and other STDs

IV. Contraindications

    A. Allergy to spermicide
    B. Allergy to sponge material
    C. Partner allergy to sponge or spermicide
    D. Cannot be used during menses
    E. History of toxic shock syndrome
    H. Current infection of vagina or cervix, PID

V. How to Use

    A. Patient should read instructions carefully prior to using the sponge.

    B. The sponge can be left in place for up to 24 hours and offers protection for each act of intercourse.

VI. Follow-up

Yearly physical examination including Papanicolaou smear is recommended. Web site: http://www.todaysponge.com.

CONTRACEPTIVE SPERMICIDES AND CONDOMS

Spermicides

I. Definition

Spermicides are substances used alone or with a vaginal barrier to prevent sperm from reaching the uterus. All contain an inert base or carrier substance and an active ingredient, most commonly the surfactant nonoxynol-9, which disrupts the integrity of the sperm cell membrane.

II. Effectiveness and Benefits

    A. Method: 96% effectiveness rate

    B. User: 60% effectiveness rate

    C. Inexpensive and readily available

III. Side Effects and Disadvantages

    A. Local irritation from spermicide or allergy to spermicide or carrier substance

    B. Can necessitate interruption of lovemaking for application

    C. Emotional reaction to touching one's own body

IV. Types

    A. Creams, jellies, gels; some are flavored and nontoxic if ingested; some are colored

    B. Foams

    C. Foaming tablets

    D. Suppositories

    E. Vaginal contraceptive film

    F. Bioadhesive gel

    G. Water soluble lubricant with spermicide

V. How to Use

    A. Instructions should be read carefully prior to using any spermicide. Method of insertion, time of effectiveness, time needed prior to intercourse, etc., vary with each type. Concentration of the spermicide varies among products.

    B. A new insertion of spermicide is needed before each act of intercourse.

    C. Wash the applicator with soap and water after each use.

    D. When the woman uses a spermicide alone, the partner should always use a condom.

    E. Frequent use of Nonoxynol-9 can cause genital and rectal lesions and increase the risk of HIV and other STDs.

VI. Follow-up

Yearly physical examination including Papanicolaou smear is recommended. See Appendix A for patient handout on spermicides and condoms and Bibliography for references.

Condoms

I. Definition

Condoms are thin sheaths, most commonly made of latex but also made of sheep intestine or polyurethane, which prevent the transmission of sperm from the penis to the vagina. The female condom (vaginal pouch) is made of polyurethane.

II. Effectiveness

    A. Method: 97–98% effectiveness rate

    B. User: 70–94% effectiveness rate; 85% for female condom (range 74.0–91.1%)

    C. Inexpensive and readily available

    D. Offer protection against sexually transmitted diseases, including the AIDS virus (HIV)

    E. Encourage male participation with birth control (conventional male condom)

    F. Female condom is polyurethane (fewer allergic reactions as compared with latex)

    G. Use of both vaginal spermicides and condoms has an effectiveness rate in the high nineties when both methods are used correctly.

III. Side Effects and Disadvantages

    A. Allergic reactions to latex (rare) or lubricant or spermicide on products with either of these in place.

    B. Use necessitates interruption of lovemaking for application.

    C. May decrease tactile sensation.

    D. Psychological impotency may occur.

    E. Only latex condoms can be considered effective protection against the AIDS virus (HIV); the polyurethane vaginal pouch (female condom) is twice as thick as latex, and viral permeability may be less than latex.

    F. Polyurethane male condoms are more likely than latex to break or slip off, but they are useful for persons who don't like latex condoms or are latex sensitive.

IV. Types

Condoms (male) vary in color, texture (smooth, studded, or ribbed), shape, size, and price. They come lubricated or nonlubricated, impregnated with spermicide, flavored, or plain. Some are extra strength, some are sheerer and thinner, and some are uniquely shaped or scented. The new eZ•on male condom is made of polyurethane, a thin, strong, 100% latex-free material. It is designed to go on in either direction and has no reservoir tip.

V. How to Use

    A. Male Condom
       1. The male condom should always be put on an erect penis before there is any sexual contact and used in every act of intercourse.
       2. The male condom should not be pulled tightly over the end of the penis; about one inch should be left for ejaculation fluid and to avoid breakage; some condoms have a reservoir tip.
       3. The penis should be withdrawn before it becomes limp, and the open end of the male condom should be held tightly while withdrawing to prevent spilling the contents.
       4. The partner should always use a contraceptive spermicide when a male condom is used.
       5. Condoms should be used only once.
    B. Female Condom (comes prelubricated)
       1. Pinch ring at closed end of pouch and insert like a diaphragm, covering the cervix; adding 1 or 2 drops of additional

lubricant makes insertion easier and decreases or eliminates squeaking noise and dislocation during intercourse.
2. Adjust other ring over labia.
3. Can be inserted several minutes to 8 hours prior to intercourse.
4. Remove after intercourse before standing up by squeezing and twisting the outer ring and pulling out gently.

VI. Follow-up

A. Annual examination, Papanicolaou smear, mammogram as appropriate to age.
NOTE: Clinicians should remind patients that if a condom breaks or slips off, emergency contraception is available.
Appendix A has information on contraceptive spermicides and condoms that you may wish to photocopy for distribution to your patients. See Bibliography.

NATURAL FAMILY PLANNING[4]

I. Definition

Natural family planning is an umbrella term for methods that use naturally occurring fertility signs to determine the fertile and infertile days of the menstrual cycle.

II. Etiology

Effects of hormones on basal body temperature, cervical mucus, the position of the cervix, the cyclical nature of the ovulatory and endometrial cycles, and the physical process of the release of an egg make possible knowledge of occurrence of ovulation.

III. Background for Electing the Method

A. What the patient presents with
1. Motivation to learn natural signs and symptoms of ovulation for purposes of fertility regulation
2. Often a history of previous use of other methods of family planning
3. Failure, dissatisfaction, or lack of harmony in values with other methods
4. Cultural, ethnic, religious values, and personal beliefs harmonious with natural family planning

   5. Medical contraindications to the use of one or more other
      methods
B. Additional background information to be obtained from the patient
   1. Medical/surgical history
   2. Obstetrical history
   3. Gynecological history including menstrual cycle history
   4. Family planning method currently being used
   5. The patient's knowledge about the female human body, espe-
      cially the ovulation cycle
   6. Family history

IV. Physical Examination

   A. Vital signs
      1. Temperature
      2. Pulse
      3. Blood pressure
   B. Complete physical examination
   C. External examination of genitalia
   D. Vaginal examination utilizing a speculum to observe position of
      cervix and mucus
   E. Bimanual examination, noting
      1. Adnexal pain
      2. Masses
      3. Tenderness

V. Laboratory Test

   A. Papanicolaou smear if none within past year; cultures, wet
      mount as appropriate or per protocol
   B. Mammography as recommended

VI. Differential Diagnosis

   A. Preference for other methods

VII. Teaching About Natural Family Planning

   A. Fertility awareness
   B. General introduction to natural family planning
   C. Basic information about natural family planning and methods
      1. Cervical mucus method
      2. Basal body temperature method (BBT)
      3. Symptothermal method

4. Keeping and interpreting a chart
D. Interpersonal and intimate relationships and natural family planning methods

See Appendix A, Natural Family Planning.

VIII. Complications

A. Inability of patient to interpret signs and symptoms
B. Lack of acceptability of method to partner
C. Unplanned pregnancy

IX. Consultation/Referral

A. To specialist or program for teaching of natural family planning

X. Follow-up

A. Annual examination and Papanicolaou smear
B. Evaluation of effectiveness of the method
C. Evaluation of patient satisfaction

See Appendix A. See Bibliography. Web site: http://www.cyclebeads.com.

EMERGENCY CONTRACEPTION

I. Definition

Emergency contraception (EC), often known as the "morning after pill," is pharmacologic or mechanical intervention after exposure to the possibility of conception with no or uncertain contraceptive protection. Such intervention is based on inhibiting fertilization or implantation. The means for intervention are either mechanical (an intrauterine device) or hormonal (high dose, short-term oral contraceptives, or progestational agents).

II. Etiology

A. Disruption of fertilization or of implantation beginning within 120 hours after unprotected intercourse is based on several theoretical premises:
1. Progestational agents will change or interfere with sperm migration or the capacity of a sperm to penetrate the egg.
2. Progestational agents are thought to inhibit motility of the fallopian tubes; also to affect follicle growth and development of the corpus luteum.

3. Estrogen, specifically ethinyl estradiol, is thought to reduce plasma level of progesterone and may, therefore, interfere with the function of the corpus luteum or possibly the function of luteinizing hormone, thereby disrupting ovulation.
4. Progestational agents and estrogen (estradiol) are known to shorten the luteal phase of the cycle.
5. IUDs, specifically copper bearing devices, are thought to interfere with the enzyme systems of the endometrium and perhaps alter the permeability of the endometrial microvasculature, perhaps interfering with implantation.

III. Effectiveness[5]

Used within 120 hours, hormonal emergency contraception reduces risk of pregnancy by 75% for those women who would have become pregnant (8 of 100), so 2 of 100 will become pregnant. The sooner EC is used after unprotected intercourse, the more effective it is.

IV. History

A. What the patient presents with
1. Last act of unprotected intercourse within the past 120 hours
2. Desire to inhibit fertilization or implantation
B. Additional information to be obtained
1. Cycle history and any previous use of contraceptives
2. Estimated day(s) of exposure to sperm without any protection or with known method failure (i.e., condom broke or slipped off; IUD expelled; cap, shield, or diaphragm displaced; missed 7 or more combination oral contraceptives in past 2 weeks or missed two or more progestin-only OCs)
3. Contraindications to hormone or IUD use
4. Circumstance of unprotected exposure—rape, possible STD exposure, teratogen exposure
5. Other acts of unprotected intercourse during this cycle

V. Physical Examination

A. Pelvic exam—speculum and bimanual—if appropriate
B. Collect specimens per rape/sexual assault guidelines in practice setting as necessary/desired by woman; complete assessment for evidence

VI. Laboratory Diagnosis

    A. Pregnancy test

    B. STD testing as warranted by history

VII. Differential Diagnosis

    A. Consider alternatives should woman desire to keep a pregnancy if one should occur

    B. Sexual assault—consider rape counseling

    C. Pregnancy already established prior to current exposure with unprotected intercourse

VIII. Treatment

    A. Combination OCs (Yuzpe method) and progestin-only OCs must be initiated within 72 hours of exposure. See individual package inserts for use.

    B. Plan B (levonorgestrel): treatment must be initiated within 120 hours[5] (causes less nausea and vomiting); one white pill then one more white pill 12 hours later, or both pills at the same time. Plan B is now available over the counter in some parts of the United States (check individual state regulations).

    C. Mechanical agents

        1. ParaGard ® or Mirena ® insertion within 5–7 days of exposure with precautions for IUD use, STD exposure, risk factors for IUD use; some guidelines specify prophylactic antibiotics with insertion.

IX. Explanation of Method

    A. Education: for each woman specific for postcoital intervention method including side effects of intervention and danger signs; if IUD is inserted, instructions about IUD use, danger signs, and complications and potential for 5 or 10 years of protection against pregnancy.

    B. Education about resumption of menses: based on woman's cycle history, if hormones are taken during follicular phase, menses will follow about day 21; if during ovulation, around day 26, and if in the luteal phase, about day 29.

X. Complications and Side Effects

    A. Pelvic infection with IUD use (see guideline for PID)

    B. Ectopic pregnancy: possible increased risk with hormone use (up to 100% of pregnancies); copper IUD use won't inhibit tubal implantation (see information on ectopic pregnancy in the guideline "Acute Pelvic Pain")

C. Pregnancy
1. Decision-making regarding continuation or termination of pregnancy

D. Nausea and vomiting
1. Drink glass of milk or eat a snack with each oral dose to reduce risk of nausea and vomiting
2. Compazine 25 mg rectal suppository every 12 hours or 10 mg orally 4 times a day
3. Tigan, 200 mg suppository every 12 hours
4. Meclizine hydrochloride (Antivert, Dramamine II) 25 mg 1 hour before EC pills
5. Give extra tablets of oral contraceptives in event of vomiting dose; instruct woman to take repeat dose if vomiting occurs within 1 hour after taking the dose and pills are visible in vomitus

XI. Consultation and Referral

A. For pregnancy exposure as the result of sexual assault/rape, refer to rape crisis center, rape counseling, to setting with sexual assault nurse examiner (SANE)
B. For complications of postcoital intervention as necessary

XII. Follow-up

A. No menses within 3 weeks after intervention, return for evaluation for continued pregnancy (failure of emergency contraception or preexisting pregnancy); to rule out ectopic pregnancy
B. For a contraceptive method chosen by woman for use following the emergency contraception
1. Immediate use: Condoms, diaphragm, spermicides, sponge, Lea's Shield, FemCap.
2. With next menses:
OCs—Sunday start or first day quick start; injectible, contraceptive patch, vaginal ring
IUDs—insert with or after menses
NFP—initiate with menses
3. Sterilization anytime

The Emergency Contraceptive Hotline, 1-800-NOT-2-LATE, is a 24-hour toll-free service offered in English and Spanish. Callers can get names, phone numbers, and location of three local clinicians. Internet access: http://not-2-late.com, www.go2planB.com

See Appendix B and Bibliography.

STERILIZATION

I. Definition

Sterilization in women is the purposeful occlusion of the fallopian tubes by surgical disruption. Several methods are practiced through closed laparoscopy, open laparoscopy, or suprapubic mini-laparotomy. The method of tubal occlusion depends on the surgical route. These occlusion methods include excision of a portion of each tube and suturing of the ends; excision of the fimbriated end; excision of a portion and then suturing of the proximal end into the muscle of the uterus and the distal end in the broad ligament; banding with silastic bands (Falope rings, Yoon band) or clips (Hulka-Clemens Clip, Filshie Clip); ligation of a loop of the tubes with nonabsorbable suture material; occlusion by bipolar cautery. Another method is transcervical to place Essure® tubal occlusion device.

II. Background for Electing Sterilization

Decision by the woman to seek permanent sterilization through tubal ligation or occlusion as a means of fertility regulation

III. History

    A. What the woman may present with:
       1. History of use of one or more methods of contraception
       2. Dissatisfaction with available methods and/or method failure
       3. Experiencing problems with one or more methods and decision not to have any more children
       4. Medical contraindications for use of one or more methods
       5. Psychosocial contraindications for use of one or more methods
       6. Desire to have no more children or no children; need or desire for permanent method
       7. Premenopause, less than 1 year without a period
    B. Additional information to be obtained
       1. Knowledge about all family planning methods used
       2. Psychosocial and cultural aspects: size of family desired, beliefs about sterilization, family attitudes
       3. Knowledge about the sterilization procedures available and beliefs about reversibility

4. History of any previous pelvic surgery, partial or total hysterectomy, oophorectomy, salpingectomy, laparoscopy, assisted reproductive procedures, plastic surgery such as tubal reconstruction
5. Medical/surgical history, present use of medications
6. Type of anesthesia for previous surgeries; any untoward effects
7. Gynecologic and obstetric history: pregnancies, live births, abortions, ectopic pregnancies, endometriosis, uterine anomalies, presence of adhesions, uterine leiomyomas (fibroids)
8. Menstrual history to the present; last period; PMS; character of menses and menstrual cycle
9. Contraceptive use to present and reasons discontinued

IV. Physical Examination

A. Vital signs
   1. Blood pressure
   2. Pulse
B. General physical exam: lungs, heart, neck, abdomen, breasts, extremities, thyroid
C. Pelvic examination
   1. External: Skene's glands, Bartholin's glands, urethra, labia, fourchette
   2. Vaginal examination: walls, discharge, cervix; inspect for cystocele, rectocele, urethrocele
   3. Uterus: masses, tenderness, enlargement, possible pregnancy
   4. Adnexa: masses, tenderness, palpable ovaries or tubes, enlargement

V. Laboratory (for preoperative work-up only or for symptoms of problem)

A. Urinalysis, culture if signs of urinary tract infection
B. Complete blood count
C. Pregnancy test
D. Gonorrhea culture
E. Chlamydia test
F. Papanicolaou smear

VI. Differential

None

VII. Treatment

A. Teaching
   1. Methods of sterilization and possible failure

2. Chance of future reversal; choice of method of sterilization related to this
3. Information on informed consent
4. Risks and benefits
5. Discussion of regret
6. Information on waiting period
7. Postoperative implications, i.e., restrictions
8. Sexual adjustments following procedure
9. Information on possible post-tubal ligation syndrome

VIII. Complications

Conditions contraindicating procedure or choice of procedure such as previous surgery or extensive adhesions; allergy or untoward response to anesthesia

IX. Consultation/Referral

To clinician who performs tubal ligations if the procedure is not offered in the practice setting

X. Follow-up

A. Postoperative care
See Bibliography. Web site: http://www.essure.com.

Sterilization: Postoperative Care

I. Definition

Follow-up care after the completion of sterilization by tubal ligation or occlusion; time of follow-up will vary depending upon the procedure performed.

II. Etiology

A. Transabdominal surgical procedure: ligation and resection; electrocoagulation
B. Laparoscopy and electrocoagulation, clips or rings
C. Transcervical tubal occlusion: Essure micorplugs

III. History

A. Type of procedure done, when, anesthesia
B. Any sutures to be removed
C. Menstruation: last menstrual period, character
D. Resumption of sexual activity, response; change in sexual habits

E. What patient may present with
   1. Pain, fever, bleeding, or discharge from operative site
   2. Abdominal pain; pelvic pain; shoulder pain
   3. Vaginal discharge
   4. Urinary symptoms: frequency, dysuria, hematuria
   5. Any new symptoms/concerns with menstrual cycle not experienced prior to tubal ligation such as endocrine manifestations

IV. Physical Examination

A. Vital signs
   1. Blood pressure
   2. Pulse
   3. Temperature
B. Abdominal examination
   1. Inspection: incision site(s) if any
   2. Auscultation: bowel sounds, hyper- or hypoactive
   3. Palpation: tenderness, guarding, masses
C. Pelvic examination
   1. Uterus: tender, enlarged, masses, fixed or mobile; pain on cervical manipulation
   2. Adnexa: masses, tenderness

V. Laboratory

A. Cervical culture if fever, uterine, adnexal tenderness present (gonorrhea, Chlamydia)
B. Urinalysis and culture if signs of urinary tract infection
C. CBC, differential, sedimentation rate, and/or C-reactive protein if fever, tenderness
D. Pregnancy test if uterus enlarged or adnexal mass, signs of ectopic pregnancy present

VI. Differential Diagnosis

A. Urinary tract infection
B. Perforation of bowel
C. Pelvic infection
D. Salpingitis
E. Peritonitis
F. Tubal hemorrhage
G. Problems with sexual expression; lack of libido, unresponsiveness

VII. Treatment

As indicated by symptoms and diagnosis

VIII. Complications

    A. Hemorrhage
    B. Pregnancy, increased risk of ectopic
    C. Perforation of bowel
    D. Pelvic inflammatory disease
    E. Urinary tract infection syndrome
    F. Salpingitis
    G. Infection of incision site(s)
    H. Pelvic abscess
    I. Peritonitis
    J. Bladder damage burns with electrocoagulation
    K. Uterine perforation
    L. Posttubal ligation
    M. Regrets

IX. Consultation/Referral

    A. Consultation/referral to surgeon for differential diagnosis and treatment of any problem
    B. Referral for mental health counseling if experiencing sexual maladjustment, regrets

X. Follow-up

    A. Return for recheck after resolution of any complications
    B. Annual Pap smear, pelvic examination, health examination; mammography per recommendations
    See Bibliography. Web sites: http://www.womenshealth.about.com/birthcontrol/a/preventpregnanc.htm; http://www.managingcontraception.com/choice.html; Health.yahoo.com/topic/birthcontrolresources/article/healthwise/TW9250–30k.

NOTES

1. Concerns have been raised due to higher exposure to estrogen as compared to most birth control pills. FDA labeling has been changed to indicate this. At this time the patch has not been recalled nor has there been an FDA warning to discontinue patch use. Clinicians should keep up to date with ACOG news releases at www.acog.org/from_home/newsrel.cfm or check www.fda.gov/cder/drug/infopage/orthoevra/default.htm.
2. Consult individual method package insert.

3. U.S. Boxed Warning: Prolonged use of medroxyprogesterone contraceptive injection may result in a loss of bone mineral density (BMD). Loss is related to the duration of use, and may not be completely reversible on discontinuation of the drug. The impact on peak bone mass in adolescents should be considered in treatment decisions. U.S. Boxed Warning: Long-term use (i.e., > 2 years) should be limited to situations where other birth control methods are inadequate. Consider other methods of birth control in women with (or at risk for) osteoporosis. Retrieved April 15, 2007 from http://www.merck.com/mmpe/lexicomp/medroxyprogesterone.html;http://www.fda.gov/bbs/topics/ANSWERS/2004/ANS01325.html.

4. This guideline was developed by the late Eleanor Tabeek, RN, PhD, CNM, and is used with her permission and that of her family. Updates by Nancy Keaveney, RN, BS, and Mary Finnigan, BA, MA.

5. Emergency contraception is indicated for 120 hours, efficacy rates are based on pills taken within 72 hours.

CHAPTER TWO

Infertility

I. Definition

Inability to conceive after 1 year or more of unprotected intercourse.

II. Etiology

A. Factors in male infertility: faulty sperm production; reproductive tract anomaly; physical and chemical agents (coal tar, radioactive substance, orchitis, other infection, etc.); endocrine disorders; general state of health; blocked vas deferens; testicular infection; injury to reproductive organs/tract; nerve damage; impotence; lifestyle factors (smoking, alcohol, street drugs, etc.); incompatible immunologic factors for sperm—anti-spermatozoa antibodies

B. Factors in female infertility: blocked fallopian tubes; anovulatory cycles; anatomical anomalies; hormonal imbalance; polycystic ovary syndrome (PCOS); obstruction of vaginal, cervical, and/or uterine cavity; hostile cervical mucus; ovarian cyst or tumor; pituitary tumor; endometriosis; previous STDs, vaginitis, vaginosis, PID, septic abortion, history of and drug treatment for thyroid disease, depression, asthma; lifestyle factors (alcohol, smoking, street drugs, etc.)

C. Factors in couple infertility: improper technique for intercourse; infrequent intercourse; emotional state; male and female factors contributing to infertility

III. History

A. What the patient presents with
   1. History of failure to conceive for period of time with no use of contraception
   2. Desire for pregnancy

B. Additional information to be obtained
1. Complete medical and surgical history including immunizations; family history
2. Complete menstrual history including menarche, character of menses, frequency, duration, last menstrual period, postmenarche amenorrhea
3. Gynecologic history: anomalies; problems; infections; surgery including LEEP, LOOP; DES exposure; endometriosis; fibroids; abnormal Papanicolaou smears; previous treatment for menstrual disorders related to polycystic ovarian syndrome
4. Contraceptive history to the present including postmethod amenorrhea
5. Obstetrical history: any previous conceptions; number of children, abortions, stillbirths; complications
6. Partner's reproductive history; medical, surgical history
7. Employment history: exposure to radiation, viruses, other substances known to cause sterility; teratogens
8. Sexual history: techniques, frequency and timing of intercourse in relation to the menstrual cycle; use of lubricants, douches, sex stimulants, or toys; trauma
9. Report of any previous infertility testing, work-ups; diagnoses; interventions; genetic evaluation
10. Lifestyle history: use of recreational (street) drugs, prescription drugs, alcohol, tobacco, caffeine, eating habits, saunas or hot tubs, exercise (including biking and running); stress
11. Age of patient/partner may determine timing of intervention

IV. Physical Examination

A. Vital signs
1. Temperature
2. Pulse
3. Blood pressure
B. Complete physical examination; observation of secondary sex characteristics; signs/symptoms of PCOS
C. External examination (careful observation for signs of infection, lesions, or anomalies)
1. Clitoris
2. Labia
3. Skene's glands
4. Bartholin's glands
5. Vulva

   6. Perineum
 D. Pelvic examination
   1. Length of vagina
   2. Position and character of cervix
   3. Any anomalies
 E. Bimanual examination (examine for palpable masses, tenderness, anomalies, signs of trauma)
   1. Uterus
   2. Ovaries
   3. Adnexa

V. Laboratory

 A. Papanicolaou smear, maturation index; mammogram as appropriate
 B. N. gonorrhea culture; RPR status (syphilis), TB status, HIV, hepatitis status, Rubella titre, varicella titre
 C. Chlamydia smear
 D. Pregnancy test in amenorrhea
 E. Complete blood count; erythrocyte sedimentation rate
 F. Mycoplasma and ureaplasma culture
 G. Endometrial biopsy during luteal phase
 H. Serum progesterone level days 21–23 of cycle
 I. Wet mounts, vaginal cultures
 J. Prolactin level, FSH, LH, TSH, Rh factor, blood type

VI. Differential Diagnosis

 A. Partner infertility or sterility
 B. Sterility
 C. Anomaly, absence of reproductive organs

VII. Treatment

 A. Infertility work-up for the woman
   1. Basal body temperature charts, may use test for LH surge instead
   2. Commercially available ovulation tests or devices and fertility monitoring devices[1]
   3. Postcoital test—serial if antispermatozoa antibodies
   4. Cervical mucus test; sperm antibody level; sperm agglutination test; sperm immobilization test; endometrial biopsy 2–3 days before menstruation
   5. Hysterosalpingogram after menses, before ovulation

    6. Hormonal assay (serum) such as FSH, LH, prolactin, estrogen DHEA-S, testosterone, urinary LH 4–5 days at midcycle
    7. Tuboscopy
    8. Ultrasound
    9. Laparoscopy with chromotubation, hydrotubation; hysteroscopy; salpingoscopy
  B. Work-up of partner involving tests done by specialist
  C. For complete work-up, referral may be in order

VIII. Complications

  A. Risks associated with certain tests; costs of testing
  B. Persistent infertility, discovery of sterility
  C. Effects on couple's relationship

IX. Consultation/Referral

To gynecologist or infertility specialist; reproductive technology centers; genetic counseling

X. Follow-up

Long-term process for work-up that is staged, so patient would be asked to return for next phase of testing if conception not achieved.

    See Bibliography and Web site: http://www.4woman.gov/COE/pubs/pamphlets/Infertility.pdf.

NOTE

1. Examples are OvuGen; Clear Plan Easy, First Response; OVu Quick Self Test for detecting luteinizing hormone (LH) in urine; Clear Plan Easy Fertility Monitor; Fertile CM; Clear Blue Fertility Monitor Complete Kit; Ovulite; OvaCue, Fertile Focus.

CHAPTER THREE

Vaginal Discharge, Vaginitis, Vaginosis, Sexually Transmitted Diseases, Hepatitis, and HIV/AIDS

CHECKLIST FOR VAGINAL DISCHARGE WORK-UP

I. Subjective Data

    A.   Social history
        1. Age
        2. Occupation
        3. Partner status
            a. Frequency of sexual contact
            b. Last sexual act and type
            c. Age of first intercourse
        4. Pregnancy history including elective or spontaneous abortion
        5. Sexual preference
        6. Number of sexual partners over lifetime; known partner history; history of new partner within past month
        7. Documented STD history including HIV status
        8. Recent weight change
    B.   Previous gynecologic surgery including abortion, tubal ligation, D&C, cesarean section, cone biopsy, LEEP, LOOP

C. Past or current medical illness; chronic diseases
D. Family history of diabetes, personal history of Type 1, 2
E. Diet, alcohol, cigarettes, recent change in habits; use of street drugs including injectables; use of sex toys, stimulants, genital jewelry
F. Medications (past and present); recent antibiotics; use of vaginal medications (OTC and prescription)
G. Past history of similar problems
   1. Dates
   2. Treatment
   3. Follow-up
H. Vaginal discharge
   1. Onset
   2. Color
   3. Odor
   4. Consistency
   5. Amount
   6. Constant vs. intermittent
   7. Related to sexual contact
   8. Relationship to menses
   9. Relation to other life events
   10. Wear pads, tampons
I. Papanicolaou history: last Pap, any history of abnormal Paps, and any interventions
J. Sores anywhere on the body; rashes
K. Genital itching, swelling, or burning; genital sores or tears
L. Abdominal or pelvic pain
M. Fever, chills
N. Achy joints
O. Nausea and vomiting; diarrhea
P. Dyspareunia
Q. Known contact with sexually transmitted disease; AIDS risk (See Appendix E for AIDS risk assessment tool)
R. Birth control (including recent changes in method or products used)
   1. Hormonal contraception, vaginal ring, patch, implant, IUD, pills; type and length of use
   2. Intrauterine device: type, how long in place
   3. Diaphragm; cervical cap; Lea's Shield; FemCap
   4. Depo-Provera®
   5. Condom (male or female); foam, jelly, gel, cream, vaginal film, tablets, suppositories, gels, sponge
S. History of douching; use of soaps, chemicals

T. Personal hygiene
   1. Use of feminine hygiene sprays or deodorant tampons, panty liners, or pads
   2. Poor personal hygiene
U. Clothing: consistent wearing of tight-crotched pants; type of underwear; pantyhose
V. Last menstrual period; last normal menstrual period
W. Urinary problems
   1. Frequency
   2. Dysuria
   3. Urgency
   4. Hematuria: other debris in urine
   5. Odor
   6. Dark or cloudy urine; color
X. Allergies to drugs: reactions
Y. Partner problems, symptoms

II. Objective Data

A. Vital signs: blood pressure, pulse, respiration, temperature
B. Inguinal lymph nodes
C. Abdominal examination: rebound, bowel sounds, suprapubic tenderness, masses, organomegaly, enlarged bladder, costovertebral angle (CVA) tenderness
D. External genitalia: Bartholin's glands, Skene's glands, sores, rash, genital warts, swollen reddened urethra, urethral discharge; lesions on labia, between labial folds
E. Vaginal examination (speculum)
   1. Inspection of vaginal walls, vaginal lesions, tears, discharge
   2. Inspection of cervix: friability, ectropion, cervical erosion, discharge from os, cervical tenderness; color
   3. Discharge: if present, characteristically is thick, mucus at cervical os, difficult to remove
F. Bimanual examination: pain on cervical motion, fullness or pain in adnexa, tenderness of uterus, size and shape of uterus

III. Assessment and Plan

A. Normal discharge: usually clear or white, nonirritating or nonpruritic, pH 3.8–4.2, doesn't pool, has body, can write initials in it
B. Diagnosis
   1. Wet prep will be negative
   2. Gram stain will be negative

    3. pH within normal range

    4. Card test for elevated ph and trimethylamine and for prolin-eamino-peptidase (Fem Exam, Pip Activity test card)

C. Treatment: none required

D. Patient education

    1. Reassurance

    2. If clinical and/or laboratory findings are not within normal limits, refer to protocol for suspected organism(s) for further work-up

IV. Hints on Preparation of a Wet Smear[1]

A. Collect a copious amount of vaginal discharge from the lateral walls with a wooden Pap spatula (some say a cotton swab moistened with saline); repeat so you have two samples to work with.

B. Place a drop of the specimen mixture at each end of a clean glass slide, or on two separate slides, when you are ready to read the slides; or place a drop of saline on one slide and a drop of KOH on a second before collecting specimens; place in cardboard slide holders if available.

C. Add a drop of KOH[2] (10%) to one specimen or stir one specimen into the KOH on the slide and sniff immediately for the characteristic "fishy" odor of bacterial vaginosis (+whiff test).

D. Cover both specimens with cover slips once you reach the microscope. Plan to view the plain saline specimen first to allow time for the KOH to lyse cells prior to looking for Candida noting that Candida torulopsis does not have the same characteristics as Candida albicans, so KOH will be negative. If you suspect trichomonas, you may want to examine slide without a cover slip, as the slip can sometimes immobilize the trich. Warming the slide will also increase the possibility of seeing trichomonads.

E. With the 10x objective in place on the microscope, the light on low power, and the condenser in the lowest position, place the slide on the stage and lower the objective until it is as close to the slide as possible.

F. Adjust the eyepieces until a single round field is seen. Turn the coarse focus knob until the specimen is focused. Use the fine focus knob to bring the specimen into sharp focus.

G. Be sure to use subdued light and a lowered condenser for a wet specimen. Try increasing the light and raising the condenser while viewing the specimen to see how the cells and bacteria disappear from view.

H. Move the slide until you have a general impression of the number of squamous cells. Switch to high power (40x); it may be necessary to increase the amount of light slightly.

I. Evaluate the slide for bacteria, WBCs, clue cells, trichomonads, hyphae, and yeast buds. Even if one organism is identified, continue to scan the slide systematically to fully evaluate the specimen. Vaginitis/vaginosis may have multiple causes.

J. Move the KOH slide into position; switch back to low power to scan the slide for Candida. If hyphae are noted, switch to high power to confirm the impression.

K. Be sure to wipe spilled fluid from the stage. If the objective becomes contaminated, clean it only with special lens paper.

L. To perform gram staining:

1. Spread a *thin* smear of the specimen on a glass slide. Air dry the slide completely, or dry it carefully high above a flame.

2. After the specimen is dry, fix it by passing it through a flame several times (with the specimen side away from the flame). Allow it to cool completely; otherwise the reagents used in the staining process may precipitate on the slide.

3. Flood the slide with Gram crystal violet. Wait 10 seconds, then rinse with tap water.

4. Flood the slide with Gram iodine. Wait 10 seconds, then rinse with tap water.

5. Wash the slide with decolorizer just until the fluid dripping from the slide changes from blue to colorless, then immediately rinse the slide with tap water. This step is crucial to ensure correct decolorizing.

6. Flood the slide with Gram sufranin. Wait 10 seconds, then rinse the slide with tap water.

7. Allow the slide to air dry, or blot dry. Place the slide on the microscope stage and put a small drop of oil on the stained specimen. With the oil power objective in place, the condenser tip and the diaphragm open (for bright field illumination), focus and examine several fields on the slide.

8. When finished, remove the oil from the lens with lens paper.

Appendix A contains information on vaginal discharge to copy or adapt for your patients. See Bibliography.

WORK-UP FOR VAGINAL DISCHARGE AND ODOR

I. Definition

Vaginal discharge that may or may not have a distinctive odor may be a vaginitis or vaginosis.

Vaginitis: Inflammation of the vagina, characterized by an increased vaginal discharge containing many white blood cells (WBCs).
Vaginosis: Characterized by increased discharge without inflammatory cells (WBCs).

II. Etiology

    A. Foreign body (i.e., forgotten tampon, retained cap, condom, or diaphragm)
    B. Allergy to soap or feminine hygiene spray
    C. Deodorants
    D. Scented toilet tissue; scented or deodorant menstrual products
    E. Vaginal contamination through oral or rectal intercourse
    F. Poor personal hygiene
    G. Sensitivity to contraceptive spermicides or lubricants
    H. Condom allergy. (Hint: If woman is allergic to latex, then use latex condom with animal skin or polyurethane condom over; if man is allergic to latex, use animal skin condom or polyurethane with a latex condom over.)
    I. Presence of a pathogen

III. History

    A. What patient may present with
       1. Vaginal discharge, may be chronic
       2. Vaginal odor
       3. Vulvar/vaginal irritation, pruritus, and/or burning made worse by urination, intercourse
       4. Postcoital bleeding
       5. Difficulty urinating or pain with urination
    B. Additional information to be considered
       1. Relationship of discharge to birth control method; any ended
       3. Relationship of discharge to sexual contact: recency; partner affected; recent change in partners
       4. Relationship of discharge to personal hygiene: any recent change in hygiene products or toiletries; douching

5. Any history of vaginal infection associated with sexually transmitted disease or pelvic inflammatory disease
6. History of
   a. Previous infection or STD
   b. Chronic cervicitis
   c. Cervical surgery
   d. Abnormal Papanicolaou smear
   e. Diethylstilbestrol (DES) exposure
7. Description of discharge
   a. Color
   b. Onset
   c. Odor
   d. Consistency
   e. Constant vs. intermittent
   f. Color of discharge on under-wear; changes

IV. Physical Examination

   A. External examination: external genitalia
      1. Erythema
      2. Excoriations
      3. Lesions
      4. Edema
   B. Vaginal examination (speculum)
      1. Presence of foreign body
      2. Erythema and edema of the vaginal vault
      3. Inspection of cervix
         a. Erythema
         b. Erosion
         c. Severe physiological ectropion
         d. Friability
         e. Serous sanguineous discharge
         f. Lesions
   C. Bimanual examination if indicated

V. Laboratory Examination

   A. As indicated by findings
      1. Wet saline prep; KOH slide
      2. Card test for elevated pH and trimethylamine[3] and prolinea-minopeptidase[4]
      3. Gram stain
      4. Gonorrhea culture if indicated
      5. Chlamydia test if indicated

6. Urinalysis if indicated
7. Herpes culture if indicated
8. Cervical culture
9. pH with nitrazine paper; QuickVue Advance pH & Amines Test; Quick Vue Advance G. Vaginalis Test[5]
10. HIV testing

VI. Differential Diagnosis

A. Normal physiological discharge
B. Diethylstilbestrol (DES) exposure
C. Chlamydia
D. N. gonorrhea
E. Candida albicans or other Candida infection; bacterial vaginosis
F. Urinary tract infection
G. Condylomata
H. Herpes simplex
I. Contact dermatitis
J. Tinea or other fungus

VII. Treatment

A. General measures
1. Removal of causative factor
2. Education as to
a. Personal hygiene
b. Avoidance through use of alternatives to causative factors
B. Medications
1. No treatment, depending on evaluation of clinical data
2. If a pathogen is identified, treat via appropriate protocol
3. If after 1 week of no treatment, try Aci-jel®, one application intravaginally at bedtime for 7–14 days or until tube is used up

VIII. Complications

Abnormal Papanicolaou smear resulting from continuing irritation; reparative process

IX. Consultation/Referral

In case of unresolved symptomatology

X. Follow-up

A. 1 week if indicated, then as needed
B. If no improvement at 1 week after treatment of Aci-jel®, referral to physician

See Appendix A and Bibliography.

CANDIDIASIS

I. Definition

Candidiasis, or monilia, is a microscopic yeast-like fungal infection of the vagina usually caused by Candida albicans (90+%). Candida tropicalis, Torulopsis glabrata, Candida Krusei, Candida parapsilosis, and other lesser known Candida species are also clinically implicated.

II. Etiology

A. A fungus of the genus Candida, species albicans, tropicalis, or Torulopsis glabrata, part of the normal flora of the mouth, gastrointestinal tract, and vagina; may become pathogenic under variable conditions, such as change in the vaginal pH, which encourage an overgrowth of the organism
B. Incubation period: about 96 hours

III. History

A. What patient may present with
  1. Pruritus
  2. Vulvar and vaginal swelling
  3. Vulvar excoriation
  4. Vulvar burning with urination
  5. Dyspareunia or burning during and/or after intercourse
B. Additional information to be considered
  1. Previous vaginal infections or vaginosis; diagnosis, treatment, and compliance with treatment
  2. Chronic illness (diabetes); immunocompromised
  3. Sexual activity including oral and anal sex
  4. History of sexually transmitted disease or pelvic inflammatory disease
  5. Last intercourse; changes in frequency; new partner
  6. Last menstrual period

    7. Method(s) of birth control
    8. Other medications
      a. Antibiotics
      b. Steroids
      c. Estrogens
    9. Description of discharge
      a. Color
      b. Onset
      c. Odor
      d. Consistency
  10. Constant vs. intermittent
      a. Relationship to sexual contact
      b. Relationship to menses
      c. Use of vaginal deodorant sprays, deodorant or scented tampons, panty liners, or pads, douches, perfumed toilet tissue
      d. Change in laundry soaps, fabric softener, body soap (amount of soap used and application inside labia)
      e. Clothing: consistent wearing of tight-crotched pants; wearing nylon underwear; panty hose under slacks; wearing underwear to bed
  11. "Jock" itch (partner), athlete's foot (self or partner), itchy rash on thighs, buttocks, under breasts; oral candidiasis (thrush)
  12. Diet high in refined sugar

IV. Physical Examination

  A. External examination
    1. Observe perineum for excoriation, erythema, edema, ulcerations, lesions
  B. Vaginal examination (speculum)
    1. Inspection of vaginal mucosa: may be erythematous, irritated, with white patches along side walls
    2. Cervix
    3. Discharge: characteristically thick, odorless, white, curd-like, resembling cottage cheese, with pH remaining in the normal range of 3.8–4.2 (nitrazine paper)
  C. Bimanual examination

V. Laboratory Examination[6]

  A. Wet prep microscopic examination to visualize hyphae, pseudohyphae, spores, or buds

B. Consider vaginal or cervical culture
C. Consider fasting blood sugar and 2 hour postprandial on women with chronic yeast infections
D. Further laboratory work as indicated by history including HIV testing

VI. Differential Diagnosis

A. Herpes genitalis
B. Chemical vaginitis
C. Contact dermatitis
D. Normal physiologic discharge
E. Candidiasis 2° to diabetes, pregnancy, + HIV status
F. Candida Torulopsis glabrata or Candida tropicalis or lesser known species (C. Krusei, C. parapsilosis, other C. species)
G. Trichomonas, bacterial vaginosis, Chlamydia, or gonococcal infection

VII. Treatment

A. Medications (some of these are now over the counter)[7]
   1. Butoconazole 2% cream 5 grams intravaginally × 3 days (Femstat3®) OR
   2. Butoconazole1 2% cream (Gynazole1)®, 5 grams (sustained release) 1 applicator full (pregnancy category C) OR
   3. Clotrimazole (Gyne-Lotrimin®, Lotrimin®, Mycelex®, Mycelex-GS) 1% cream 5 grams (1 applicator full) intravaginally at bedtime × 7–14 days OR
   4. Clotrimazole 100 mg vaginal tablet daily at bedtime × 7 days OR
   5. Clotrimazole 100 mg vaginal tablet, 2 tablets for 3 days OR
   6. Clotrimazole 500 mg vaginal tablet 1 dose OR
   7. Clotrimazole (Gyne-Lotrimin) suppositories 100 mg at bedtime × 7 nights OR
   8. Miconazole (Monistat®) 2% cream 5 grams (1 applicator full) intravaginally × 7 days OR
   9. Miconazole 200 mg vaginal suppository 1 each for 3 days OR
   10. Miconazole (Monistat®) ovule 1200 mg single dose OR
   11. Miconazole 100 mg vaginal suppository 1 each for 7 days OR
   12. Nystatin® 100,000 unit vaginal tablet 1 tablet once a day for 14 days OR

13. Tioconazole (Vagistat-1®) 6.5% ointment 5 grams intravaginally single dose at bedtime (pregnancy category C) OR
14. Terconazole (Terazol®) 0.4% cream 5 grams (1 applicator full) intravaginally x 7 days OR
15. Terconazole 0.8% cream 5 grams (1 applicator full) intravaginally x 3 days OR
16. Terconazole 80 mg suppository 1 each x 3 days
17. Oral therapy: Fluconazole (Diflucan®) 150 mg oral tablet, one tablet in a single dose (pregnancy category C)
18. In pregnancy: use only topical azole therapies; most effective in pregnancy are butoconazole, clotrimazole, miconazole, and terconazole; most experts recommend 7-day therapy
19. Miconazole cream (Monistat-Derm®) or clotrimazole cream (Mycelex®) can be used for external irritation
20. If treatment is unsuccessful, may refill script x 1; if still unsuccessful, consider treating partner and/or fasting blood sugar and 2 hour postprandial; review history carefully with woman
21. If fasting blood sugar and 2 hour postprandial are within normal limits several options may be considered:
    a. Clotrimazole® 1 applicator full intravaginally every other week x 2 months. If patient remains symptom free, reduce treatment to every month, the week prior to menses.
    b. If a. is not successful, Candida torulopsis glabrata or Candida Tropicalis should be considered. If lab confirms diagnosis, treat with gentian violet one tampon at bedtime x 12 days; triazole compounds have also been found to be effective (Terazol®—terconazole).
    c. Boric acid capsules. 600 mg 1 capsule 2 x/week intravaginally for recurrent candida vaginitis (4 or > episodes year) as organism may be Torulopsis glabrata (less sensitive to fluconazole or imidazoles).
    d. Clove of garlic in gauze placed in vagina for 10–12 hours; other complementary therapies (see guideline and Bibliography).
B. General measures
    1. No intercourse until symptoms subside; then use condoms until end of treatment
    2. No douching
    3. Stress importance of continuing medication even if menses begin
    4. Do not use tampons during treatment
    5. Stress hygiene, cotton underwear, loose clothing, no underpants while sleeping, wipe front first and then back

6. Do not use feminine hygiene sprays, deodorants, etc.
7. Treat athlete's foot, "jock" itch, or rash with OTC antifungals (such as Lotrimin®, Tinactin®) or prescription Dual-action Lotrisone®
8. Consider the use of vitamin C 500 mg twice to four times a day to acidity of vaginal secretions or oral acidophilous tablets 40 million to 1 billion units daily (1 tablet); eat live culture yogurt several times a week

VIII. Complications

Drug interactions; adverse reactions to treatment

IX. Consultation/Referral

A. No response to treatment as outlined above
B. Elevated fasting blood sugar or 2 hour postprandial
C. Presence of concurrent systemic disease

X. Follow-up

A. None necessary unless
   1. Symptoms persist after treatment
   2. Symptoms recur or exacerbate

Appendix A has information on candidiasis that you may wish to photocopy or adapt for your patients.

See Bibliography. Web site: http://www.cdc.gov/ncidod/dbmd/diseaseinfo/candidiasis_gen_g.htm.

TRICHOMONIASIS

I. Definition

Infection with the organism Trichomonas, usually sexually transmitted; found in the vagina and urethra of women and the urethra of males.

II. Etiology

The parasitic protozoan flagellate, Trichomonas vaginalis

III. History

A. What the patient may present with
   1. Foul-smelling vaginal discharge, often fishy
   2. Burning and soreness of vulva, perineum, thighs

    3. Vaginal and perineal itching

    4. Dyspareunia, dysuria

    5. Postcoital bleeding

    6. Possibly no objective symptoms

  B. Additional information to be considered

    1. Previous vaginal infection, vaginosis; diagnosis, treatment; compliance with treatment

    2. Sexual activity; partner preference (do not disregard possibility of women having sex with women)

    3. History of sexually transmitted disease or pelvic inflammatory disease

    4. Last menstrual period

    5. Last intercourse, sexual contact

    6. Method of birth control; other medications

    7. History of chronic illness (especially seizure disorders)

    8. Description of discharge

      a. Color

      b. Onset

      c. Odor

      d. Consistency

      e. Amount

      f. Constant vs. intermittent

      g. Relationship to menses

      h. Relationship to sexual contact

    9. Whether or not partner has symptoms

IV. Physical Examination

  A. External examination

Observe perineum for excoriation, erythema, edema, ulceration, or lesions.

  B. Vaginal examination (speculum)

    1. Inspection of vaginal walls; red papules may appear

    2. Inspection of cervix: strawberry appearance of cervix and upper vagina due to petechiae

    3. Discharge: greenish, yellow, malodorous, frothy with > 4.5 pH (5.0–7.0)

  C. Bimanual examination

V. Laboratory Examination

  A. Wet prep microscopic examination; should see highly motile cells, slightly larger than leukocytes, smaller than epithelial cells; > 10 WBCs/high power field

B. Gonococcus culture, Chlamydia test, serology testing for syphilis if history indicates; culture for T. vaginalis; DNA probe for T. vaginalis

C. CBC should be done if more than two courses of Metronidazole® taken within 2-month period

D. KOH "whiff" test: sometimes fishy but not always

E. Trichomonas Rapid Test—dipstick of vaginal swab; 83% sensitivity

VI. Differential Diagnosis

A. Candidiasis
B. Bacterial vaginosis
C. Urinary tract infection
D. Gonorrhea
E. Chlamydia infection

VII. Treatment[8]

A. Medications
1. Metronidazole (Flagyl®, Metryl®, Protostat®, Satric®) 2 grams orally in single dose (review history for seizure disorder)
2. Metronidazole 500 mg twice a day x 7 days (recommended for treatment failures)
3. Metronidazole capsules 375 mg twice a day x 7 days
4. Tindamax (tinidazole) tablets single 2 gram dose with food (tablets come in 250 and 500 mg) (pregnancy category C)
5. In pregnancy, Metronidazole 2 grams orally in single dose
6. Lactation: Tindamax single dose; interruption of breast feeding for 72 hours following treatment

B. General Measures
1. Stress importance of not drinking alcohol during treatment or for 48 hours after treatment; with Tindamax 72 hours
2. Metronidazole® can cause gastrointestinal upset; also causes urine to darken
3. Stress avoidance of intercourse during treatment; if intercourse does occur, condoms should be used
4. Stress importance of completing medication
5. Stress personal hygiene; cotton underpants, no underpants while sleeping, wipe front first, and then back
6. Patient should be given informational handout to deliver to sexual partner advising need for partner's treatment
7. Comfort measures for severe symptoms: sitz baths

8. Stress that if partner is not treated before next act of unprotected intercourse, reinfection can occur

VIII. Complications

  A. Of the disease
      1. Spread of the infection to urethra, or prostate in the male
      2. Untreated Trichomonas vaginalis may result in atypia on Papanicolaou smear; may also be associated with adverse pregnancy outcomes (premature rupture of membranes, and premature delivery); increased susceptibility to HIV acquisition
  B. Of the treatment
      1. Nausea
      2. Neurological symptoms: seizures
      3. Vomiting (may be severe) if alcohol is consumed while on treatment or within 48 hours after treatment
      4. Possibility of blood dyscrasia posttreatment

IX. Consultation/Referral

  A. Refer to physician if woman has seizure disorder prior to initiating therapy
  B. Consult if treatment (VII A. 1. and 2.) fails

X. Follow-up

None necessary unless symptoms persist or recur after treatment.
    See Appendix A and Bibliography. Web site: http://www.cdc.gov/NCIDOD/dpd/parasites/trichomonas/default.htm.

BACTERIAL VAGINOSIS

I. Definition

A clinical syndrome characterized by an overgrowth of anaerobic bacteria (bacteroides, peptostreptococcus, mobiluncus curtesii, eubacterium, and prevoltella) and facultative bacteria (gardnerella vaginalis, mycoplasma hominis, Ureaplasma urealyticum, enterococcus, group B Streptococcus, and decrease in H_2O_2–producing lactobacilli).

II. Etiology

  A. Bacterial vaginosis (BV) is a vaginosis rather than vaginitis. As such, there is usually little or no inflammation of epithelium associated with the syndrome (relative absence of polymorphonuclear leukocytes). It is not caused by a single pathogen, but is probably a disturbance of the vaginal microbial ecology, with a displacement of normal lactobacillary flora by anerobic microorganisms.

B. It is a sexually associated rather than a sexually transmitted syndrome. (Bacterial vaginosis is found more often in sexually active women.) A male version of BV has not been identified.

III. History

A. What the patient may present with
   1. Vaginal odor (fishy)
   2. Increased vaginal discharge—milky white, thin adherent discharge, or dark or dull gray discharge
   3. Vaginal burning after intercourse; vulvar pruritis (15% of women)
   4. No symptoms in many patients
B. Additional information to be considered
   1. Previous vaginal infections; diagnosis, treatment; compliance with treatment
   2. Chronic illness; careful history of seizure disorders
   3. Sexual activity; partner preference
   4. History of sexually transmitted disease or pelvic inflammatory disease
   5. Last intercourse
   6. Last menstrual period; pregnancy
   7. Method of birth control; other medications
   8. Description of discharge
      a. Onset
      b. Color
      c. Odor stronger during intercourse
      d. Consistency
      e. Constant vs. intermittent
      f. Relationship of symptoms to sexual contact
      g. Relationship of symptoms to menses
      h. Amount
   9. Use of vaginal deodorant sprays, deodorant tampons, pantyliners or pads, douches, or perfumed toilet tissue
   10. Change in laundry soaps, fabric softener, body soap
   11. Clothing: consistent wearing of tight-crotched pants; nylon underwear, underwear to bed
   12. Personal hygiene
   13. Recent change in lifestyle (stress, personal crisis)
   14. Partner symptoms

IV. Physical Examination

    A. External examination
    Perineum usually has a normal appearance; occasional irritation
    B. Vaginal examination (speculum)
        1. Inspection of vaginal walls
        2. Inspection of cervix
        3. Discharge: characteristically adherent homogenous, whitish in color, and of a fishy, musty odor with pH > 4.5. Take smear from lateral walls of vagina, not cervix, for accurate pH (use nitrazine paper for test)
    C. Bimanual examination if indicated

V. Laboratory Examination May Include

    A. Diagnosis (3 of 4 Amsel criteria)
        1. White, thin adherent discharge
        2. ph > 4.5
        3. +whiff test (fishy amine odor from vaginal fluid mixed with 10% KOH)
        4. Clue cells on wet mount: epithelial cells dotted with large numbers of bacteria that obscure cell borders, should see > 20% clue cells
    B. Card Test (FemExam, Pip Activity Test Card); OSOM BV Blue test—vaginal swab in test tube with reagent—+ for BV if it turns blue or green
    C. Few WBCs seen on wet mount; decreased Lactobacilli
    D. Further laboratory work as indicated by history or wet prep/ card, BV blue test results

VI. Differential Diagnosis

    A. Trichomoniasis
    B. Presence of foreign body

VII. Treatment: Acute BV

    A. Medications
        1. Vaginal preparation
            a. Metronidazole gel (MetroGel®) 0.75% one applicatorful (5 grams) intravaginally twice a day x 5 days or one applicatorful at bedtime x 5 days (if additional treatment is necessary within 2 months, a CBC will be necessary).
            b. Clindamycin phosphate cream (Cleocin® vaginal cream 2% one applicatorful, 5 grams) intravaginally at

bedtime x 7 nights. Clindamycin is contraindicated with colitis, other chronic bowel disease. Use cautiously in patients with asthma or impaired renal or hepatic function. *Note:* the mineral oil in Cleocin® vaginal cream may weaken latex or rubber products such as condoms or vaginal diaphragms. Use of these products within 72 hours following treatment is not recommended.

   c. Clindamycin (Cleocin®) vaginal ovules 100 mg at bedtime x 3 nights.

   d. Clindesse (clindamycin phosphate) vaginal cream 2% intravaginally once (one dose). Same precaution with latex or rubber products as Clindamycin (pregnancy category B, not recommended with breastfeeding).

   e. Vandazole (metronidazole vaginal gel 0.75%) intravaginally one applicatorful at bedtime x 5 nights (pregnancy category B, not recommended with breastfeeding).

2. Oral preparation
   a. Metronidazole (Flagyl®) 500 mg orally twice a day x 7 days

3. Alternative treatment
   a. Metronidazole 2 grams orally single dose OR
   b. Clindamycin 300 mg orally twice a day x 7 days OR

4. In pregnancy: symptomatic women require treatment of:
   a. Metronidazole 500 mg orally three times a day for 7 days OR
   b. Metronidazole 250 mg orally three times a day for 7 days OR
   c. Clindamycin 300 mg orally twice a day for 7 days

5. In pregnancy: asymptomatic women at low risk for preterm delivery
   a. Controversial as to treat or not to treat: data with treatment < 20 weeks gestation = reduction in preterm birth.
   b. Treatment at 16–32 weeks = increase in adverse events. Conclusion: use Clindamycin only in first half of pregnancy per CDC 2006 recommendations.

5. Treatment for partner not recommended by CDC (no decrease in recurrences with partner treatment and no effect on cure rates)

6. Note: If bacterial vaginosis coexists with candidiasis:
   a. Treat a predominant organism first. If symptoms persist, recheck and treat as indicated.
   b. Consider local treatment for candidiasis concurrently with oral treatment for bacteria vaginosis as above

     c. Cleocin® also kills lactobacilli, so candidiasis is common after treatment. Consider sequential treatment.

     d. If bacterial vaginosis coexists with Strep B, treat concurrently.

B. General measures

  1. Stress avoidance of intercourse until symptoms subside, then use condoms until end of treatment; condom therapy for 4–6 weeks (without antibiotic treatment) often results in resolution of BV.

  2. Stress no douching during treatment or after.

  3. Stress necessity of completing course of medication.

  4. Nausea, vomiting, and cramps can occur (if patient is on Metronidazole®). Stress no alcohol intake during treatment and for 48 hours after completing medications.

  5. Stress appropriate choice of medications if pregnant, if possibly pregnant, or if nursing.

  6. Stress hygiene: cotton underwear, loose clothing, no underpants while sleeping, wipe front first and then back, no feminine deodorants or hygiene sprays.

  7. Carefully review history for seizure disorders.

  8. Metronidazole® can cause GI upset even with no alcohol.

XIII. Treatment: Chronic, Recurring

A. For recurring BV, consider treatment with a different regimen.

B. If no relief, consider consultation with a specialist.

C. Try Metronidazole gel 0.75% twice a week for 6 months after completion of recommended regimen as above, per CDC 2006.

IX. Complications

Bacterial vaginosis has been associated with PID, endometritis, cervicitis, inflammation or ASC on Pap smears, possible link to LGSIL on Pap smears, preterm rupture of membranes, preterm labor, preterm birth, low birth weight, chorioamnitis, postpartum endometritis, and increased risk of HIV acquisition.

X. Consultation/Referral

If no response to treatment as discussed above.

XI. Follow-up

A. None necessary unless:

  1. Symptoms persist after treatment

  2. Symptoms recur

3. Pregnancy—asymptomatic women at high risk consider evaluation 1 month after completion of treatment

See Appendix A and Bibliography. Web site: http://www.cdc.gov/ STD/BV/STDFact-Bacterial-Vaginosis.htm.

CHLAMYDIA TRACHOMATIS INFECTION

I. Definition

Chlamydia trachomatis infection is a parasitic sexually transmitted disease of the reproductive tract mucous membrane of either sex.

II. Etiology

    A. The causative organism is a small, obligate, intracellular, bacterium-like parasite (Chlamydia trachomatis, or C. trachomatis) that develops within inclusion bodies in the cytoplasm of the host cells.

    B. The incubation period is unknown.

III. History

    A. What the patient may present with
        1. Female
            a. Vaginal discharge
            b. Dysuria
            c. Pelvic pain
            d. Changes in menses
            e. Intermenstrual spotting in cervical os
            f. Postcoital bleeding
            g. Frequently asymptomatic
            h. Mucopurulent discharge
        2. Male
            a. Dysuria
            b. Thick, cloudy penile discharge
            c. Rarely asymptomatic
    B. Additional information to be considered
        1. Previous vaginal infections; diagnosis, treatment; compliance with treatment
        2. Chronic illness
        3. Sexual activity; new partner(s)
        4. History of sexually transmitted disease or pelvic inflammatory disease
        5. Known contact

6. Last intercourse, sexual contact, sex toys
7. Method(s) of birth control, other medications
8. Description of discharge
   a. Onset
   b. Color
   c. Odor
   d. Consistency
   e. Amount
   f. Constant vs intermittent
   g. Relationship to sexual contact
   h. Relationship to menses
9. Use of vaginal deodorant sprays, deodorant tampons, panty liners, pads, perfumed toilet tissue, douches
10. Change in laundry soaps, fabric softener, body soap
11. Clothing: consistent wearing of tight-crotched pants
12. Personal hygiene
13. Any drug allergies
14. Travel to Asia, Africa, Europe—LGV chlamydia (not detected by usual laboratory tests in the United States)—see guideline on lymphogranuloma venereum for symptoms, treatment

IV. Physical Examination

A. Vital signs
   1. Blood pressure
   2. Temperature
B. Abdominal examination: check for guarded referred pain, rebound pain
C. External examination: observe perineum for edema, ulcerations, lesions, excoriations, erythema, enlarged, tender Bartholin's glands
D. Vaginal examination (speculum)
   1. Inspection of vaginal walls
   2. Cervix (cervicitis), friability
   3. Discharge: if present, is characteristically mucopurulent
E. Bimanual examination: cervical motion tenderness, fullness in adnexa, tender uterus

V. Laboratory Examination

A. DFA: secretions fixed on slide and stained with fluorescein labelled monoclonal antibody specific for chlamydial antigens
B. Laboratory test for chlamydia (sensitivities and specificities vary):

    1. Enzyme-linked immunoassays (EIA) detection of chlamydial antigens
    2. DNA probe (Genprobe®) (PRC + LCR = amplified tests done on Genprobe®)
    3. Polymerase chain reaction (PCR)
    4. Ligase chain reaction (LCR)
    5. Rapid test with endocervical swab or brush—12 minutes for results 92% sensitivity, 99% specificity
C. Endocervical culture (only 100% specific test in transport media—do in medicolegal cases—rape, child sexual abuse)
D. Serology test for syphilis if history indicates
E. Consider HIV testing
F. Consider hepatitis B & C testing
G. GC culture

VI. Differential Diagnosis

A. Gonorrhea
B. Appendicitis
C. Cystitis

VII. Treatment

A. Medication
    1. Azithromycin 1 gram orally in a single dose OR Doxycycline 100 mg orally twice a day x 7 days
    2. Alternative regimens
        a. Erythromycin base 500 mg orally 4 times a day x 7 days OR
        b. Erythromycin ethylsuccinate 800 mg orally 4 times a day x 7 days OR
        c. Ofloxacin 300 mg orally twice a day x 7 days OR
        d. Levofloxacin 500 mg orally daily for 7 days
    3. In pregnancy
        a. Erythromycin base 500 mg orally 4 times a day x 7 days
        b. Amoxicillin 500 mg orally three times a day x 7–10 days (for erythromycin intolerance)
    4. Alternative regimens in pregnancy
        a. Erythromycin base 250 mg orally 4 times a day x 14 days
        b. Erythromycin ethylsuccinate 800 mg 4 times a day, x 7 days
        c. Erythromycin ethylsuccinate 400 mg orally 4 times a day x 14 days
        d. Azithromycin 1 gram orally in single dose

   B. For sexual contacts during 60 days preceding onset of symptoms
       or diagnosis of Chlamydia
       1. Offer Chlamydia test prior to treatment.
       2. Start treatment prior to results of testing.
       3. Treat same as for woman; do follow-up if symptoms persist
           and rescreening per CDC 2006 Guidelines
   C. General measures.
       1. Stress partner should be treated.
       2. No intercourse until both partners are treated, or use con-
           doms, but abstinence is preferred.
       3. Condom for back-up birth control method for remainder of
           cycle if on oral contraceptives.
       4. Stress importance of completing medication for woman and
           partner.
       5. Stress no use of feminine hygiene sprays, deodorants, or
           douches.
       6. Stress possibility of increased photosensitivity with Doxycy-
           cline®.
       7. Inform patient taking tetracycline that medication should be
           taken 1 hour before or 2 hours after meals and/or consumption
           of dairy products, antacids, or mineral-containing products.
       8. Return for reevaluation if symptoms persist or return after
           treatment.

VIII. Complications

   A. Women
       1. Pelvic inflammatory disease
           a. Pelvic abscess (ovarian)
           b. Infertility; chronic pelvic pain; ectopic pregnancy
       2. Abnormal Papanicolaou smear with cervicitis (30–50%)
       3. Postpartum endometritis
   B. Men
       1. Epididymitis, prostatitis
       2. Reiter's syndrome
   C. Risk of acquiring HIV
   D. Newborn
       1. Conjunctivitis
       2. Pneumonia
       3. Urogenital tract, rectal infection
   E. Urethritis

IX. Consultation/Referral

   A. If no response to treatment as discussed previously
   B. If complications develop

X. Follow-up

  A. If no response to treatment or possibility of reinfection.
  B. Test of cure not routinely required per CDC 2006 Guidelines. If symptoms persist or reinfection is suspected, consider retesting women after treatment (rate of reinfection). Consider rescreening all women with Chlamydia infection 3–4 months after treatment. Rescreen all women treated when they next present for care within 12 months.
  C. Consider retesting 3 weeks after completion of treatment with erythromycin.
  D. Repeat Pap if abnormal prior to treatment.
  E. Gonorrhea cultures if not done.
  F. Serology test for syphilis.
  G. In some states, Chlamydia is a reportable disease.

Appendix A has information on chlamydia trachomatis infection to photocopy or adapt for your patients. See Bibliography.

Web site: http://www.cdc.gov/std/Chlamydia/STDFact-Chlamydia.htm.

GENITAL HERPES SIMPLEX

I. Definition

Genital herpes simplex is a recurrent viral infection of the skin and mucous membranes of the genitalia, characterized by eruptions on a lightly raised erythematous base.

II. Etiology

  A. Herpes simplex virus (HSV). There are two HSV strains:
    1. HSV Type 1 (HSV-1): commonly causes herpes labialis (cold sores) and herpes keratitis
      a. Usually seen in childhood (as acute gingivostomatitis)
      b. May be seen in adults who engage in oral sex, kissing
      c. Incubation period 3–7 days, course 1–3 weeks
      d. May be recurrent and has no cure
      e. Offers no protection against getting HSV-2 but makes HSV-2 more likely to be subclinical
    2. HSV Type 2 (HSV-2)
      a. Genital counterpart of acute gingivostomatitis; primarily sexually transmitted
      b. Incubation period 4–7 days up to 4 weeks, course may last 2–3 weeks
      c. HSV-2 remains dormant in dorsal nerve ganglia, may be recurrent, and has no cure

    d. May be present for many years with no symptoms or no recognizable symptoms

    e. HSV-2 does provide immunity against HSV-1

    f. 25% of population has HSV-2

3. Both HSV-1 (10%) and 2 (90%) have been implicated in genital infections, but rarely is HSV-2 found orally

III. History

  A. Genital herpes

    1. Primary infection (may actually be caused by HSV-1 or 2); mean duration 12 days

      a. Multiple lesions

        1) Male: penis, buttocks, thighs

        2) Female: labia, fourchette, cervix, buttocks, thigh, nipples

      b. Myalgia

      c. Arthralgia

      d. Malaise

      e. Fever, lymphadenopathy

      f. Dysuria, male and female (urinary retention may occur, especially in women with lesions close to meatus)

      g. Dyspareunia

      h. Headache (can be sign of herpes meningitis)

    2. Recurrent genital lesions

      a. Lesions less painful

      b. Less or no systemic symptoms

      c. Unilateral

      d. Prodromal symptoms (itching, burning, and/or tingling at site where lesions then appear)

  B. Additional information to be considered

    1. Genital herpes: primary infection

      a. Known exposure

      b. Sexual preference

      c. Recent participation in oral sex with partner having herpes labialis

    2. Genital herpes: recurrent infection

      a. History of recent exposure to reactivating factors: physical trauma, exposure to sunlight, stress, menses

      b. Prodrome

        1) Pruritus

        2) Burning at site of previous lesion(s)

        3) Tingling at site of previous lesion(s)

4) Symptoms as in 1, 2, and/or 3 across nerve tract serving site of previous lesion(s); i.e., sciatic pain with lesion on labia

IV. Physical Examination

A. Genital herpes
   1. Primary infection
      a. Temperature, blood pressure
      b. Examination of genitalia: vesicular lesions containing cloudy liquid on erythematous base. Vesicles break, lesions coalesce forming ulcerative lesions with irregular borders, macerated if in moist areas
         1) Female: lesions (painful), examination will be difficult; use of speculum may be impossible. Lesions present as described in III.A. Cervicitis may be present.
         2) Male: lesions (painful) present in areas previously described in III.A. Urethral discharge may be present.
      c. Groin: inguinal adenopathy may be present
      d. Abdomen: bladder distension, secondary to urinary retention may be present; more common in women
      e. Check for atypical presentation as cystitis, meningitis, encephalitis, urethritis, ocular lesions
   2. Recurrent infection genital herpes
      a. As above (III.B.2.) but clinical picture is less severe

V. Laboratory Examination May Include HSV Types 1 and 2

A. Scrape lesion for samples for
   1. Virology culture with typing (within 7 days of 1st episode, 2 days of recurrence)
   2. Genital lesions: consider gonococcus culture, serology test for syphilis, chlamydia test (may need to wait until follow-up visit if infection is severe)
   3. Antibody E detection (such as HerpeSelect-1 & HerpeSelect-2 ELISA IgG; Herpe-Select-1 & 2 Immunoblot IgG; POCKit-HSV-2 assay[9])

B. Consider HIV testing

VI. Differential Diagnosis

A. Syphilis
B. Chancroid
C. Lymphogranuloma inguinale
D. Granuloma inguinale

VII. Treatment of Genital Herpes

A. General therapy
  1. Consider immune status of patient with frequent outbreaks and/or long duration outbreaks, plus the degree of systemic involvement
  2. Consider also the potential for asymptomatic shedding
  3. Comfort measures
     a. Tepid water sitz baths, plain or with Betadine solution; dry carefully with cool air hair dryer making sure to hold it away from body
     b. If voiding over lesions is painful, instruct patient to void while sitting in water in bathtub
     c. Stress avoidance of tight, restricting clothing. The vulva should be exposed to air flow as much as possible (patient may wear a skirt or robe without underpants when at home)
     d. Peri-irrigation for comfort
  4. Patient education
     a. Explain the disease process and route of transmission to the patient (i.e., oral/genital sex during outbreaks)
        1) 90% of those infected don't know
        2) Majority of transmission occurs without symptoms in the infected person
        3) Viral shedding occurs 5–70% of day
        4) Condom use protects women not men
     b. Patients should be advised to abstain from sexual activity while lesions are present
     c. Explain the dangers associated with herpes during pregnancy
     d. Discuss possible factors involved with recurrences
     e. Discuss need for yearly Papanicolaou smear
     f. Support group: alt.support.herpes (usenet news group)
B. Medication
  1. Initial genital outbreak
     a. Acyclovir 400 mg orally 3 times a day x 7–10 days OR
     b. Acyclovir 200 mg orally 5 times day x 7–10 days OR
     c. Famciclovir (Famvir®) 250 mg orally 3 times a day x 7–10 days OR
     d. Valacyclovir (Valtrex®) 1 gm orally twice a day x 7–10 days OR
     e. Zovirax (acyclovir) ointment 5% for initial genital herpes and limited non–life-threatening mucocutaneous infections in immunocompromised patients (pregnancy category B)

    f. Zylocaine 2% gel or cream; apply 3–4 times daily (do not use around urethra) for comfort measure

    g. Bacitracin ointment, apply locally, for secondary infection only 2–5 x daily

    h. Add Gramicidin, a topical antibiotic, to suppress replication of HSV-1 and HSV-2.

2. Episodic recurrent infection—infrequent outbreaks 6 times or fewer a year; therapy should be initiated within 1 day of lesion onset or during prodrome for best effect
    a. Acyclovir 400 mg orally 3 times a day x 5 days OR
    b. Acyclovir 800 mg orally twice a day x 5 days OR
    c. Acyclovir 800 mg orally three times a day x 2 days OR
    d. Famciclovir 125 mg orally twice a day x 5 days OR
    e. Famciclovir 1000 mg orally twice daily x 1 day OR
    f. Valacyclovir 500 mg orally twice a day x 3 days OR
    g. Valacyclovir 1.0 gram orally daily x 5 days

3. Episodic infection in persons infected with HIV
    a. Acyclovir 400 mg orally 3 times a day x 5–10 days OR
    b. Famciclovir 500 mg orally twice a day x 5–10 days OR
    c. Valacyclovir 1.0 gram orally twice a day x 5–10 days

4. Suppressive therapy: Evidence is growing showing benefits of beginning suppressive therapy with first episode, not waiting for chronic outbreaks to be established. Early intervention will decrease recurrences during the first year when outbreaks are the most frequent as well as decrease the likelihood of viral shedding. Safety has been established for up to 15 years of continuous use.
    a. Acyclovir 400 mg orally twice a day OR
    b. Famciclovir 250 mg orally twice a day OR
    c. Valacyclovir 500 mg orally daily for persons with ≤ 9 outbreaks per year OR
    d. Valacyclovir 1 gram orally daily for persons with ≥ 10 per year

5. Suppressive therapy in persons infected with HIV
    a. Acyclovir 400–800 mg orally twice to 3 times a day OR
    b. Famciclovir 500 mg orally twice a day OR
    c. Valacyclovir 500 mg twice a day

6. In pregnancy (see CDC 2006 Guidelines)
    a. First clinical episode or severe recurrent—treat with oral acyclovir
    b. In life-threatening, severe maternal HSV infection, treat with IV acyclovir

       7. Unresolved herpes—herpes outbreaks lasting several weeks or more

         a. Immunological status should be evaluated with physician consultation

VIII. Complications

    A. Secondary infection of lesion
    B. Keratitis (keep fingers away from eyes)
    C. Generalized herpetic skin eruptions
    D. Meningitis
    E. Encephalitis
    F. Pneumonitis
    G. Hepatitis
    H. Fetal–neonatal infection
    I. Spread to other persons at risk of developing disseminated herpes

       1. Immunosuppressed or deficient individuals including persons with HIV
       2. Patients with open skin lesions, e.g., burns, atopic dermatitis
       3. Infants, small children

IX. Consultation/Referral

    A. Secondary infections
    B. Urinary retention if unable to void in bathtub
    C. Suspected ocular lesion
    D. Severe primary episode
    E. Poor fluid intake associated with severe primary episode
    F. Persistent headache, nausea, vomiting, photophobia, convulsions, pain in upper right quadrant, chest pain, shortness of breath (SOB)
    G. Unresolved outbreaks lasting several weeks or more
    H. Life-threatening episode in pregnant woman

X. Follow-up

As needed or See Appendix A for information you may want to photocopy or adapt for your patients. See Bibliography.

    Herpes Resources online: http://www.herpes.com; http://www.ashastd.org/herpes/hrc.html; http://www.webmd.com; America on-line keyword Better Health; http://www.thrive.com; http://www.viridas.com; http://www.diagnology; American Social Health Assoc. (ASHA) booklets, books, handouts; The Helper, 800-230-6039; ASHA patient herpes hotline, 919-361-8488.

CONDYLOMATA ACUMINATA (GENITAL WARTS)

Human Papilloma Virus

I. Definition

Condylomata acuminata is a sexually transmitted condition (but it may also be a fomite) caused by one or more members of the Human Papilloma Virus (HPV) group numbering more than 150 types, and characterized by the formation of warty excrescences on the external genitalia, and on the cervix, vagina, anal area, nipples, umbilicus, and pharynx. The virus does not always cause a lesion; subclinical infection occurs on cervix and externally.

II. Etiology

    A. The cause of the condition is a DNA virus of the Papilloma group (HPV); more than 30 types of HPV can affect the genital tract; 17 are considered high-risk types.

    B. Incubation period: 1 to 6 months; may be much longer (up to 30 years); up to 70% may regress spontaneously.

    C. Period of communicability is unknown.

III. History

    A. What the patient may present with
       1. "Feeling a lump" in vulvar area
       2. Increased vaginal discharge
       3. Vulvar itch, burning, pain, bleeding

    B. Additional information to be considered
       1. Previous vaginitis/vaginosis; diagnosis, treatment
       2. Sexual activity, last intercourse, sexual contact
       3. Last menstrual period: any chance of pregnancy
       4. Method of birth control
       5. Previous history of condylomata, herpes simplex
       6. Known contact; consider any contact with person with condylomata on any body part
       7. History of sexually transmitted disease or pelvic inflammatory disease
       8. Description of discharge (odor, consistency, amount, color)
       9. Any drug allergies
      10. History of abnormal Papanicolaou smear, colposcopy, treatment
      11. Reactivation of subclinical infection with sexual activity
      12. Self-infection from condyloma on any body part
      13. Lifestyle: smoking, sexual practices such as anal intercourse, sex toys, exposure to utraviolet light, nutrition

IV. Physical Examination

A. External examination
    1. Small, pink, or flesh colored, soft papillomatous, or raised "warty" lesion visualized in
        a. Periclitoral area
        b. Vestibule
        c. Posterior perineal and perianal areas
        d. Extragenital areas
    2. Confluence of many individual warts may give impression of a single, fleshy, proliferative lesion
    3. Secondary infection of lesions (from scratching)
    4. On hair-bearing skin, keratotic appearance
B. Vaginal examination (speculum); observe for same lesions as described previously
    1. Vaginal walls
    2. Cervix (more often subclinical and no visible lesions on inspection)

V. Laboratory Examination May Include

A. Visual examination (classic appearance, as described previously); often visible after application of 5% acetic acid (white vinegar)
B. Gonococcal culture
C. Chlamydia smear
D. Serology test for syphilis
E. Other laboratory work as indicated by history and examination
F. Colposcopy
G. Papanicolaou test
H. DNA testing—such as the Hybrid Capture Tube Test®
I. Biopsy of cervix or unresponsive or unusual lesion on vulva for histologic examination
J. HIV testing

VI. Differential Diagnosis

Condylomata lata (associated with syphilis), molluscum contagiosum, lipomas, fibroma, adenomas, squamous cell carcinoma, nevi, seborrheic keratoses, psoriatic plaques, carcinoma in situ, micropapillometosis labialis, giant condyloma (Buschke-Löwenstein tumor), Bowenoid papulosis, malignant melanoma, skin tags, lichen nitidus, lichen planus, sebaceous Tyson's glands, herpes simplex, angiokeratoma

VII. Treatment
  A. Medical treatment
    1. Patient applied
        a. Podofilox (Condylox®) 0.5% solution or gel twice a day for 3 days; no therapy 4 days; repeat as needed up to 4 cycles
        b. Imiquinod (Aldara®) (an immune response modifier inducing cytokines), 5% cream 3 times a week at bedtime for up to 16 weeks (may weaken rubber in diaphragms, condoms); needs to be washed off after 6–10 hours
    2. Provider applied for visible genital warts
        a. Apply trichloracetic acid (TCA) or bichloracetic (BCA) acid (80–90%)[10] (topical) or podophyllin resin (podophyllin), 10–25% in tincture of benzoin (10%) and isopropyl alcohol: allow to dry (apply vaseline collar with podophyllin[11]); no need to wash trichloracetic acid off; wash podophyllin off in 1–4 hours; may burn on application; if excess amount of TCA or BCA is applied, powder treatment area with talc, Na bicarb, or liquid soap to remove unreacted acid; only use once a week x 8–12 weeks
        b. Cryotherapy with liquid nitrogen or cryoprobe every 1–2 weeks
        c. Podophyllin resin 10–25% in tincture of benzoin weekly as needed
        d. Inject intralesional interferon
    3. Cervical warts—colpo/consultation; Vaginal warts—cryotherapy, TCA, or BCA repeat weekly; Urethral meatus—cryotherapy OR podophyllin; Oral & Anal—cryotherapy, BCA, or TCA or surgical removal
    4. Pregnancy: Podofilox, imiquimod, and podophyllin should NOT be used in pregnancy.
  B. Surgical treatment
    1. Cryotherapy with liquid nitrogen or cryoprobe; dimethylether (Histofreezer®) repeat every 1–2 weeks
    2. CO_2 laser vaporization
    3. Surgical excision
    4. LEEP (loop electrosurgical excision procedure)
  C. General measures
    1. Sexual partner(s) should be checked if lesions are present; CDC 2006 guidelines note that the role of reinfection in recurrences is probably minimal.
    2. Stress importance of personal hygiene.

    D. Use of condoms to help prevent further infection with partners likely to be uninfected (note precaution with imiquimod)

    E. Education that even after treatment and elimination of visible warts, the potential for transmission exists

VIII. Complications

    A. Lesions can become numerous and large requiring more extensive treatment.

    B. Visible genital warts and benign low-grade cervical changes are usually caused by HPV types 6, 11, 40, 42, 43, 44, 54, 61, 70, 72, 81. Other HPV types in the anogenital region (types 16, 18, 31, 33, 35, 39, 45, 51, 52, 56, 58, 59, 68, 73, 82) have been strongly associated with low grade and high grade cervical changes, cervical neoplasia, and anogenital and other cancers.

    C. Laryngeal papillomatosis in infant.

    D. Men with HPV are at increased risk for dysplastic changes and cancers in the penile and anorectal areas.

IX. Consultation/Referral

    A. Refer to or consult with physician
       1. After 8–12 treatments for evaluation
       2. If warts are present on vaginal walls or cervix or rectal mucosa (see VII.C.)
       3. Extensive or deep anorectal warts for proctologic examination; urethroscopy as indicated
       4. If any wart is over 2 cm in size or for large cluster of warts
       5. Abnormal Pap smear (per guidelines)
       6. For possible biopsy in older age groups; atypical appearance of lesions, poor response to treatment in younger patients
       7. Pregnant women

X. Follow-up

    A. Weekly x 8–12 weeks

    B. Patient advised to check self periodically and return if warts recur

    C. Stress importance of repeating the Papanicolaou smear in woman treated for condylomata every 6 months (some settings repeat every 3 months x 1 year, then every 6 months x 1 year; if normal, then yearly, and some now say yearly if none over 1 year are abnormal). See Papanicolaou guidelines.

    D. Consider use of HPV vaccine Gardasil® (quadrivalent vaccine against HPV 6, 11, 16, 18) in preadolescent girls, adolescent girls, and young women ages 9–26 per FDA approval

See Appendix A on condylomata acuminata and for information you may want to photocopy or adapt for your patients. See Bibliography. Web sites: National Cancer Institute, http://www.nci.nih.gov; http://www.ashastd.org; http://www.cdc.gov/std/hpv/; http://www.cdc.gov/std/hpv/STDFact-HPV-vaccine-hcp.htm.

GONORRHEA

I. Definition

Gonorrhea is a sexually transmitted bacterial infection of the urethra, rectum, and/or cervix; the causative organism can also be cultured in the nasopharynx. As many as 80% of infected women may be asymptomatic.

II. Etiology

The causative organism is Neisseria gonorrhoea, a gram negative, intracellular, nonmotile diplococcus. Increasingly, plasmid-mediated penicillinase-producing N. gonorrhoea (PPNG), plasmid-mediated tetracycline resistant (TRNG), chromosomally mediated resistant (CMRNG), Spectinomycin-resistant, and quinolone resistant strains exist. Incubation: 1–13 days.

III. History

    A. What patient may present with
        1. Females: a large percentage (perhaps 80%) of infected women are asymptomatic in the early disease stage
            a. Early symptoms
                1) Dysuria, dyspareunia
                2) Leukorrhea; change in vaginal discharge
                3) Unilateral labial pain and swelling
                4) Lower abdominal discomfort
                5) Pharyngitis
            b. Later symptoms
                1) Purulent, irritating vaginal discharge
                2) Fever (possibly high)
                3) Rectal pain and discharge
                4) Abnormal menstrual bleeding
                5) Increased dysmenorrhea
                6) Nausea, vomiting
                7) Lesions in genital area; labia pain
                8) Joint pain and swelling

         9) Upper abdominal pain (perihepatitis)

       10) Pain, tenderness in pelvic organs; urethral pain

  2. Males: usually symptomatic (up to 10% asymptomatic)

    a. Early symptoms

      1) Dysuria with frequency

      2) Whitish discharge from penis

      3) Pharyngitis

    b. Later symptoms

      1) Yellow or greenish discharge from penis

      2) Epididymitis

      3) Proctitis

B. Additional information to be considered

  1. Previous vaginal infections, diagnosis and treatment

  2. Chronic illness

  3. Sexual activity; number, new sexual partner(s)

  4. History of sexually transmitted disease or pelvic inflammatory disease

  5. Known contact

  6. Last intercourse, sexual contact

  7. Method of birth control, other medications

  8. History of cervical ectopy, friability in known patient

  9. Post-coital bleeding

  10. Description of discharge

    a. Onset

    b. Color

    c. Odor

    d. Consistency

    e. Amount

    f. Relationship to sexual contact

  11. Any change in menses (increased flow or dysmenorrhea)

  12. Any drug allergies

  13. HIV risk or exposure

  14. Travel to Asia, Africa, the Pacific, U.S. West Coast

IV. Physical Examination

  A. Vital signs

    1. Blood Pressure

    2. Temperature

    3. Pulse

  B. Abdominal examination

    1. Guarding

    2. Referred pain

3. Rebound pain
4. Upper bilateral quadrant pain
5. Bowel sounds indicating intestinal hyperactivity

C. External examination
1. Inspection of Skene's glands
2. Inspection of urethra
3. Inspection of Bartholin's glands

D. Vaginal examination (speculum)
1. Vaginal walls: discharge, redness
2. Cervix: mucopurulent discharge, ectopy, friability
3. Vaginal discharge

E. Bimanual examination
1. Pain when cervix is moved by examiner
2. Uterine tenderness
3. Adnexal tenderness
4. Adnexal mass

F. Throat examination
1. Erythema including tonsils
2. Edema of posterior pharynx
3. Erythema

V. Laboratory Examination

A. Gonococcus culture/Chlamydia test (Thayer-Martin still the gold standard for GC); polymerase chain reaction (PCR) and ligase chain reaction (LCR) tests useful; for rectal and throat need to culture (Thayer-Martin); gram stain > 20 polys (in males sufficient for diagnosis)

B. Serology test for syphilis

VI. Differential Diagnosis

A. Chlamydia
B. Appendicitis
C. Ectopic pregnancy

VII. Treatment: Cervix, Urethra, Rectum

A. Medication
1. Ceftriaxone 125 mg IM single dose, OR Cefixime 400 mg orally in single dose (not in women < 18) OR Ofloxacin 400 mg orally single dose OR Levofloxacin 250 mg orally single dose (for Chlamydia coverage if not ruled out)
   a. Azithromycin 1 gram orally in a single dose OR
   b. Doxycycline 100 mg orally twice a day x 7 days

2. Alternative regimens
   a. Spectinomycin 2 grams IM in a single dose OR
   b. Ceftizoxime 500 mg IM single dose OR
   c. Cefoxitin 2 grams IM single dose with probenecid 1 gram orally OR
   d. Cefotaxime 500 mg IM single dose
   e. Gatifloxacin 400 mg orally single dose OR
   f. Norfloxacin 800 mg orally single dose OR
   g. Lomefloxacin 400 mg orally single dose
   h. PLUS Chlamydia regimen
3. Pregnancy: Cephalosporins such as Ceftriaxone 125 mg IM single dose; if not tolerated use Spectinomycin 2 grams IM single dose
   a. PLUS Chlamydia regimen for pregnancy
   b. Do not use quinolones (Ciprofloxacin, Ofloxacin, Gatifloxacin, Lomefloxacin, Norfloxacin) or tetracyclines in pregnancy)
4. Pharynx
   a. Ceftriaxone 125 mg IM single dose
   b. Ciprofloxacin 500 mg PO single dose
   c. PLUS Chlamydia regimen
5. Conjunctiva 1 gram IM Ceftriaxone plus lavage infected eye with saline solution x 1
6. For contacts: verify if partner had diagnosed infection; also try to ascertain if culture was betalactinase positive or negative, then after appropriate culture treat with same regimen as patient depending on history of sensitivities

B. General measures
   1. All sexual partners should be treated if last sexual contact was within 60 days of onset of symptoms in patient or diagnosis of infection. If > 60 days, treat patient's most recent sexual partner.
   2. No intercourse until both partners are treated, or use condoms, but abstinence is preferred.
   3. Stress importance of completing medication.
   4. Stress personal hygiene.
   5. Stress need for follow-up culture if symptoms persist, recur, or exacerbate.

VIII. Complications

A. Females
   1. Pelvic inflammatory disease
      a. Pelvic abscess or Bartholin's abscess
      b. Infertility
   2. Disseminated gonococcal infection—gonococcal bacteremia

3. In pregnancy: spontaneous abortion, premature rupture of membranes, premature delivery, chorioamnionitis

B. Males
   1. Proctitis
   2. Infertility due to epididymitis, prostatitis, and/or seminal vesiculitis
   3. Urethral stricture
   4. Disseminated gonococcal infection—gonococcal bacteremia

C. Newborns: ophthalmia neonatorum, sepsis, arthritis, meningitis, rhinitis, urethritis, vaginitis, inflammation at sites of fetal monitoring

D. Males and females
   1. Meningitis
   2. Endocarditis
   3. Gonococcal conjunctivitis

IX. Consultation/Referral

A. If no response to treatment as discussed previously
B. If complications develop

X. Follow-up

A. Test of cure not recommended by CDC (2006) unless symptoms recur, exacerbate, or do not resolve.
B. Serology test for syphilis in 30 days.
C. Chlamydia test if not done at initial visit prior to treatment.
D. Consider HIV and hepatitis B and C screening.

Appendix A has information about gonorrhea that you can photocopy or adapt for your patients. See Bibliography.

CDC Web site: http://www.cdc.gov/std/Gonorrhea/STDFact-gonorrhea.htm.

SYPHILIS

I. Definition

Syphilis is a sexually transmitted disease characterized by periods of active florid manifestations and periods of symptomless latency. It can affect any tissue or vascular organ of the body and can be passed on from mother to fetus.

II. Etiology

A. The causative organism is a motile spirochete, Treponema pallidum (T. pallidum)
B. Incubation period, 10–90 days; average 21 days

III. History

    A. What the patient may present with
        1. Primary symptoms
           a. Painless lesion (chancre) at site of entry of T. pallidum. Chancre appears on average about 3 wks after sexual contact and heals in 3–6 wks with a small inculum—this incubation period may be as long as 90 days. Sites include vulva, labia, fourchette, clitoris, cervix, nipple, lip, roof of mouth, tonsils, bite area, finger, urethra, rectum, and smooth, firm borders of ulcer.
           b. Enlarged inguinal or regional nodes; trochlear.
        2. Secondary symptoms that may or may not occur in untreated patients within 4–10 weeks of resolution of primary symptoms
           a. Generalized symmetrical papillo-squamous eruption of palms, soles or mucous membrane (condylomata lata)
           b. Alopecia; may have moth-eaten look
           c. Loss of lateral 1/3 of eyebrow
           d. Generalized nontender lymphadenopathy with firm, rubbery feel
           e. Symptoms of upper respiratory tract infection
           f. Low grade fever
           g. Malaise, anorexia, and arthralgia
           h. Mild hepatitis, splenomegaly, or nephrotic syndrome in about 10% of cases
           i. Mucus patches on tongue, under foreskin, and in intertriginous areas
        3. Latent stage: No clinical symptoms although 25% may have recurrence of cutaneous lesion; however demonstrate seriologic evidence
           a. Early latency: infection within the preceding year
           b. Late latency: over a year from date of initial infection. Patient may remain in latent stage for remainder of his/her life; however, 1/3 will develop the tertiary form of disease
           c. Tertiary stage: Osseous or cutaneous structures, cardiovascular system or nervous system become involved; most common developments are cardiovascular syphilis and neurosyphilis
           d. Neurosyphilis (exceedingly uncommon today) can occur at any stage from 1–30 or more years after original infection
    B. Additional information to be considered
        1. Sexual preference
        2. Current sexual activity
        3. Last sexual contact

4. Birth control method(s)
5. History of known contacts
6. History of previous sexually transmitted disease
7. History of recurrent infectious illness (e.g., mononucleosis)
8. History of fever, malaise, arthralgia, or rash of unknown etiology
9. History of cognitive dysfunction, sensory deficits, other neurological symptoms
10. Current medical therapy
11. Risk for HIV exposure

IV. Physical Examination

   A. Vital signs
      1. Temperature
      2. Blood pressure
      3. Pulse
   B. General examination of skin
      1. Alopecia
      2. Rash including soles of feet, palms, condyloma lata
   C. Pharyngeal examination
   D. Examine for enlarged inguinal nodes
   E. External examination of genitalia; vulvar lesions; chancre at point of inoculation
   F. Internal examination (speculum)
      1. Inspection of vaginal walls for lesions
      2. Inspection of cervix for lesions
      3. Inspection of discharge
   G. Bimanual examination
   H. Neurological examination per history and clinical findings

V. Laboratory Examination

   A. Nontreponemal: venereal disease research laboratory (VDRL) and rapid plasma reagin (RPR) (these are nonspecific serum tests) detect cross-reaction of antibody to syphilis with cardiolipin. Reported as reactive or nonreactive. Reactive test is reported by a quantitative titre, and reactive tests should be confirmed with treponemal testing. Use of only one type of serologic test is insufficient for diagnosis.
      1. Biological false positives occur with cardiolipin antigens sometimes present in drug abuse and in such diseases and conditions as:
         a. Lupus erythematosus
         b. Mononucleosis

      c. Malaria

      d. Leprosy

      e. Viral pneumonia

      f. After smallpox vaccinations or other recent vaccinations

      g. Persons with HIV

      h. Narcotic addiction

      i. Arthritis

      j. Scleroderma

      k. Tuberculosis

      l. Chronic fatigue syndrome

      m. Pregnancy

B. Specific serum treponemal antibody tests (correlate poorly with disease activity; persons who have a reactive test will have it for life unless diagnosis and treatment are very early)

    1. Fluorescent Treponemal Antibody-Absorption Test (FTA-ABS)

    2. T. Pallidum particle agglutination (TP-PA)

C. Gonococcus culture

D. Chlamydia test

E. Biopsy of the lesion

F. Darkfield microscopy exam (rarely available in free-standing clinics or offices)—most useful for males

G. Consider HIV testing; testing for Hepatitis B, C

VI. Differential Diagnosis

A. Herpes simplex

B. Condylomata acuminata

C. Granuloma inguinale

D. Chancroid

E. Lymphogranuloma venereum

F. Carcinoma

G. Pyoderma

VII. Treatment (with physician consult in some settings)

A. Medication (for primary and secondary syphilis)

    1. Benzathine penicillin G (BiCillin®) 2.4 million units IM single dose immediately.[12] Caution re: Jarisch-Herxheimer Reaction: in 50% of cases, 6–12 hours after injection, patient develops high fever, malaise, and exacerbation of symptoms lasting 24 hours. (This is a sign that the spirochete is breaking down.)

      2. For penicillin allergy: Doxycycline 100 mg orally twice a day x 14 days OR Tetracycline 500 mg orally 4 times a day x 14 days.

  B. For early latent syphilis (<1 year)

      1. Benzathine penicillin G, 2.4 million units IM single dose

  C. For late latent syphilis or unknown duration

      1. Benzathine penicillin G, 7.2 million units total, in 3 doses of 2.4 million units IM each at 7–day intervals

  D. For late syphilis or unknown duration

      1. Benzathine penicillin G, 7.2 million units total, in 3 doses of 2.4 million units IM each at 7–day intervals

  E. In pregnancy

      1. Treat with penicillin regimen appropriate for stage of syphilis.

      2. Hospitalize pregnant patients with history of penicillin allergies to undergo skin testing. If positive, should be desensitized and treated with penicillin. See 2006 CDC guidelines.

  F. General measures

      1. Support, especially in regard to possible Jarisch-Herxheimer Reaction

      2. Stress importance of completing all medication

      3. Partner should be treated concurrently; all contacts exposed within 90 days of diagnosis of primary, secondary, or early latent syphilis

VIII. Complications

  A. Progression of disease to tertiary stage

  B. 100% transmission to fetus with primary and secondary in pregnancy; 50% fetal mortality and 50% congenital syphilis. Early latent: 80% fetal infection (20% premature, 20% fetal death, 40% congenital syphilis). Late latent: 30% fetal transmission, 11% fetal death.

IX. Consultation/Referral

Positive diagnosis of disease

X. Follow-up

Quantitative serology tests for primary and secondary syphilis (nontreponemal serologic) should be obtained at 6 and 12 months (falling titer should be demonstrated if treatment is adequate—at least a 4–fold drop by 6 months using same test). If repeat titre does not decrease, patient should be followed with titres, or re-treated. For persons with persistent signs and symptoms, symptoms that recur, or 4-fold increase in nontreponemal test titre, re-treat and re-evaluate for HIV. For latent syphilis, repeat testing at 6, 12, and 24 months.

See Appendix A and Bibliography. Web site: http://www.cdc.gov/node.do/id/0900f3ec80007600.

CHANCROID

I. Definition

Chancroid is a bacterial infection of the genitourinary tract in which a rapidly growing ulcerated lesion forms on external genitalia. Definitive diagnosis requires the identification of H. ducreyi using special culture media. Even with the use of these media, sensitivity is < 80%. Diagnosis is usually based on clinical findings.

II. Etiology

    A. Causative agent is Haemophilus ducreyi, a short gram negative bacillus with rounded ends, usually found in chains and groups.

    B. Incubation period is 4–7 days after exposure (rare <3 or >10 days); lesion appears 3–14 days after exposure.

III. History

    A. What patient may present with
        1. History of (1–3) painful macules on the external genitalia, which rapidly changed to a pustule and then to an ulcerated lesion; may have "kissing ulcers" from autoinoculation; can also be painless
        2. Enlarged inguinal nodes
        3. Abscess in inguinal region
        4. A sinus formed over the healed lesion
        5. New lesions forming when exposed to lesions already present
        6. Pain on voiding or defecating
        7. Rectal bleeding
        8. Dyspareunia
    B. Additional information to be obtained
        1. History of sexually transmitted disease or pelvic inflammatory disease
        2. Previous vaginal infections; diagnosis, treatment

3. Previous urinary tract infections
4. Sexually active
5. Last sexual contact; new partner
6. If partner complained of sores
7. Last menstrual period
8. Method of birth control; other medications (antibiotics may mask symptoms)
9. Any associated vaginal discharge; duration of ulcers
10. Any associated pain
11. Travel to Asia (Thailand especially), Africa, South America, or Philippines in past month

IV. Physical Examination

   A. Vital signs
      1. Temperature
      2. Blood pressure
      3. Pulse
   B. Inguinal nodes
      1. Size
      2. Tenderness
      3. Nodes matted together forming a fluctuant abscess (buboes) in groin; usually unilateral inguinal lymphadenopathy
   C. External examination
      1. Observe labia, fourchette, clitoris, vagina, anal area for macules, papules
      2. Observe for shallow, nonindurated, painful ulcers with ragged, undetermined edges, varying in size and often coalesced; base of ulcers may be gray/bluish gray; surrounding red halo
      3. Observe for sinuses that may have formed when skin over abscesses has broken down
      4. Look for new lesions that may be forming as a result of autoinoculation
   D. Vaginal examination (speculum); observe for lesions in vagina, on cervix
   E. Bimanual examination

V. Laboratory Examination

   A. Usually based on clinical findings and history
   B. Cultures to laboratory; use media containing fresh defibrinated rabbit's blood or patient's own serum
   C. Darkfield exam for T. pallidum or serologic test for syphilis performed at least 7 days after onset of lesions and repeated in 3 months

D. Gonococcus culture, Chlamydia test
E. Herpes antibodies
F. HIV testing should be done at the time of this diagnosis and again in 3 months if initial results are negative
G. Further laboratory work as indicated
H. PCR testing for H. ducreyi is available in clinical laboratories that have conducted CLIA verification studies

VI. Differential Diagnosis

A. Herpes simplex
B. Syphilis

VII. Treatment

A. Medications
    1. Azithromycin 1 gram orally single dose OR
    2. Ceftriaxone 250 mg IM single dose OR
    3. Ciprofloxacin 500 mg orally twice a day x 3 days (safety in children < 18 years of age or in pregnancy or lactation has not been established) OR
    4. Erythromycin base 500 mg orally 4 times a day x 7 days
B. Medications in pregnancy
    1. Ceftriaxone 250 mg IM single dose OR
    2. Erythromycin base 500 mg orally 4 times a day x 7 days
C. General measures
    1. Buboes should be aspirated through adjacent intact skin, not incised
    2. No sexual contact until course of medication is finished
    3. Stress importance of completing course of medication
    4. Comfort measures
        a. Tepid water sitz baths; dry carefully with cool air hair dryer making sure to hold it away from body
        b. Avoid tight, restricting clothing
        c. Expose perineum to air flow as much as possible (wear a skirt without underpants when at home)
        d. Recommend peri-irrigation set for comfort
    5. Patient education
        a. Explain disease process and route of transmission
        b. Stress that sexual partner(s) need to be checked regularly (see X.C.)

VIII. Complications

A. Phimosis in the male
B. Urethral stricture

C. Urethral fistula
D. Severe tissue destruction
E. Ulcers may take years to heal
F. Perineal fistulas

IX. Consultation/Referral

A. If infection is suspected
B. If no response after 7 days of treatment, treatment as outlined above
C. Secondary infections
D. All HIV positive persons diagnosed with chancroid

X. Follow-up

A. Patient should be reexamined 3–7 days after initiation of therapy. If treatment is successful, there should be symptomatic improvement within 3 days of starting therapy. Clinical improvement should be evident within 7 days. If no improvement, consultation as described previously.
B. It should be noted that it may take > 2 weeks for complete healing of ulcers. The amount of time is related to the size of the ulcer.
C. All sexual partners who have had sexual contact within 10 days preceding symptoms with a person diagnosed with chancroid should be evaluated and treated even in the absence of symptoms.

See Bibliography. Web site: http://www.health.state.ny.us/diseases/communicable/chancroid/fact_sheet.htm.

LYMPHOGRANULOMA VENEREUM

I. Definition

Lymphogranuloma venereum is a sexually transmitted disease characterized by a transitory primary lesion followed by suppurative lymphangitis and serious local complications.

II. Etiology

A. Causative agent: Chlamydia trachomatis, serotypes, L1, L2, L3
B. Incubation period: 3–12 days up to 3 weeks
C. Found mainly in tropical or subtropical climates (Asia, Africa, South America); rare in the United States

III. History

    A. What the patient may present with

        1. "Sore" in genital area, mouth, anus, penis (of short duration, may go unnoticed); usually single and painless vesicle or nonindurated

        2. Fever

        3. Malaise

        4. Headaches

        5. Joint pain

        6. Anorexia

        7. Vomiting

        8. Unilateral tender enlargement of inguinal lymph node; stiffness, aching of groin

        9. Abscess in groin after 2–3 weeks

      10. Sinuses, scars in lower vagina or around introitus, or (in males) on penis

      11. Rectal discharge; perirectal/perianal fistulas and strictures

      12. Vaginal discharge

    B. Additional information to be considered

        1. Sexual preference; sexual practices

        2. Last sexual contact; new partner

        3. Known contact

        4. History of sexually transmitted disease or pelvic inflammatory disease

        5. Last menstrual period

        6. Method of birth control; other medications (antibiotics may mask symptoms)

        7. History of chronic infections

        8. Recent trip out of country or new immigrant from a country where LGV is common

        9. Duration of lesion

IV. Physical Examination

    A. Vital signs

        1. Blood pressure

        2. Pulse

        3. Respiration

        4. Temperature

    B. Inguinal nodes

        1. First symptoms unilateral tender enlargement of nodes

        2. Disease progresses for 2–3 weeks to form a large, tender, fluctuant mass that adheres to deep tissues and has overlying reddened skin (bubo)

      3. Multiple sinuses develop with purulent or serosanguineous discharge

      4. Healing occurs with scar formation, but sinuses persist or recur

      5. Chronic inflammation causes blockage of the lymphatic vessels leading to edema, ulceration, and fistula formation

  C. Vaginal examination (speculum)

      1. Vaginal walls: initial lesion may be on upper vaginal wall, resulting in enlargement and suppuration of perirectal and pelvic lymphatic vessels

      2. Cervix: initial lesion could be on the cervix

  D. Bimanual examination: tenderness in groin, vulva

  E. Rectovaginal examination: rectal wall may be involved, resulting in ulcerative proctitis with serosanguineous rectal discharge

V. Laboratory Examination and Diagnosis

  A. Genital and lymph node swabs of lesion or bubo aspirate can be tested by culture, immunofluorescence, or nucleic acid detection

  B. Chlamydia serology complement fixation test: fourfold rise or single titer of > 1:64 can support diagnosis

  C. Serology test for syphilis, gonorrhea culture

  D. Biopsy of chronic anorectal lesions and lymph nodes to rule out carcinoma

  E. Diagnosis made on clinical suspicion, epidemiologic information, and exculsion of other etiologies along with C. trachomatis testing

VI. Differential Diagnosis

  A. Syphilis

  B. Herpes simplex

  C. Carcinoma

  D. Chancroid

  E. Granuloma inguinale

  F. Chlamydia

  G. Hodgkin's disease

  H. Proctocolitis

  I. Inguinal lymphadenopathy

  J. Genital or rectal ulcers

VII. Treatment

  A. Medications

      1. Doxycycline 100 mg orally twice a day x 21 days

      2. Alternative regimens: Erythromycin base 500 mg orally 3 times a day x 21 days; Azithromycin 1 gram orally once weekly x 3 weeks is likely effective but clinical data are lacking

   B. Medications in pregnancy and lactation
      1. Erythromycin base 500 mg orally 3 times a day x 21 days
   C. General measures
      1. Sitz bath.
      2. Stress importance of completing the course of medication.
      3. All sexual partners should be treated if contact within 30 days before onset of symptoms; examine and test for Chlamydia/gonorrhea in urethra, cervix.
      4. Comfort measures
         a. Tepid water sitz baths; dry carefully with cool air hair dryer making sure to hold it sufficiently away from body.
         b. Avoid tight, restricting clothing.
         c. Expose perineum to air flow as much as possible (wear a skirt or robe without underpants at home).
         d. Recommend peri-irrigation set.
      5. Patient education
         a. Explain disease process and route of transmission.
         b. Stress importance of sexual partner(s) within 60 days of onset of symptoms being checked for urethral or cervical chlamydia.

VIII. Complications

   A. Scar formation
   B. Sinuses causing blockage of the lymphatic vessels, which leads to edema
   C. Fistula formation: rectovaginal, vulvar, other
   D. Suppuration of perirectal and lymphatic vessels
   E. Rectal stricture
   F. Systemic: phlebitis, hepatomegaly, nephropathy

IX. Consultation/Referral

   A. With physician prior to treatment if infection is suspected
   B. If no response to treatment as outlined previously
   C. If any of the above complications occur

X. Follow-up

   A. Reevaluate 3–5 days after treatment.
   B. Then evaluate every 1–2 weeks until healing is complete.
See Bibliography. Web site: http://www.health.state.ny.us/diseases/communicable/.

GRANULOMA INGUINALE

I. Definition

Granuloma inguinale (Donovanosis) is a chronic granulomatous bacterial infection with the intracellular gram-negative bacterium Klebsiella granulomatis usually involving the genitalia and surrounding tissues, and probably spread by sexual contact.

II. Etiology

    A. Usually found in tropical and subtropical areas such as India, Papua New Guinea, Central Australia, and southern Africa

    B. Calymmato bacterium granulomatis (a difficult-to-grow encapsulated bacillus organism)

    C. Incubation period: 5–6 weeks (some say anywhere from 1–12 weeks)

III. History

    A. What the patient presents with

        1. Female

            a. Painless papular or nodular ulcerative lesions arising on the vulva, in the vagina, urethra, anal area, inguinal region, or on the perineum with proliferation of granulation tissue and local destruction with scar tissue formation; single or multiple

            b. Beefy red proliferative lesion of fourchette with elevated rolled borders; bleeds easily

            c. Inguinal adenopathy (due to secondary infection)—bilateral

            d. Malodorous vaginal discharge

        2. Male

            a. Lesion same as in the female and appearing on penis, scrotum, groin, or thighs

            b. In homosexual males, lesions on anus and buttocks

    B. Additional information to be obtained

        1. History of sexually transmitted disease or pelvic inflammatory disease

        2. History of chronic illness

        3. Has patient recently been out of country? Where? (Especially India, Papua New Guinea, central Australia, southern Africa.) Is patient or patient's partner from, or has either visited, southeastern United States?

        4. Sexual preference; sexual practices (anal intercourse; sex toys)

     5. Last sexual contact
     6. Birth control method, current medications
     7. Last menstrual period

IV. Physical Examination

   A. Vital signs
     1. Temperature
     2. Blood pressure
     3. Pulse
     4. Respirations
   B. External examination
     1. Observe vulva for lesions (papular, nodular, or vesicular), beefy red nodules that develop into a rounded, elevated, velvety granulomatous mass; sharply defined rolled borders; signs of secondary infection
   C. Vaginal examination (speculum)
     1. Inspect vaginal walls for lesions
     2. Inspect cervix for lesions
   D. Bimanual examination

V. Laboratory Diagnosis

   A. Giemsa-stained smears of ulcer (diagnosis is confirmed by visualization of the Donovan bodies, large mononuclear cells with intracytoplasmic vacuoles containing the organism)—scrape at base of ulcer to get the tissue crush preparation or biopsy; no FDA-cleared PCR tests available
   B. Syphilis serology
   C. HSV culture

VI. Differential Diagnosis

   A. Syphilis
   B. Herpes simplex
   C. Lymphogranuloma venereum
   D. Chancroid
   E. Carcinoma
   F. Fungal infection
   G. Genital Amoebiasis

VII. Treatment

   A. Medication
     1. Doxycycline 100 mg orally twice a day for at least 3 weeks OR

B. Alternative regimens
1. Azithromycin 1 gram orally once a week for at least 3 weeks and until all lesions have completely healed
2. Ciprofloxacin 750 mg twice a day for at least 3 weeks OR
3. Erythromycin base 500 mg orally 4 times a day for at least 3 weeks OR
4. Trimethoprim-sulfamethoxazole one double-strength tablet (800 mg/160 mg) orally twice a day for at least 3 weeks and until all lesions have completely healed
C. In pregnancy and lactation
1. Erythromycin base 500 mg orally 4 times a day for minimum of 3 weeks plus strongly consider gentamicin parenterally (or other parenteral aminoglycoside)
D. Additional therapy for all adults
1. Gentamicin 1 mg/kg IV every 8 hours if lesions do not respond within first few days of therapy (or other parenteral aminoglycoside)
E. General measures
1. No sexual contact until treatment is completed.
2. Stress importance of completing course of medication.
3. Stress importance of examination of sexual contacts (within 60 days preceding onset of symptoms).

VIII. Complications

A. Scar tissue secondary to slow healing formation
B. Secondary infection, a common occurrence that results in gross tissue necrosis of genitalia
C. Deformity of genitalia
D. Dyspareunia
E. Systemic infection
F. Massive edema of vulva; penis (may be chronic)

IX. Consultation/Referral

A. With physician prior to treatment if disease is suspected
B. If no response to treatment as discussed above in 7 days—contact CDC or state health department

X. Follow-up

A. After completion of 2 to 5 days of medication.
B. Follow clinically until signs and symptoms have resolved.
C. Annual follow-up visits as disease can reappear, and there is a possibility of scar carcinoma.

See Bibliography. Web site: http://www.health.state.ny.us/diseases/communicable/granuloma_inguinale/fact_sheet.htm.

MOLLUSCUM CONTAGIOSUM

I. Definition

Molluscum contagiosum is an infectious disease of the skin affecting the face, arms, genitals, abdomen, and thighs. It is caused by a virus (molluscipox virus) and is seen in all age groups and in both sexes.

II. Etiology

    A. Unknown
    B. Probably transmitted through direct skin contact
    C. Incubation: 1 week–6 months (usual 2–7 weeks)

III. History

    A. What the patient may present with
        1. Fleshy growths (1–20), dome-shaped, waxy, or pearly white papules with central caseous white core, primarily in genital area, but may be found on other body surfaces; may be 1–5 mm in diameter (but up to 15 mm), may be pedunculated; can be single or grouped.
        2. No other symptoms or complaints but occasional pruritus, tenderness, and/or pain.
    B. Additional information to be considered
        1. Previous episode of similar lesions
        2. History of sexually transmitted disease
        3. Sexual activity, last intercourse
        4. Known contact
        5. Method of birth control; other medications
        6. Any drug allergies
        7. HIV risk/exposure, especially with widespread lesions 100 or more

IV. Physical Examination

    A. Observe perineum for fleshy, usually papular, skin-colored lesions with indented centers that contain white, curd-like material.
    B. Observe any other involved body area.

V. Laboratory Examination

    A. Visual examination

    B. Pathology report on crushed excised lesion using Papanicolaou smear, Wright's, Giemsa's, or Gram stain

    C. Serology test for syphilis

    D. Gonococcus culture/Chlamydia test

    E. Further laboratory work as indicated by history

    F. Consider HIV screen especially with 100 or more lesions

VI. Differential Diagnosis

    A. Genital warts (condylomata acuminata)

    B. Herpes simplex

    C. Pyogenic granuloma

    D. Folliculitis

    E. Small epidermal cysts

    F. Closed comedones

    G. Basal cell carcinoma

    H. Furunculosis

VII. Treatment

    A. Removal of lesion
       1. Cytotoxic agents—TCA (trichloracetic acid), BCA (bichloracetic acid), podophyllin
       2. Excision of lesions by curettage with topical anesthetic followed by application of silver nitrate
       3. Destruction of lesions by cryotherapy; consider MD consult
       4. Topical 5% imiquimod daily x 5 days/week at bedtime

    B. General measures
       1. Return for weekly or biweekly evaluation and treatment until lesions have healed.
       2. Refer sexual partner(s) for evaluation.

VIII. Complications

    A. Secondary staphylococcus infection

IX. Consultation/Referral

    A. For treatment stated previously.

    B. Patients with extensive molluscum, lesions on face, or repeated recurrence after treatment should be reevaluated for HIV infection.

X. Follow-up

Return for reevaluation if lesions persist/recur after treatment.
See Bibliography. Web site: http://dermatology.cdlib.org/92/reviews/molluscum/diven.html.

HEPATITIS

I. Definition

Hepatitis is an acute or chronic inflammation of the liver with or without permanent tissue damage and can be caused by many viruses including influenza viruses, mononucleosis, and CMV; there are also hepatitis viruses whose only target is the liver. At least 6 are known at present and are designated by the letters A, B, C, D, E, and G.

II. Etiology

    A. Causative organisms include hepatitis viruses A to E and G, mononucleosis virus, CMV, and various influenza viruses.
        1. Hepatitis A (HAV) is transmitted enterically—fecal oral route (rarely parenterally) with an incubation of 15–50 days, 28 day average.
        2. Hepatitis B (HBV) is transmitted parenterally, sexually via body fluids, perinatally, or from saliva from human bites; incubation 6 weeks to 6 months.
        3. Hepatitis C (HCV) is transmitted parenterally and permucosally, with an incubation average of 1–3 weeks for detection of HCV RNA in blood and 8–9 weeks to seroconversion for the antibody; major cause of posttransfusion hepatitis. It is thought that sexual and perinatal transmission may be possible, but latter is rare unless mother is co-infected with HIV.
        4. Hepatitis D (HDV), known as Delta virus, only affects persons who have active hepatitis B; transmitted parenterally, sexually, and perinatally. Incubation 3–13 weeks.
        5. Hepatitis E (HEV) is transmitted enterically (rarely parenterally) with 15–60 days, mean 40 days incubation.
        6. Hepatitis G: Percutaneous route; associated with chronic Hepatitis C; noted especially in drug users.

III. History

    A. What the patient may present with
        1. Right upper quadrant pain (may be intermittent)
        2. Loss of appetite

      3. Malaise, fatigue (increased sleep, activity level, libido)

      4. Fever, often low grade

      5. Flu-like symptoms, including headache

      6. Adenopathy

      7. Jaundice

      8. Nausea and vomiting

      9. Rash, hives

   10. Joint and muscle pain

   11. Darkened urine

   12. Light-colored stools

   13. Taste and smell peculiarities

   14. Intolerance of fatty foods, cigarettes

B. Additional information to consider

      1. Use of recreational drugs

      2. Alcohol use, quantity and frequency

      3. Medication use (including nontraditional remedies, herbal preparations)

      4. Partner an injectable drug user

      5. Recent transfusion of blood or blood products

      6. Recent surgery

      7. Eating raw or undercooked shellfish

      8. Daycare worker or has child/children in day care

      9. Occupational risks including exposure to body fluids, excrement; blood, blood products

   10. Sexual history and habits, especially anal intercourse; number of partners; use of sex toys; human bites

   11. History of sexually transmitted diseases

   12. Sexual partner and/or household member with symptoms

   13. Known exposure to someone with hepatitis

   14. Military or civilian service in the Middle East; travel to Africa, Asia, Central & South America, Eastern Europe, Alaska

   15. History of hepatitis B

   16. Visited or from disease-endemic areas of world

   17. Hemodialysis patient; transplant recipient; hemophiliac

   18. Inmate of correctional institution

   19. Contraceptive history

   20. History of needlestick injury, tattoos, body piercing; acupuncture, sharing toothbrushes, razors, nail files, clippers

   21. Infants of HBV & HCV mothers

IV. Physical Examination

A. Vital signs

      1. Temperature

      2. Pulse

     3. Respirations
     4. Blood pressure
  B. Abdomen
     1. Liver percussion, palpation
     2. Observation of skin color, turgor
     3. Organomegaly, tenderness
     4. Masses
     5. Adenopathy
  C. Complete physical examination with careful attention to
     1. Skin: rash, hives, color, turgor
     2. Joints: joint pain on range of motion; muscle pain
     3. Adenopathy

V. Laboratory Examination

  A. Feces for virus
  B. Liver function tests
  C. Mononucleosis screen
  D. Serology to determine type of hepatitis HAV: IgM anti-HAV in serum with acute or convalescent phase (5–10 days into incubation up to 6 months); HBV: several including HBsAg (HBV surface antigen), IgM Anti-HBc; HCV: test for antibody with EIA or inhanced chemiluminescence assay, possible supplemental antibody test; HDV: HBsAg, Anti-HDV; HEV: Ig Manti-HEV, IgG anti-HEV; HGV: PCR testing, test for HAV, HBV, HCV, HDV, HEV
  E. CMV
  F. HIV testing
  G. In severe hepatitis, serum albumin, prothrombin, and partial thromboplastin times, electrolytes, glucose, CBC, platelets
  H. Pregnancy test

VI. Differential Diagnosis

Infectious mononucleosis, primary or secondary hepatic malignancy, ischemic hepatitis, drug-induced hepatitis, alcoholic hepatitis, acute fatty liver (acute fatty metamorphosis) of pregnancy.

VII. Treatment

  A. As needed according to laboratory report and etiology; generally referral for medical management and follow-up
  B. Supportive for symptoms
     1. No alcohol during acute phase of hepatitis and for 6–12 months thereafter
     2. Adequate calories; balanced diet

C. Interferon is being used for HBV, HCV

D. Gamma globulin to household and daycare center contacts for hepatitis A within 2 weeks of exposure

E. Prevention for hepatitis B: for exposed persons HBV hyperimmune globulin and then hepatitis B vaccination after antibody testing

F. Prevention for hepatitis D: hepatitis B vaccination; TWINRIX

G. HAV recovery not aided by activity limitation; isolate food handlers with HAV; prevention for HAV with HAVRIX® or TWINRIX vaccine

VIII. Complications

A. Hepatitis A: rarely fatal, no chronic form, fulminant hepatitis, relapse

B. Hepatitis B: death; chronic disease in 5–10% of victims; of these, 50% get chronic liver disease leading to hepatocellular carcinoma in half of the cases; fulminant hepatitis, transmission to fetus 10–85%

C. Hepatitis C: > 50% of cases become chronic; cirrhosis; hepatocellular carcinoma; perinatal transmission

D. Hepatitis D: chronic liver disease, fulminant hepatitis

E. Hepatitis E: high mortality in pregnancy (fetus and mother); no reported chronic cases

F. Hepatitis G: little information to date

IX. Consultation/Referral

A. For medical treatment and follow-up

X. Follow-up

A. As appropriate for type of hepatitis

B. Encourage hepatitis B vaccination (HBV) of those who have not had disease; schedule 3 dose administration; okay in pregnancy and lactation

C. Repeat laboratory work as indicated for monitoring liver function after illness

D. Test for chronic HBV with serum assay for HBsAg

E. Encourage HAV vaccination for persons at increased risk

F. Note availability of TWINRIX—HAV and HAB Combined 3 dose vaccine

See Bibliography. Web site: http://www.cdc.gov/ncidod/diseases/hepatitis; http://www.cdc.gov/hepatitis/.

HIV/AIDS

Information on AIDS/HIV continues to increase and change. Because our role as clinicians in ambulatory settings is to identify, educate, and refer persons at high risk for the disease, the purpose of this guideline is to serve as a reference in those three areas only. Because AIDS has become the leading cause of death among young women, it has become increasingly important that women's health care clinicians keep abreast of current information by consulting professional journals and attending seminars on the subject.

I. Definition

AIDS is the commonly used acronym for acquired immune deficiency syndrome, which is the name for a complex of health problems first reported in 1981.

II. Etiology

Caused by the human immune deficiency virus (HIV); infection mainly by sexual contact (anal, vaginal, oral); contaminated blood and blood products, including needle and syringe sharing; contaminated semen used for artificial insemination; intrauterine acquisition (baby of woman with AIDS); and rarely breast milk. Majority of cases in the United States are HIV-1; HIV-2 infection is endemic in West Africa.

III. History

    A. What the patient may present with
        1. Rapid weight loss without known factor (> 10%)
        2. Extreme fatigue; unexplained, increasing tiredness
        3. Chronic diarrhea (> 1 month)
        4. Persistent dry cough, shortness of breath, dyspnea on exertion
        5. Prolonged fever, soaking night sweats, shaking chills
        6. Loss of appetite
        7. Purple or pink flat or raised lesions on skin or under skin, inside mouth, nose, eyelids, anus
        8. Changes in neurological and/or cognitive function
        9. Generalized adenopathy
      10. Chronic herpes simplex
      11. Recurrent herpes zoster
      12. Generalized dermatitis pruritic
      13. Oral and pharyngeal candidiasis; fungal infection of nails
      14. Persistent muscle pain

15. Fear of exposure to AIDS through sexual partner or high-risk behavior or work-related accident (needlestick, contact with infected blood)
16. Chronic sinusitis
17. History of abnormal Papanicolaou smears
18. Persistent vulvar, vaginal, and anal condyloma

B. Additional information to be considered
   1. Sexual history
      a. Homosexual encounters; anal penetration
      b. Use of condoms, other methods of contraception, anal intercourse as contraception
      c. High-risk partners
      d. High-risk sexual practices
      e. History of previous sexually transmitted disease
      f. Contact with prostitute
      g. Multiple partners or partner with multiple partners
   2. Use of injectable drugs by self or partner
   3. High-risk occupation
   4. History of blood transfusions or recipient of blood products particularly from 1980–1985
   5. Duration and frequency of any presenting symptoms
   6. Reason for fear of exposure to AIDS
   7. Gynecological history
      a. Recurrent sexually transmitted diseases, vaginitis, vaginosis
      b. Widespread molluscum contagiosum 100 or more lesions
      c. Infected with several sexually transmitted diseases concurrently (may include gonorrhea, syphilis, Chlamydia)
      d. Rapidly progressing cervical dysplasia
      e. Papillomavirus on Papanicolaou smear
      f. Recurrent, recalcitrant vaginal candidiasis
      g. External condyloma unresponsive to treatment
      h. Existing pregnancy
      i. Anal discharge
      j. Pelvic, abdominal pain
   8. Travel outside the United States, especially to West Africa

IV. Physical Examination

   A. As appropriate to presenting complaint

V. Laboratory Examination

   A. Per protocol for presenting complaint, symptoms, risk status, exposure.

B. HIV testing if indicated or requested; if setting offers testing, resources must be in place for both pretest and posttest counseling for positive or negative results and follow-up; retest as needed.

C. CDC recommends HIV testing for all persons seeking evaluation for STDs; consider rapid testing if patients unlikely to return for results.

D. All pregnant women should have HIV screening and encourage for women planning a pregnancy (per new CDC guidelines, 2006).

E. Workplace exposures.

F. Consider other bloodborne screening including HAB, HAC.

VI. Differential Diagnosis

A. Widely different depending on presenting complaint

VII. Treatment

A. General measures
   1. Counseling to avoid or minimize high-risk behaviors
      a. Instruction and counseling regarding safer sexual practices to protect self and partner from exchange of body fluids (e.g., by using latex condoms, female condoms, dental dams, Saran Wrap™); by avoiding anal intercourse and oral-genital contact; avoiding sharing sex toys such as vibrators and dildos (or clean them with bleach or alcohol).
      b. Decreased number of sexual partners; mutual monogamy; abstinence.
      c. Discourage use of injectable drugs; if patient is using injectable drugs, stress the need to avoid needle, works, or cooker sharing; offer resources on drug rehabilitation programs.
      d. Avoid unsafe sexual contact with persons who are injectable drug users or fall into other high-risk groups.
      e. Sexual activities with partner with AIDS that do not involve direct passage of body fluids, such as light kissing, caressing, mutual masturbation.
      f. Empowering women to maintain equal decision-making power in their relationship(s).
      g. Avoid sharing razors, toothbrushes, nail files and clippers, and other items that could be contaminated with blood.

B. Specific treatment
1. Per guideline for specific presenting complaint.
2. Refer those patients falling into high-risk groups for further counseling and appropriate testing and follow-up if setting does not offer such services.
3. Referral for exposure so prophylactic therapy can be instituted.

VIII. Complications

A. Opportunistic infections.
B. AIDS may be fatal to some of its victims within two years of diagnosis.
C. Transmission to unborn child (infant's true HIV status based on antibody testing will not be accurate until 6–10 months); for a child < 18 months, definitive tests include evidence of HIV in blood or tissues by culture, nucleic acid, or antigen detection.

IX. Consultations and Referral

A. All patients falling into high-risk groups in need of testing for presence of HIV virus unless setting offers testing and counseling.
B. Referral for all patients testing positive to HIV antibody for appropriate treatment.
C. Referral per guideline for all occupational exposures.

X. Follow-up

A. Per referral
B. Contraceptive and gynecological services for women with AIDS
See Appendix E for self-assessment of AIDS (HIV) risk list, which can be photocopied or adapted for your patients. See Bibliography. Web sites: http://www.cdc.gov/nchstp/hiv_aids/hivinfo.htm; http://www.cdc.gov/hiv/pubs/facts.htm.

SAFE PRACTICES FOR CLINICIANS

A. Dispose of all needles, scalpels, capillary tubes, glass slides, lancets, and other sharp items in puncture-resistant containers. Handle as little as possible (i.e., do not recap needles); use safety needles when available.
B. Wear gloves *when anticipating* exposure to body fluids, including for phlebotomy and for handling specimens (urine, blood,

stool, sputum, vaginal secretions), and for contact with any mucus membranes (vaginal, oral, nasal, rectal) and open wounds. Don't substitute gloves for handwashing, however.

C. Wear gloves, gowns, masks, and goggles as appropriate when there is to be extensive contact with body fluids as during surgery or delivery; wear double gloves for surgical procedures when possible. Change any blood-stained clothing as soon as possible.

D. Wash thoroughly (with copious amounts of soap and water) following any skin contact with patient's body fluids.

E. Wear gloves on both hands for vaginal and rectal exams; use careful technique to keep one hand clean when handling clean materials such as fixative spray for Pap smears or examination lights; wash after examination is completed. Goggles are now recommended for vaginal examinations and phlebotomy in ambulatory as well as inpatient settings.

F. Change gloves for rectal examination after vaginal examination or for fitting a diaphragm or cervical cap after pelvic examination.

G. Avoid contamination of surfaces in the examining room or laboratory with body fluids from patients.

H. Use chlorine bleach solution 1:10 in a spray bottle to clean examining table and other surfaces and items contaminated with body fluids. Several other commercial products with longer shelf life are available for this use. Wear gloves for clean-up.

I. Keep hands from becoming dry and cracked.

J. Follow Centers for Disease Control (CDC) and OSHA recommendations and updates for protection of self and patients (CDC: http://www.cdc.gov; OSHA: http://www.osha.gov).

K. Assume every patient has the potential to be infected with AIDS or to be HIV positive and protect him/her and yourself with good technique.

L. Educate staff and patients about modes of infection, protection, and address myths to dispel unwarranted fears.

See Bibliography. Web site: http://www.osha.gov/pls/oshaweb/owadisp.show_document?p_table=STANDARDS&p_id=10051.

NOTES

1. Adapted from material developed by R. Mimi Secor (1997) Vaginal microscopy, *Clinical Excellence for Nurse Practitioners, 1*(1), 29–34.
2. Note that KOH should be used with care since it is very damaging to the microscope.
3. Fem Exam (Cooper Surgical), Shelton, CT.

4. Pip Activity Test Card (Litmus Concepts), Santa Clara, CA.
5. Quidel Corporation, San Diego, CA.
6. Biomed Diagnostic has introduced In Tray Colorex Yeast Test to differentiate the 4 species www.biomeddiagnostics.com/pilot.asp?pg=yeast.
7. Imidazole drugs (Miconazole, Clorimazole, Econazole, Butaconazole) are not as effective for non-Candida albicans as are triazole compounds including terconazole and tioconazole. Note serious adverse effects can occur; use with caution when patient is taking other drugs, so check carefully for drug interactions before recommending or prescribing.
8. Vaginal gel Metronidazole is not recommended for trichomoniasis as the protozoa are multifocal including the urethra, Skene's glands, and so on.
9. Many new blood tests for HSV are available depending on geographic location.
10. No data on BCA efficacy are available.
11. Podophyllin is now considered ineffective: its use has been discontinued in many settings. Use should be limited > 0.5ML or < 10CW^2/session to decrease potential systemic effects.
12. In Massachusetts the regimen is 2 doses, one week apart (Massachusetts Department of Public Health, Division of STD Prevention, 2006 STD Treatment Guidelines).

CHAPTER FOUR

Miscellaneous Gynecological Aberrations

BARTHOLIN'S CYST, BARTHOLINITIS

I. Definition

Bartholin's duct cyst is a postinflammatory pseudocyst that forms proximally to the obstructed duct of a Bartholin's gland. The obstruction leads to dilatation of the duct. Bartholinitis is inflammation of one or both of the Bartholin's glands.

II. Etiology

    A. Responsible organisms include:
        1. Staphylococcus aureus
        2. Streptococcus fecalis
        3. Escherichia coli (E. coli)
        4. Pseudomonas may also be cultured from abscess
        5. Gonococcus
        6. Chlamydia trachomatis
        7. Trichomoniasis
        8. Bacteroides

III. History

    A. What the patient may present with
        1. Painful, swollen lump in posterior vaginal area—can be unilateral or bilateral

    2. Difficulty sitting and walking due to severe pain and swelling

B. Additional information to be considered

    1. Previous infection of a Bartholin's gland or duct; if yes, how was it treated?

    2. History of sexually transmitted disease

IV. Physical Examination

A. Vital signs
    1. Temperature
    2. Blood pressure

B. Visual examination of external genitalia
    1. Cyst is characteristically located in the lower half of the labia with its inner wall immediately adjacent to the lower vaginal canal
    2. Lesions may vary in size from 1 to 10 cm
    3. The involved area may be painfully tender
    4. There may be no subjective symptoms

V. Laboratory Examination

A. Culture lesion at time of incision and drainage

B. Consider cervical cultures for Chlamydia and gonorrhea

VI. Differential Diagnosis

A. Lipoma

B. Fibroma

C. Hydrocele

D. Carcinoma of Bartholin's gland (extremely rare)

E. Inclusion cysts, sebaceous cysts

F. Congenital anomaly

G. Secondary metastatic malignancy

H. Hernia

VII. Treatment

A. Sitz baths 4 times a day × 2–3 days, then reexamine. If size has increased or there is no change, perform incision and drainage or refer to physician for possible marsupialization. If cyst or gland is extremely painful or large, immediate physician referral.

B. Antibiotics as appropriate to organism; most common ampicillin 500 mg 4 times a day × 7 days; Ceftriaxone 125 mg IM single dose; Cefixime 400 mg orally in single dose; Azithromycin 1 gram orally in a single dose or Doxycycline 100 mg orally twice a day × 7 days.

VIII. Complications

Recurrence

IX. Consultation/Referral

See VII. A. and B.

X. Follow-up

At clinician's discretion after incision and drainage or marsupialization.

See Bibliography. Web site: http://www.mayoclinic.com/health/bartholin-cyst/DS00667.

VULVAR CONDITIONS[1]

I. Definition

Primary vulvar conditions are those that arise from abnormal epithelial growth that can be inflammatory, dermatologic, or congenital in origin or from neoplastic alterations. Because the vulva includes the labia majora and minora, the mons veneris, fourchette, and vestibule and encompasses the urethral and vaginal orifices and the ducts of the Skene's and Bartholin's glands, vulvar conditions are varied both in origin and in clinical manifestations. Please refer to separate guidelines for sexually transmitted diseases that can cause clinical signs and symptoms on the vulva and guidelines for Bartholin's cyst, molluscum contagiosum, herpes, and condyloma.

II. Etiology

    A. Nonneoplastic epithelial disorders
        1. Squamous cell hyperplasia
        2. Lichen simplex chronicus
        3. Lichen sclerosis
        4. Pigmented lesions
        5. Systemic diseases
    B. Neoplastic disorder (vulvar intracellular neoplasia—VIN)
        1. Vulvar intraepithelial neoplasia
            a. Low grade squamous intraepithelial lesion (SIL) mild dysplasia
            b. High grade SIL moderate to severe dysplasia
            c. Carcinoma in situ
            d. VIN 2 to 3

  e. Invasive VIN
2. Other neoplastic disorders
  a. Paget's versus vulvar vaginal candidiasis (VVC)
  b. Melanoma (5% is vulvar)

III. History

A. What the patient may present with
    1. Pruritus, rash
    2. Hypo- or hyperpigmentation
    3. Bullae
    4. Weeping, scaling, crusting
    5. Excoriation
    6. Maceration
    7. Thickening
    8. Hyperkeratosis
    9. Fissures
    10. Abscesses
    11. Lesions: macules, papules, vesicles, warty, pedunculated, domed, flat, plaques
    12. Lichenification
    13. Change in color of vulva
    14. Dyspareunia
    15. Burning
B. Additional information to be considered
    1. Type of clothing commonly worn
    2. Type of underwear: cotton, synthetic
    3. Use of feminine deodorant products
    4. Use of scented, deodorant tampons, pads, panty liners
    5. Douching; shaving of perineum
    6. Detergents, bathing soap, fabric softeners
    7. Bubble bath or oils, body washes, lotions, creams
    8. Family or personal history of diabetes
    9. Sexual partners, activity; contraception; STD history
    10. Fungal infection of hands and feet, self or partner; oral candidiasis
    11. Last menstrual period
    12. Perimenopausal symptoms
    13. History of dermatologic conditions: HPV, psoriasis, eczema, seborrheic dermatitis
    14. Fever, malaise, flu-like symptoms
    15. Character and changes in lesions
    16. Partner with symptoms
    17. History of Crohn's disease; other systemic disease

18. Genital HPV history, history of Papanicolaou smear with HPV, any abnormal Papanicolaou history
19. Any other possible allergens: plant, make-up, nail polish, depillatories, piercings, & jewelry

IV. Physical Examination

A. Vulva
   1. Skin appearance: inflammation, edema, dry or moist, thickening hyperkeratosis
   2. Lesions present
   3. Weeping, scaling, crusting
   4. Fissuring
   5. Lichenification
   6. Excoriation
   7. Hypopigmentation
   8. Hyperpigmentation
B. Adenopathy
C. Groin, inner thighs, buttocks
   1. Lesions
D. Other systems as indicated by history and drugs

V. Laboratory Examination as Indicated by History and Appearance of Lesions

A. Bacterial cultures and sensitivities
B. Wood's lamp examination
C. Grain-stain scraping from lesions
D. Scrapings in KOH
E. Punch biopsy of lesions
F. Colposcopic examination
G. Staining with 1% toluidine blue
H. Fasting blood sugar
I. HPV testing

VI. Differential Diagnosis

A. Allergic vulvitis, cellulitis
B. Inflammatory conditions and reactions
C. Bacterial, viral, fungal infections
D. Lichen sclerosis
E. Necrotizing fasciitis
F. Pigmentation disorders
   1. Hyperpigmentation
   2. Congenital hypopigmentation
G. Benign epithelial changes

H. Neoplasms: vulvar intraepithelial neoplasia, Paget's disease, melanoma
I. Lesions from Crohn's disease
J. Trauma
K. Infestation

VII. Treatment

A. Medication
   1. Contact dermatitis: Burow's compresses; 1% cortisone cream
   2. Bacterial infections: Erythromycin 250 mg 4 times a day × 14 days; tetracycline 250 mg 4 times a day × 10–14 days or until resolved
   3. Tinea: topical antifungals such as GyneLotrimin, Mycelex, or Monistat Derm
   4. Analgesics for pain
   5. Topical antibiotics
B. Lifestyle changes and self-care measures
   1. Wear loose, cotton underwear; don't wear underwear in bed
   2. Keep area dry and clean
   3. Discontinue use of irritant or allergen
   4. Hot packs
   5. Sitz baths
C. Teaching and reassurance

VIII. Complications

A. Secondary infection
B. Progressive disease
C. Masking more serious disease

IX. Consultation/Referral

A. Unable to identify lesion or condition
B. No response to treatment
C. Progression of disease
D. For biopsy, diagnostic work-up
E. For surgical excision or other surgical intervention
F. To specialist for systemic disease or dermatoses beyond the vulva
G. To specialist for vulvar vestibulitis and vulvodynia

X. Follow-up

As indicated by therapy or for further diagnostic work.

See Bibliography. Web site: http://www.ivf.com/vse.html for vulvar self-examination.

DYSESTHETIC VULVODYNIA

I. Definition

Chronic mild to severe vulvar pain that is described as burning, stinging, irritating, and/or rawness that occurs alone or in conjunction with other vulvar pain syndromes or dermatoses and may occur with or without an identifiable provocation. The name is derived from the Greek word *odynia,* which means *pain.* The vulvar discomfort may involve the urethra, perianal area, and the thighs as well as the generalized vulvar area. Accounts for 15% of gynecology visits and includes all ages of women.

II. Etiology

    A. May not be one single etiology but rather a mixed pathology.

    B. Chronic infection could be the precipitating factor, careful diagnosis of candida by positive wet mount or fungal culture, whereby the vulva becomes permanently sensitized from infection.

    C. Cutaneous perception or sensory nerve damage—neuropathic pain.

        1. The vulva is rich with nerve fibers that may be disrupted or altered by inflammation and cause a sustained prolonged firing along the nerve even after the initial causative agent is removed or treated (i.e., infection).

            a. C fibers in the vestibule that are unmyelinated and are mechanosensitive and thermosensitive nociceptors.

            b. The remainder of the vulva is rich with A delta fibers that are mechanosensitive and myelinated and sensitive to light touch and thermosensitive nociceptors + C fibers.

        2. Sensitization occurs with chronic stimulation or irritation resulting in allodynia (pain from a non-noxious stimulus).

        3. Pain or hypersensitivity in radiating areas such as the thighs and perianal area may be suggestive of pudendal neuralgia.

        4. Hyperpathia—stimulus causes greater pain than would be expected.

        5. Central sensitization—related to lower parts of the brain and the cortex as well as centers of the spine. This sensitization is caused by a persistent signal to the nerve center that causes sensitization. Neurotransmitters activate these pain centers

as well and are the same chemicals that are increased in stress and anxiety. Lower peripheral pain thresholds in other sites such as the thumb and shin have been noted in women with vulvodynia that help to support this theory.

6. Dysesthetic vulvodynia is associated with cutaneous pain perception unrelated to touch.

7. Neuroimmunologic mechanisms involved in the allodynia/hyperpathia process in vulvodynia. These proposed mechanisms are under study.

D. Embryogenic correlation with interstitial cystitis—tissue from two anatomic sites that have a common embryonic origin, the urogenital sinus; because of this common origin, may have a similar pathology response when provoked.

E. Inflammatory dermatosis—related to prolonged topical steroid use, where temporary relief rebounded with more severe discomfort upon discontinuing the topical, or associated with benzylkonium chloride in pads and tampons or meds like benzocaine and lidocaine, or lotrisone.

F. Genetic relationship—check to see if other female family members have had problems with tampon use or dyspareunia.

G. Pelvic floor dysfunction—the muscles involved in the pelvic floor are both tight and weak, the increase in muscle tone decreases blood flow to the vulvar tissue with decreases in nutrients and build up of lactic acid causing tightness and pain. The resting tone of the muscle is most associated with the pain and secondly the variability of the contractile signal.

III. History

A. What the patient may present with
   1. High incidence of anxiety and emotional distress as a result of the vulvar pain
   2. Experiencing the pain for years
   3. In a stable relationship
   4. Having been examined by several clinicians
   5. History of one or more chronic pain conditions
      a. Migraines
      b. Fibromyalgia
      c. Irritable bowel syndrome
      d. Low back pain
      e. Interstitial cystitis
      f. Chronic fatigue syndrome
      g. Other

B. Begin with a thorough history
   1. Use open-ended questions about the pain and associated factors
      a. Location and duration of pain
      b. Any initiating factors
      c. Medications used and their effects on the pain
      d. Family history of similar pain
      e. Use of soaps, detergents, feminine products
      f. Contraceptive use
      g. History of trauma—vulvar surgery, episiotomy
      h. Discomfort with intercourse or pelvic exams
      i. Impact on daily living
      j. Any associated symptoms—urinary, bowel
      k. Pain or discomfort for hours or days following a pelvic exam or intercourse
      l. Constant or intermittent discomfort not related to touch or pressure
      m. History of seeing many clinicians without successful therapy

IV. Physical Examination

A. As appropriate to the history
B. Pelvic exam
   1. Inspection: erythema, erosions, ulcers, vesicles, whitened epithelium, any vulvar lesions or alterations in the vulvar architecture
   2. Cotton Q-tip test, light pressure, indent 5 mm to labia, urethra, hymenal remnants, and thighs, especially the posterior introitus and posterior hymenal remnants and note areas of tenderness—vulvodynia patients will have more generalized pain not necessarily made worse by touch or any pressure
   3. Signs and symptoms of infection
   4. May be no objective findings or some mild erythema noted
   5. Pelvic exam—note any associated pelvic pain and vaginal muscle tone
   6. Check for vaginismus

V. Laboratory Examination as Indicated by History and Physical Examination

A. Bacterial cultures and wet mount
B. If wet mount is negative for candida, do a fungal culture
C. HSV culture if erosions, fissures, or vesicles are present
D. Vulvar biopsy if there is a suspicious vulvar lesion

VI. Differential Diagnosis

    A. Infection—candida or other fungal, herpes or other viral, bacterial
    B. Inflammatory dermatoses—contact dermatitis, immunobullous disorders, lichen planus, lichen sclerosus, erosive lichen planus
    C. Neoplastic—squamous cell carcinoma, Paget's, VIN neoplasm
    D. Neurologic—HSV neuralgia, spinal nerve compression, pudendal nerve compression

VII. Treatment

    A. Chronic pain model emphasizing ameliorating pain rather than cure.
    B. Patient education: good vulvar care—avoid tight clothes, 100% cotton underwear as well as tampons or pads. Use of hypoallergenic detergents and stress reduction methods; avoid chemical irritants—soaps, feminine sprays.
    C. Multidisciplinary team approach; consider gynecologist, dermatologist, urologist, gastroenterologist, physical therapist, and pain specialist per individual situation and accompanying symptoms.
    D. Establish a sound, communicative, and trusting relationship.
    E. Establish one clinician as coordinator for the multidiscipline team (NP ideal).
    F. Treat any identified infections first, vaginal atrophy, or HSV with appropriate medication.
    G. Begin with local topical anesthetics such as Lidocaine 5% ointment, applied to a cotton ball and placed at the vestibule overnight.
    H. Medications for neuropathic pain include:
        1. Tricyclics—Amitriptyline, nortriptyline with gradual dose increases to numb the nerves by decreasing the electrical signals
        2. Neurontin (gabapentin) anti-seizure medication that is used for neuropathic pain
        3. SSRIs such as Cymbalta, Effexor
        4. None of these medications are FDA approved for use in neuropathic pain
            a. Refer to an appropriate clinician with experience with these drugs, or
            b. Work with an appropriate clinician in treating the patients
            c. Doses and effectiveness will vary as will adverse events
            d. Closely monitor
        5. Alpha interferon injections intralesionally to the vestibule in vestibulodynia only

I. Advise a low oxalate diet with calcium citrate.

J. Refer to physical therapy for biofeedback to train the muscles to relax and teach the patients some control of these muscles.

1. Specific sEMG to identify pelvic floor muscle abnormality and treatment to those muscles (cranio-sacral, myofascial)

2. Trigger point muscle massage—work with a physical therapist or massage therapist trained in women's health

3. Muscle stabilizing program, based on each woman's individual needs (6–8 months of PT)

K. Suggest acupuncture and/or hypnosis.

L. Suggest personal counseling to decrease the woman's personal distress related to vulvar pain when necessary.

M. Suggest marital counseling and sexual counseling when appropriate for issues related to intimacy discomforts that may arise with vulvodynia. As a woman's pain decreases so may her sexual discomforts, distress, and anxiety, because these are correlated.

VIII. Complications

A. Development of additional symptoms following institution of treatment

B. Side effects of any medications

C. Co-existence of life-threatening condition

IX. Consultation/Referral

A. Specialist in vulvodynia, dermatologist

B. Psychotherapy, marital, sexual counseling

C. Physical therapy, massage therapy, other complementary and alternative therapies

D. Nutritional therapy

E. Gastroenterologist

F. Pain specialist or pain clinic

X. Follow-up

A. Return for recheck after treatment is initiated

B. Team review as warranted by patient's response to interventions

C. As indicated by therapy or for further diagnostic work and consultation

Web site: http://www.mayoclinic.com/health/vulvodynia/DS00159.

Guideline developed by Linda Hansen Rodier, MS, RN, WHCNP, Dermatology Nurse Practitioner, Dartmouth-Hitchcock Dermatology Clinic, Manchester, New Hampshire.

ACUTE PELVIC PAIN

I. Definition

Acute pelvic pain can be defined as sudden onset of severe lower abdominal pain assessed to be gynecologic in nature.

II. Etiology

    A. Physiologic causes
1. Infection from a variety of organisms resulting in pelvic inflammatory disease
2. Extrauterine pregnancy
3. Ovarian pathology
4. Uterine perforation
5. Ruptured pelvic abscess in a variety of sites
6. Aberrant uterine leiomyomata
7. Bladder pathology; bowel pathology
8. Ureteral pathology
9. Proliferate endometrium beyond the uterine corpus
10. Postsurgical sequelae
11. Mittelschmerz
12. Trauma, abuse, sexual assault
13. Age-related physiologic change
14. Acute cholecystitis
15. Pancreatitis
16. Appendicitis
17. Vascular

    B. Psychologic causes
1. Secondary to pelvic surgery
2. Secondary to pregnancy whatever the outcome
3. Secondary to resolved pelvic pathology
4. Primary or secondary as a focal site for stress; post-traumatic stress disorder secondary to sexual abuse, assault

III. History

    A. What the patient may present with
1. Sudden onset of symptoms
2. Chills, fever, body aches
3. May have nausea, vomiting, and/or diarrhea
4. May have constipation
5. Increased vaginal discharge
6. Acute, continuous, or intermittent cramping
7. Urinary symptoms including frequency and pain

      8. Missed menses
      9. Menses at time of onset
   10. History of pelvic surgery
   11. History of ovarian cysts
   12. History of extrauterine pregnancy
   13. History of PID
   14. History of urinary tract infection
   15. History of endometriosis
   16. History of gonorrhea or Chlamydia infection
   17. History of rape, sexual assault, incest
   18. History of bowel disease

B. Additional information to be considered

1. Location of pain: whether it stays in any one place or is variable; whether the patient has ever had this pain before
2. Description of pain: sharp, dull, throbbing; rate pain
3. When does pain occur; does it wake patient up
4. Does anything induce the pain such as eating, defecating, urinating, sexual intercourse, sexual stimulation; beliefs about cause of pain
5. What, if anything, relieves the pain
6. Any weight gain or loss
7. Associated symptoms such as diarrhea, blood in stool or urine, increase in vaginal discharge, or vaginal bleeding
8. Timing in relation to menses, if any association
9. Duration of symptoms: days, weeks, months; regularity of symptoms
10. Sexual history: exposure to sexually transmitted disease, unprotected intercourse, new partner, change in contraception, methods used in recent past and currently; use of sex toys
11. Psychosocial history: unusual stressors at time of onset when pain occurs; life changes such as moving, new job, new relationship, end of relationship
12. Pelvic surgery in the past 12–24 months such as hysterectomy, laparotomy, tubal ligation
13. Diagnostic pelvic work-up such as laparoscopy, endometrial biopsy, colonoscopy, infertility work-up
14. Change in character of menses: heavier, lighter, more or less frequent

IV. Physical Examination

A. Vital signs as appropriate
    a. Temperature
    b. Blood pressure

       c. Pulse

       d. Respirations

B. Abdominal examination

  1. Bowel sounds: normal, hyperactive, sluggish, absent, any adventitious sounds, any bruits

  2. Generalized or localized lower abdominal tenderness

  3. Any guarding, pulsations observed

  4. Any rebound tenderness

  5. Any old scars

  6. Any distention

  7. Patient's perception of location of pain

  8. On percussion, are liver or spleen enlarged or is bladder distended

  9. Any pain elicited with light touch, with deep palpation

  10. Any organomegaly or masses

C. Vaginal examination

  1. Examine cervix for discharge

  2. Examine vagina for lesions, discharge, and any unusual odor

D. Bimanual examination

  1. Examine cervix for cervical motion tenderness

  2. Examine uterus for tenderness

  3. Examine adnexa for ovarian tenderness, masses, or tenderness in rest of adnexa

E. Rectal examination

  1. Pain or tenderness

  2. Masses

  3. Melena

F. Elicit psoas sign; perform obturator maneuver

V. Laboratory Examination

A. Cultures as indicated might include gonococcus culture, Chlamydia smear; wet mount; pH of vaginal fluids; vaginal & cervical cultures

B. Complete blood count/differential

C. Sedimentation rate; C-Reactive protein

D. Urinary tract infection screen

E. Pregnancy test—urine, UCG quantitative; do serial if positive

F. Ultrasound transvaginal, pelvic, abdominal

G. Flat plate of abdomen; renal ultrasonography

H. Other tests as symptoms and/or history indicate

I. Consider CA125 if age, history, family history, and/or physical findings indicate

VI. Differential Diagnosis

    A. Septic abortion

    B. Ectopic pregnancy

    C. Uterine leiomyomas with hemorrhage or infarction

    D. Ovarian cyst with rupture extruding blood, cyst fluid, and dermoid contents into pelvic cavity

    E. Uterine perforation

    F. Ruptured abscess from ovary, uterus, bowel; tubo-ovarian abscess

    G. Urinary tract infection: cystitis or pyelonephritis; kidney stones; interstitial cystitis

    H. Appendicitis

    I. Adhesions

    J. Solid ovarian tumor

    K. Irritable bowel syndrome; diverticulitis, acute bowel

    L. Primary dysmenorrhea, especially in women over 35

    M. Pelvic inflammatory disease

    N. Mittelschmerz, especially in women under 35

    O. Endometriosis

    P. Adenomatosis

    Q. Complications of intrauterine device

    R. Posttubal ligation syndrome; pelvic pain syndrome

    S. Constipation

    T. Lower bowel tumor

    U. Uterovaginal prolapse

    V. Sexual/physical abuse

VII. Treatment

    A. Medication as indicated for diagnosis

    B. Physician consult for suspected ectopic pregnancy, appendicitis, ovarian pathology, abscess, complications of uterine leiomyomas, suspected pelvic adhesions, irritable bowel syndrome, suspected bowel or other tumors

    C. Treatment for primary dysmenorrhea per guideline

    D. Removal of IUD; consult as needed for complications

    E. Teaching and comfort measures for Mittelschmerz

VIII. Complications

    A. Generalized sepsis

    B. Hemorrhage

    C. Perforation of bowel

    D. Rupture of abscess

    E. Rupture of site of extrauterine pregnancy
    F. Shock
    G. Bowel obstruction

IX. Consultation/Referral

    A. Unable to find cause
    B. Physician consult for medical or surgical intervention
    C. For hospitalization if no admitting privileges
    D. If symptoms worsen or recur after treatment
    E. No response to treatment
    F. Unable to remove IUD or find IUD or differentiate cause of problem with method

X. Follow-up

    A. Consider reevaluation in 48 hours as warranted by clinical findings
    B. Consider repeating bimanual and/or abdominal examination in 1 week and review status
    C. Seek immediate clinical consultation if symptoms worsen
    D. Follow up as appropriate for specific conditions such as PID
    See Bibliography. Web sites: http://womenshealth.about.com/cs/pelvicpain/a/pelvicpainpt2.htm; http://www.familydoctor.org/X2593.xml; http://www.medicinenet.com/abdominal-pain/article.htm; http://www.mayoclinic.com/health/abdominal-pain/DG00013.

CHRONIC PELVIC PAIN

I. Definition

Pain in any region of the pelvis that is long-term and unresponsive to treatment of symptoms and/or undiagnosed.

II. Etiology

    A. 50% enigmatic
    B. 25% endometriosis
    C. 25% other pathology including subacute and chronic salpingitis

III. History

    A. What the patient may present with
        1. Chronic pelvic pain with or without menstrual exacerbation
        2. Dysmenorrhea
        3. Dyspareunia
        4. Dyschezia

    5. Chronicity of symptoms
    6. Absence of chills, fever associated with pain
    7. Nausea, vomiting, and/or diarrhea associated with pain
    8. Chronic constipation
    9. Chronic intermittent cramping

IV. Additional Information to Be Considered

  A. Any symptoms of chronic bowel disease; any previous assessments for such, and results
  B. Any symptoms of chronic urinary tract infection, urinary tract anomaly, kidney disease
  C. Location of pain, duration, exacerbation, and what precedes increased symptoms
  D. Description of pain: sharp, dull, aching, cramping, intermittent, continuous
  E. Pain relief measures; what helps; use of over-the-counter analgesics
  F. Any weight gain or loss
  G. Symptoms that accompany pain
  H. Sexual history including sexual responsiveness; STDs, PID; contraceptive history including IUD
  I. Surgical history including hernia repair
  J. Medical history
  K. Pelvic surgery including laparoscopy, laparotomy, tubal ligation, hysterectomy, repair of cystocele, rectocele, urethrocele, appendectomy, myomectomy, cervical cone biopsy, LEEP, LOOP
  L. Menstrual history
  M. Pregnancy history including extrauterine pregnancy(ies), infertility assessments and/or treatments
  N. Psychosocial history including life stressors, major life changes, and timing in relation to onset of symptoms; depression, anxiety disorder, personality disorder
  O. History of incest, other sexual assault or abuse

V. Physical Examination

  A. Vital signs as appropriate
  B. Abdominal examination
    1. Bowel sounds: normal, hypo- or hyperactive, sluggish, absent, adventitious sounds, bruits
    2. Lower abdominal tenderness, sites of acute, dull pain elicited on superficial and/or deep palpation
    3. Any guarding
    4. Any rebound tenderness
    5. Scars

      6. Distention, asymmetry
      7. Patient's perception of pain location
      8. On percussion, liver, spleen enlarged, bladder distended
      9. Organomegaly, masses, hernias
  C. Vaginal examination
      1. Examine cervix for discharge
      2. Examine vagina for masses, lesions, discharge, unusual odor, color
  D. Bimanual examination
      1. Examine cervix for cervical motion tenderness
      2. Examine uterus for tenderness, masses, shape, size, consistency
      3. Examine adnexa for ovarian shape, size, tenderness, masses, other adnexal masses or tenderness
  E. Rectal examination
      1. Pain, tenderness
      2. Masses
      3. Melena
      4. Rectovaginal masses, fistulas, adhesions
      5. Rectocele
  F. Elicit psoas sign; perform obturator maneuver

VI. Laboratory Examination

  A. Cultures as indicated by history, physical findings
  B. Complete blood count/differential
  C. Sedimentation rate, C-reactive protein
  D. Urinary tract infection screen
  E. Pregnancy test
  F. Ultrasound evaluation based on pelvic examination
  G. Consider consultation for CAT scan and/or MRI if pelvic examination is abnormal
  H. Consider psychological testing

VII. Differential Diagnosis

  A. Uterine
      1. Dysmenorrhea (primary or secondary)
      2. Adenomyosis
      3. Leiomyomata
      4. Positional (prolapse)
      5. Pelvic congestion
  B. Adnexal
      1. Adhesive disease (infection, postsurgical)
      2. Neoplasm

      3. Functional ovarian cysts (Mittelschmerz)
      4. Endometriosis
  C. Peritoneal
      1. Endometriosis
      2. Adhesive disease
  D. Gastrointestinal
      1. Irritable bowel syndrome
      2. Other bowel disease (e.g., Crohn's, inflammatory)
  E. Urinary
  F. Musculoskeletal
  G. Psychogenic (e.g., sexual abuse, rape)
  H. Congenital, anatomical
  I. Neurologic (neuroma)
  J. Infections

VIII. Consultation/Referral

  A. For laparoscopic diagnostic examination
  B. For medical evaluation of suspected GI, GU conditions as indicated by history and physical examination
  C. For pelvic venography
  D. To confirm a suspected diagnosis and initiate treatment as co-managers of care
  E. For psychological evaluation
  F. For ultrasound, MRI

IX. Treatment

  A. Endometriosis
      1. Create a pseudomenopause with Danocrine 200 to 800 mg orally twice a day for 6 months; or GnRH analogues for 6 months (Nafarelin nasal spray 400 to 800 gm daily) or Leuprolide acetate (Lupron depot) 1 mg IM daily for 6 months, Zoladex® (Goserlin Acetate) implant 3.6 mg administered subcutaneously every 28 days for 6 months
      2. Continuous monophasic oral contraceptives
  B. Other pathological causes
      1. Diagnose and treat cause according to established guidelines (such as salpingitis, trauma from sexual assault, incest or rape, childbirth)
  C. Enigmatic pelvic pain
      1. Follow-up to diagnostic laparoscopy as appropriate to any findings
      2. Multidisciplinary approach to pain management

    D. Consideration of empiric therapy
       1. Antidepressant
       2. GnRH agonist
       3. Musculoskeletal relaxant

X. Follow-up

    A. As appropriate for diagnosis and treatment
    B. As desired by patient if no definitive cause is found and palliative treatments are suggested
    C. If symptoms continue, introduce the team approach
       1. Mental health care specialist
       2. Physical therapist
       3. Nutritionist
       4. Urogynecologist
       5. Gastroenterologist

See Bibliography. Web site: http://www.mayoclinic.com/health/chronic-pelvic-pain/DS00571.

ABDOMINAL PAIN

I. Definition

Pain (mild to severe) in any region of the abdomen as differentiated from the pelvic area, including the area from the costal margins to the beginning of the mons pubis, including but not limited to the abdominal organs and anatomical structure.

II. Etiology

    A. Inflammation, ulceration, infection, irritation, referred pain
    B. Space occupying lesion
    C. Response to injury: intra-abdominal or extra-abdominal
    D. Sequelae of surgery: adhesions, presence of foreign body, unrepaired perforation
    E. Systemic; hematologic; metabolic/endocrine; infectious; inflammatory; toxic; functional
    F. Tension pain

III. History

    A. What the patient may present with
       1. Anorexia
       2. Vomiting

    3. Nausea

    4. Change in bowel habits, constipation

    5. Urinary symptoms; dark urine

    6. Gynecological symptoms and history (see acute and chronic pelvic pain guidelines); menstrual, contraceptive history

    7. Diaphoresis

    8. Fainting, malaise, confusion, fatigue, joint pain

    9. Distension of the abdomen

   10. Dyspnea, tachycardia, bradycardia

   11. Fever

   12. Chills

B. Additional information to be considered (patient will generally complain only of abdominal pain; history must be very thorough). Specific questioning is needed to elicit information about and sequence of symptoms.

    1. Onset (sudden, gradual, chronic, and so on)

    2. Character (e.g., throbbing, aching, burning, knife-like)

    3. Intensity: difficult to define, but can be likened to other pain such as toothache, cramps, labor pain

    4. Location: where did pain originate; quadrant; generalized; epigastric

    5. Radiation: does it travel elsewhere

    6. Pain relief measures: what helps, what makes it worse

    7. Any weight gain or loss

    8. Pregnancy history; infertility diagnostics or treatments

    9. Psychosocial history including life stressors, major life changes and timing in relation to onset of symptoms

   10. History of incest, other sexual assault or abuse, violence or battering in relationships

   11. History of bowel obstruction, polyps, hernias

   12. History of abdominal tumors benign or malignant

   13. Use of GI irritants including spicy foods, lactose, infectious agents; nonfood substances

   14. Possible contaminated drinking water source in home country and/or abroad; food allergies, food poisoning

   15. History of pelvic and/or abdominal surgery including organ transplant

   16. History of extrauterine pregnancy

   17. History of ovarian cysts, rupture of cysts

   18. History of chronic bowel syndrome, any bowel disease

   19. History of gall bladder disease

   20. History of hepatitis, jaundice, liver disease, mononucleosis, abnormal liver function

21. History of trauma to the abdomen: accident, battering
22. History of travel abroad, recent immigrant and from where
23. History of exposure to industrial toxins, pesticides
24. History of kidney anomaly or disease; other genitourinary problems
25. History of appendicitis, chronic or acute
26. History of ulcers; gastric surgery
27. History of cardiovascular, respiratory problems
28. Previous care for abdominal pain; type of pain, origin, any treatments

IV. Physical Examination

A. Vital signs as appropriate
B. Cardiovascular, respiratory examinations; general appearance
C. Abdominal examination
    1. Bowel sounds; normal, hypo- or hyperactive, sluggish, absent, adventitious sounds, bruits
    2. Abdominal tenderness, sites of acute, dull pain elicited on superficial and/or deep palpation
    3. Any guarding
    4. Any rebound tenderness
    5. Scars
    6. Distension, symmetry or asymmetry
    7. Patient's perception of pain location
    8. On percussion liver or spleen enlarged, other abdominal organs enlarged
    9. Organomegaly, masses
    10. Abdominal bruits
D. Vaginal and bimanual examination
    1. Examine cervix for presence of IUD string
    2. Examine vagina for masses, lesions, discharge, unusual odor, color
    3. Examine cervix for cervical motion tenderness, mucopurulent discharge
    4. Examine uterus for tenderness, masses, shape, size, consistency
    5. Examine adnexa for ovarian shape, size, tenderness, masses; other adnexal masses or tenderness
E. Rectal examination
    1. Pain, tenderness
    2. Masses

    3. Melena

    4. Rectovaginal masses, fistulas, adhesions

    5. Rectocele

  F. Psoas sign, obturator sign

V. Laboratory Examination

  A. Cultures as indicated by history, physical findings

  B. Complete blood count/differential, serum electrolytes

  C. Liver function studies, enzymes; H. pylori culture, stool cultures

  D. Urinary tract infection screen; hepatitis panel

  E. Pregnancy test; cervical, vaginal smears, cultures

  F. Ultrasound evaluation based on examination

  G. X-ray if indicated; abdomen, chest, posterior, anterior & lateral, KUB films

  H. May consider consultation for CAT scan and/or MRI if abdominal or pelvic examination is abnormal

  I. Sickle cell prep if indicated

  J. ESR; TB skin test, blood, sputum cultures

  K. TSH

  L. Toxicology screen

VI. Differential Diagnosis

  A. Consider possible causes under acute and chronic pelvic pain and rule out:

    1. GI and GU pathology including appendicitis, pancreatitis, bowel obstruction, ulcers, cholecystitis, cholelithiasis, renal colic, biliary colic, rupture of spleen, diverticulitis, ileitis, carcinoma, irritable bowel syndrome, ulcerative colitis, pyelonephritis, hepatitis, hernias, urinary calculus, mesenteric thrombosis, urethral syndrome, perforation, strangulation, abscess, urinary tract infections, interstitial cystitis

    2. Acute or chronic constipation

    3. Dissecting aneurysm; embolism

    4. Ectopic pregnancy or other gynecologic finding

    5. Acute gastritis

    6. Drug or toxin reaction; toxic systemic causes

    7. Injury secondary to accident, violence including organ rupture

    8. Abdominal pain, undetermined etiology

    9. Referred pain from thoracic pathology: coronary thrombosis, pleural pneumonia, pleurisy, herpes zoster

    10. Gastritis, coronitis, ileitis secondary to parasitic infection, cholera, waterborne diseases

11. Systemic diseases: hematologic, metabolic/endocrine, infectious, inflammatory, functional

VII. Consultation/Referral

A. For laparoscopic diagnostic examination
B. For medical evaluation of suspected GI, GU conditions as indicated by history and physical examination
C. To confirm a suspected diagnosis and initiate treatment as co-managers of care
D. For surgical consultation as indicated by history and findings
E. For CAT scan, MRI

VIII. Treatment

A. As indicated by findings and history
B. Etiology undetermined, pain persists
   1. Follow-up to any diagnostic work-up
   2. Multidisciplinary approach to pain or symptom management

IX. Follow-up

A. As appropriate for diagnosis and treatment
B. As desired by patient if no definitive cause is found and palliative treatments are suggested
   See Bibliography. Web sites: http://www.mayoclinic.com/health/abdominal-pain/DG00013; http://www.familydoctor.org/X2593.xml; http://www.medicinenet.com/abdominal-pain/article.htm.

PELVIC INFLAMMATORY DISEASE (PID)

I. Definition

Pelvic inflammatory disease comprises a spectrum of inflammatory disorders of the upper genital tract. This may include any combination of endometritis, salpingitis, tuboovarian abscess, and pelvic peritonitis.

II. Etiology

A. Causative organisms include
   1. Neisseria gonorrhoea
   2. Streptococcus; agalactiae
   3. Peptostreptococcus, Peptococcus
   4. Bacteroides

5. Chlamydia trachomatis
6. Escherichia coli
7. Mycoplasma hominis
8. influenza
9. urealyticum
10. Gardnerella vaginalis
11. Trichomonads
12. Staphylococcus
13. Pseudomonas
14. Diphtheroids
15. Cytomegalovirus (CMV)
16. G vaginalis
17. Haemophilus agalactiae
18. M. hominis

III. History

A. What the patient may present with (wide variation in symptomatology, making diagnosis difficult)
    1. Lower abdominal pain, usually bilateral
    2. Chills, fever
    3. May have anorexia
    4. May have nausea
    5. May have vomiting
    6. Increased vaginal discharge
    7. Heavier than usual period; abnormal bleeding
    8. Urinary symptoms: frequency, pain
    9. May complain of right upper quadrant pain; also Fitz-Hugh Curtis syndrome
    10. Dyspareunia
B. Additional information to be considered
    1. Known exposure to sexually transmitted disease
    2. Previous sexually transmitted disease
    3. Previous diagnosis of pelvic inflammatory disease
    4. Previously diagnosed endometriosis
    5. History of abdominal surgery
    6. Chronic illness
    7. Sexual activity (present and recent past)
    8. Last menstrual period; birth control method; is there an intrauterine device in place or recent insertion; recent pregnancy, childbirth, or abortion
    9. Medication allergy
    10. Currently taking any medication

11. Recent pelvic surgery (i.e., therapeutic abortion or dilatation and curettage)
12. Smoker or nonsmoker (smoking cigarettes has recently been implicated as a risk factor for PID)
13. History of douching

IV. Physical Examination

  A. Vital signs
    1. Temperature
    2. Blood pressure
    3. Pulse
    4. Respiration
  B. Abdominal examination
    1. Bowel sounds: normal, hyperactive, sluggish, absent
    2. Generalized lower abdominal tenderness
    3. Guarding
    4. Rebound tenderness
  C. External genitalia
    1. Lesions
    2. Observe and palpate Skene's and Bartholin's glands
  D. Vaginal examination (speculum)
    1. Profuse vaginal discharge (may be purulent)
    2. Examine cervix for
      a. Erosion, ectropion
      b. Friability
      c. Discharge in os
  E. Bimanual examination
    1. Examine cervix for cervical motion tenderness
    2. Examine uterus for tenderness
    3. Examine adnexa for
      a. Tenderness
      b. Mass
    4. Rectovaginal examination for tenderness; if present, describe location (i.e., cervix, uterus, adnexa)

V. Laboratory Examination

  A. Gonococcus culture
  B. Chlamydia smear
  C. Complete blood count/differential, C-reactive protein
  D. Sedimentation rate
  E. Urinary tract infection screen
  F. Serology test for syphilis

G. Human chorionic gonadotropin if history indicates: urine, serum
H. Transvaginal ultrasound
I. Magnetic resonance imaging
I. Endometrial biopsy with histological evidence of endometritis
J. Laparoscopic abnormalities consistent with PID
K. Culdocentesis (refer to physician)

VI. Criteria for Clinical Diagnosis

A. Criteria for ambulatory treatment
  1. The three minimum criteria for diagnosis of PID are:
    a. History of uterine tenderness
    b. Cervical motion tenderness
    c. Adnexal tenderness (may be unilateral)
  2. Additional criteria that will increase the specificity of diagnosis
    a. Temperature of 101 degrees F (38.3 degrees C) or greater
    b. White blood cells on saline microscopy of vaginal secretions
    c. Abnormal cervical or vaginal mucopurulent discharge
    d. Elevated C-reactive protein
    e. Culdocentesis yielding peritoneal fluid, which contains bacteria, white blood cells
    f. Presence of adnexal mass noted on bimanual examination; tubo-ovarian abscess on sonography
    g. Elevated sedimentation rate greater than 15 mm/hour
    h. Positive gonococcal culture from cervix
    i. Positive Chlamydia smear from cervix
B. Criteria for hospitalization
  1. Surgical emergencies such as appendicitis cannot be excluded
  2. The patient is pregnant
  3. The patient does not respond clinically to oral antimicrobial therapy
  4. The patient is unable to follow or tolerate an outpatient oral regimen
  5. The patient has severe illness, nausea, and vomiting or high fever
  6. The patient has a tubo-ovarian abscess
  7. The patient is immunodeficient (i.e., has HIV infection with low counts, is taking immunosuppressant therapy), or has another disease

VII. Differential Diagnosis

A. Septic abortion
B. Ectopic gestation

C. Ovarian cyst
D. Ruptured ovarian cyst
E. Cystitis
F. Pyelonephritis
G. Peptic ulcer disease
H. Hepatitis
 I. Appendicitis
 J. Adhesions
K. Endometriosis/endometritis
L. Diverticular disease
M. Pelvic neoplasms
N. Irritable bowel syndrome
O. Ovarian torsion
P. Inflammatory bowel disease

VIII. Treatment (CDC Recommendations 2006) for Uncomplicated Pelvic Inflammatory Disease

A. Medication
    1. Ofloxacin 400 mg orally twice a day for 14 days OR Levofloxacin 500 mg orally once daily for 14 days with or without Metronidazole 500 mg orally twice a day for 14 days
    2. Alternative regimens
        a. Ceftriaxone 250 mg IM once OR
        b. Cefoxitin 2 gm IM plus Probenecid 1 gram orally once OR
        c. Other parenteral 3rd generation cephalosporin (e.g., ceftizoxime or cefotaxime PLUS Doxycycline 100 mg orally twice a day for 14 days (for a, b, or c) with or without Metronidazole 500 mg orally twice a day for 14 days
    3. Pregnant women: Hospitalize and treat with parenteral antibiotics per CDC guidelines for hospitalization
    4. Refer to CDC guidelines (2006) if patient meets hospitalization criteria
B. General measures
    1. Bed rest
    2. Increased fluid intake
    3. General diet
    4. Stress importance of partner being examined and treated
    5. Stress use of condoms to prevent reinfection or future infections
    6. No douching
C. Management of sex partners
    1. Examine and treat if sexual contact with patient during 60 days prior to onset of symptoms

IX. Complications

    A. Sterility
    B. Generalized sepsis
    C. Chronic pelvic pain
    D. Tubal pregnancy
    E. Surgical interventions
    F. Dyspareunia
    G. Tubo-ovarian abscess
    H. Fitz-Hugh-Curtis Syndrome: perihepatitis

X. Consultation/Referral

    A. If failure to improve within three days (48–72 hours) after starting above treatment
    B. For hospitalization
    C. For culdocentesis or diagnostic laparoscopy if indicated

XI. Follow-up

    A. Reevaluate within 72 hours or sooner if symptoms worsen or do not improve; patients should demonstrate substantial clinical improvement within 3 days
    B. After completion of medication course (no sooner than 7 days)
       1. Bimanual
       2. Cultures if indicated (i.e., positive lab results prior to treatment); some specialists recommend rescreening for gonorrhea and Chlamydia trachomatis regardless of prior culture results 4 to 6 weeks after completion of therapy
    C. Male sex partners of women with PID should be examined and treated if sexual contact was 60 days or less preceding symptom onset
    See Bibliography. Web site: http://www.cdc.gov/node.do/id/0900f3ec800e9b48.

PELVIC MASS

I. Definition

Mass found in adnexa, cul de sac, or uterus during bimanual examination.

II. Etiology

A pelvic mass may be caused by any number of factors. This guideline is meant to assist the clinician in the screening and referral process.

III. History

 A. What the patient may present with
  1. May be asymptomatic
  2. Bloating
  3. Abdominal pain: generalized or localized/duration/onset
  4. Flatulence
  5. Dysfunctional bleeding—can be heavy
  6. Amenorrhea; number of weeks
  7. Vaginal discharge
  8. Low back pain and/or pressure
  9. Dyspareunia
  10. Bowel or bladder dysfunction; chronic bowel disease
  11. Prior abdominal surgery
  12. Prior pelvic surgery
  13. Endometriosis
  14. Pregnancy history; assisted reproduction
 B. Additional information to be obtained
  1. LMP
  2. Contraception used
  3. Menstruation, pregnancy, and infertility history
  4. Any change in bowel habits; last bowel movement
  5. History of ovarian cysts
  6. History of uterine fibroids
  7. History of pelvic inflammatory disease (PID)
  8. History of Chlamydia or gonorrhea
  9. History of IUD use
  10. History of ectopic pregnancy
  11. Family history
  12. Results of recent Papanicolaou smear; any follow-up if abnormal
  13. Diagnostic tests including colonoscopy, laparoscopy, flexible sigmoidoscopy

IV. Physical Examination

 A. Abdominal exam
  1. Bowel sounds
  2. Pain
  3. Organomegaly
 B. Vaginal examination
  1. Examine cervix for discharge and presence of IUD string
  2. Examine vagina for masses, lesions, discharge

C. Bimanual examination
  1. Examine cervix for cervical motion tenderness
  2. Examine uterus for tenderness, masses, shape, size, and consistency; prolapse
  3. Examine adnexa for masses, attempting to differentiate between ovaries and bowel
  4. Evaluate mass for shape, consistency, size, mobility, and tenderness
  5. Examine bladder; check for cystocele
  6. Cul de sac for mass
  7. Thickening or tenderness at or near utero sacral ligaments
D. Rectal examination
  1. Pain, tenderness
  2. Masses
  3. Melena
  4. Rectovaginal masses, fistulas
  5. Rectocele/occult blood

V. Laboratory Examination

  A. Cultures as indicated
  B. Wet prep as indicated
  C. Serum pregnancy test as indicated
  D. CBC with sedimentation rate; C-reactive protein
  E. Ultrasound; transvaginal and transabdominal, or with doppler as indicated
  F. CA 125, ovarian cancer tumor marker as indicated
  G. Consider carcinoembryonic antigen (CEA)
  H. Endometrial biopsy as indicated

VI. Treatment

  A. Adnexal masses
    1. If thought to be retained stool or intestinal gas, patient should have bowel prep and be reexamined.
    2. If thought to be ovarian in origin, the following differentiation may be made:
       a. Age of patient (ovulation or using ovulation inhibitor, perimenopausal or menopausal)
       b. Menstrual history
       c. Indication of infection
       d. Is pregnancy test positive?
    3. If ovulation is presumed, assess size of mass.

    a. If greater than 5 to 6 cm, MD referral is indicated.

    b. If less than 5 cm and asymptomatic, reexamine after next menses; if unchanged may (i) recommend ovulatory inhibitor × 3 months and reexamine. If remaining after 3 months, refer to MD (ii) consider ultrasound as baseline. If functional cyst is confirmed, wait 2 months and repeat ultrasound.

4. If on ovulatory inhibitor, do appropriate work-up (i.e., ultrasound) and refer, or refer immediately depending on setting.

5. If perimenopausal/menopausal:

    a. Do appropriate work-up (i.e., ultrasound); refer for MD evaluation as indicated.

B. Uterine mass

1. Do ultrasound; small, nonsymptomatic fibroids may be followed and assessed on a 6 month to 12 month basis as appropriate to setting. Large fibroids or other finding refer to MD.

C. Ectopic pregnancy

1. Do ultrasound; if ectopic confirmed, consult or refer for treatment. Current treatment includes:

    a. serial serum human gonadotropin levels (HCG level < 2000 milli-international units and < 50% rise in 48 hours)

    b. medical management (per guidelines of clinical site)

        1) methotrexate in single dose IM 50 mg/square meter of body surface calculated on body weight

        2) monitor HCG per guidelines of clinical site and possible ultrasound monitoring

    c. consult and referral for surgical management

VII. Differential Diagnosis

A. Inflammatory

1. Tubo-ovarian abscess

2. Appendiceal abscess

3. Diverticular abscess

B. Functional

1. Ovarian cysts

    a. Follicular

    b. Luteal

    c. Polycystic ovaries (PCO)

C. Neoplastic

1. Benign

2. Malignant

  D. Anatomic anomalies
      1. Pelvic kidney
      2. Bicornuate uterus
  E. Other
      1. Ectopic pregnancy
      2. Endometrioma
      3. Paratubal/ovarian cyst
      4. Hydrosalpinx

VIII. Complications

Complication of individual entity as listed in differential diagnosis.

IX. Consultation and Referral

As indicated by laboratory work-up and physical findings indicated in
VI treatment.

X. Follow-up

As indicated by diagnosis.
      See Bibliography. Web sites: http://www.mamc.amedd.army.mil/refer-
ral/guidelines/obgyn_pelvicmass.htm; http://www.merck.com/mmpr/sec18/
ch242/ch242c.html.

UTERINE LEIOMYOMATA

I. Definition

Often referred to as uterine fibroids, fibromyomas, myomas, or fibromas,
leiomyomas are benign uterine tumors arising from the smooth muscle
and having some connective tissue elements as well.

II. Etiology

  A. Physiology
      1. Appear to arise from single (monoclonal) neoplastic smooth
          muscle cells (4th and 5th decades) within the myometrium
      2. May be single or multiple
      3. May range in size from microscopic to more than 20 cm (fill-
          ing the abdomen)
      4. May occur within the uterine wall (intramural) or extend ex-
          ternally from the serosal surface (subserosal) internally into
          endometrial cavity (submucous); have both estrogen and
          progesterone receptors

5. Can also be in broad ligament, ovary, or cervix
6. Occur most commonly during a woman's fertile years, 35–50
7. Usually undergo regression with menopause; rare before menarche
8. Sometimes increase in size with hormonal contraceptives or pregnancy

III. History

    A. What the patient may present with
      1. May be asymptomatic
      2. Pelvic pain (acute or chronic) 1:3 women
      3. Abnormal vaginal bleeding (30%)
      4. Urinary frequency, retention, incontinence, urgency
      5. Constipation
      6. Pelvic pressure
      7. Dyspareunia
      8. Backache
    B. Additional information to be considered
      1. Menstrual history, menorrhagia, dysmenorrhea
      2. History of infertility
      3. Habitual spontaneous abortions
      4. Menopausal symptoms
      5. Last menstrual period; methods of birth control; intrauterine device in place or history of intrauterine device use
      6. Any pelvic surgery
      7. Pregnancy history; parity
      8. Use of hormones: oral contraceptives, hormone therapy, infertility drugs
      9. Family history; ethnic background
     10. Obesity (elevated BMI)

IV. Physical Examination

    A. Vital signs as indicated
    B. Abdominal examination
      1. Any abdominal guarding or tenderness
      2. Location of any pain
      3. Bladder palpable or distended
    C. Vaginal examination
      1. Examine cervix for any extraneous tissue, distortion of configuration
      2. Palpate vagina for any masses
      3. Examine any bleeding or discharge

D. Bimanual examination
  1. Examine uterus for tenderness, masses
  2. Examine adnexa for masses, tenderness
  3. Locate any pain if possible
E. Rectovaginal examination for tenderness, masses

V. Laboratory Examination

A. Ultrasound
B. Pregnancy test if pre- or perimenopausal
C. CBC
D. MRI
E. Endoscopic visualization
F. Hysterosalpingography
G. Sonohysterography

VI. Differential Diagnosis

A. Uterine pregnancy
B. Malignant uterine tumor
C. Ovarian cyst or tumor
D. Extrauterine pelvic mass
E. Bowel tumor
F. Bladder tumor
G. Tumor of ureter, kidney
H. Pelvic abscess
I. Extrauterine pregnancy
J. Bicornuate uterus

VII. Treatment

A. As indicated by ultrasound
  1. Watch size of leiomyomata with bimanual examination and repeat ultrasound
  2. Consultation for medical management: progestins, gonadotropin releasing hormone (GnRH) agonists (e.g., leuprolide 3.75 mg 1×/month)
  3. Consultation for surgical management: hysterectomy, myomectomy, hysteroscope, resectoscope, laser ablation; myolysis or myoma coagulation; cryomyolysis; fibroid embolization

VIII. Complications

A. Torsion of pedunculated leiomyomata resulting in necrosis
B. Uterine abscess

    C. Infarction
    D. Hemorrhage
    E. Degeneration: hyalinization, cystic, calcification, fatty

IX. Consultation/Referral

    A. Rapid change in size
    B. Signs of complications
    C. Menorrhagia
    D. Compromise of adjacent organs
    E. Intractable pelvic pressure or pain

X. Follow-up

    A. Reevaluate every 6 to 12 months or as indicated
    B. As indicated under medical management with medication
        1. Long-term GnRH agonists > 6 months add estrogen for osteoporosis, menopausal symptoms
See Bibliography. Web sites: http://www.mayoclinic.com/health/uterine-fibroids/DS00078; http://www.womenshealth.about.com/cs/fibroidtumors/a/fibroidtumors.htm; http://www.med.umich.edu/ilibr/wha/wha-lapfibtu_crs.htm.

SCABIES

I. Definition

A highly contagious papulo-follicular skin rash whose chief symptom is pruritus. Rash and itching are thought to be hypersensitivity reactions to the mites and are not confined to the locations of mite burrows. With first exposure, sensitization can take several weeks. After reinfestation, pruritus can occur within 24 hours. Scabies among adults may be sexually transmitted.

II. Etiology

Sarcoptes scabiei mite. The mite burrows into skin and deposits eggs along a tunnel. Larvae hatch in 3 to 5 days and gather around hair follicles. Newly hatched female burrows into the skin, maturing in 10 to 19 days, then mates and starts a new cycle. Crusted scabies (Norwegian scabies) is an aggressive infestation.

III. History

    A. What the patient may present with:

1. Pruritus—worse at night or at times when body temperature is raised, i.e., after exercise. Pruritus exists prior to physical manifestations.
2. Lesions are usually on interdigital webs of hands, flexor aspects of wrists, extensor surfaces of the elbows, areas surrounding the nipples, anterior axillary folds, umbilicus, belt line, lower abdomen, genitalia and gluteal cleft; male genitals; can be all over body especially with immunosuppression.

B. Additional information to be considered
1. Known contact with scabies. Incubation period in persons without previous exposure is usually 4 to 6 weeks (mean 3 weeks). Persons who were previously infected develop symptoms 1 to 3 days after repeat exposure to the mite. These reinfections are usually milder.
2. Lifestyle. Persons living in close proximity with others, dormitories, crowded living conditions, shared clothing, shelters, are at increased risk for nonsexual exposures.
3. History of atopic dermatitis, +HIV, or other immunosuppressed condition; hematologic malignancies.
4. At high risk for crusted scabies.

IV. Physical Examination

A. Skin: Thorough examination of lesions and of those areas most frequently involved
1. Linear burrows about 1.5 to 2 cm. in length terminating in a papule or vesicle
2. Lesions: papules or vesicles
3. Scaling, crustation lesions, furuncles, excoriations may be present with secondary infection

B. Lymph nodes exhibit generalized lymphadenopathy

V. Laboratory

A. KOH prep of scraping from several of the excoriated lesions, examined under low power. It may be difficult to find mite. Application of water, alcohol, or mineral oil to the skin facilitates collection of the scraping.

B. Diagnosis is usually made on the basis of clinical presentation.

VI. Differential Diagnosis

A. Atopic dermatitis
B. Impetigo
C. Urticaria

    D. Psoriasis

    E. Drug-induced eruption

    F. Insect bites

VII. Treatment

    A. Medication

        1. 5% permethrin cream (Elimite®), applied to all areas of the body from neck down and washed off after 8 to 14 hours; OR

        2. Ivermectin 200 μg/kg orally, repeated in 2 weeks (safety in children < 15 years of age not determined)

        3. In pregnancy and lactation and for children under 2 use only permethrin. Do not use ivermectin or lindane.

        4. Lindane is not recommended as first line therapy due to toxicity. Only use as alternative in patients who cannot tolerate other therapies or those therapies have failed. Lindane 1% lotion or 30 mg of cream applied in a thin layer to all areas of the body from the neck down and thoroughly washed off after 8 hours. It should not be used immediately after a bath or shower or by persons with extensive dermatitis.

    B. Symptomatic treatment

        1. Antihistamines may be given to relieve pruritus.

        2. Patient should be informed that pruritus may persist for several weeks. If patient does not respond to therapy and itching is still persistent after one week, she/he should be instructed to contact health care provider to decide if further therapy is necessary.

    C. General measures

        1. Clothing, towels, and bed linens should be laundered at 60 degrees C (hot cycle) or dry cleaned on the day of treatment.

        2. If clothing items can't be washed or dry cleaned, these should be separated from washed clothes and not worn for at least 72 hours. Mites cannot exist for more than 2 to 3 days away from the body.

        3. Sexual partners and close personal or household contacts within the past month should be informed, examined, and treated if necessary.

        4. Patient should be instructed to follow treatment regimen carefully.

        5. Although fumigation of living areas is not necessary, some patients may wish to decontaminate mattresses, sofas, and other inanimate objects that cannot be washed. OTC sprays and powders are available for this purpose.

VIII. Complications

    A. Secondary infection (may require systemic antibiotics)
    B. Reaction to lindane (Kwell®, Scaben®)
       1. Dermatitis
       2. CNS toxicity

IX. Consultation and Referral

    A. Secondary infection
    B. Generalized widespread inflammatory response
    C. Failure to respond to therapy
    D. Reaction to lindane (Kwell®, Scabene®)
    E. Patients with coexisting dermatitis or other dermatologic condition
    F. Patients with coexisting HIV infection or who are otherwise immunosuppressed; those with crusted scabies

X. Follow-up

    A. Failure to respond to therapy. Some experts recommend re-treatment after 1 to 2 weeks for patients who are still symptomatic; others recommend re-treatment only if live mites can be observed. Re-treatment should be with an alternative regimen.
    B. Recurrence.
    Appendix A may be copied/adapted for your patients.
    Web site: www.cdc.gov/NCIDOD/DPD/parasites/scabies/factsht_scabies.htm.

PEDICULOSIS

I. Definition

Pediculosis is the state of being infested with lice that may be found on the skin, particularly the hairy areas such as the scalp and pubis, and may cause intense pruritus.

II. Etiology

    A. Two species that look like each other but have different feeding habits are:
       1. Pediculus humanus var capitis: inhabits the skin of the head or body; transmitted by shared clothing, towels, brushes, combs, batting helmets, stuffed animals, car seats, bedding, headphones, hats; P. humanus var corporis body louse lives in clothes.

2. Phthirus pubis ("crab louse," pubic louse); inhabits the genital area but may colonize other areas including axillae, eyelashes, head hair; transmitted by close personal contact, bedding.

B. Nits hatch in 5–10 days incubation; adult pubic lice probably survive no more than 24 hours off their host; nits can survive in hot and humid climates up to 10 days.

III. History

A. What the patient may present with
   1. Pruritus
   2. Visual identification of the parasite or feces on bed pillow
   3. Known exposure to household member or intimate partner with head, body, or pubic lice
   4. Rarely lymphadenopathy at back of neck; an allergic reaction to saliva and feces of lice
B. Additional information to be considered
   1. Lifestyle: shared clothing, towels, beds, pillows; shag rugs or carpets, upholstered furniture

IV. Physical Examination

A. Pediculosis capitis (infestation with head lice); examine for:
   1. The parasite
   2. Greenish-white oval attachments to hair shaft (nits)
   3. Secondary impetigo and furunculosis
   4. Cervical lymphadenopathy
B. Pediculosis corporis (infestation with body lice); examine for:
   1. Parallel linear scratch marks on back, shoulders, trunk, buttocks (areas easily reached for scratching)
   2. Impetigo lesions and furuncles associated with scratch marks secondary to scratching
   3. Lice on clothing, especially the seams, as lice are very rarely found on the body
C. Pediculosis pubis (infestation with pubic (crab) lice); examine for:
   1. The parasite (rarely found)
   2. Oval attachments on pubic hair (nits)
   3. Black dots (representing excreta) on surrounding skin and underclothing
   4. Nits in eyebrows, eyelashes, scalp hair, axillary hair, and other body hair
   5. Crusts or scabs in pubic area

V. Laboratory Examination

None

VI. Differential Diagnosis

See Etiology.

VII. Treatment

   A. General measures
      1. Wash with hot water, dry clean, or run through a dryer on heat cycle all contaminated clothing, hats, towels, bedclothes, etc., to destroy nits and lice; wash combs and hairbrushes in hot soapy water letting them soak for at least 15 minutes.
      2. Spray couches, chairs, car seats, and items that can't be washed or dry cleaned with OTC product (A-200 Pyrinate® (pyrethrin), Triplex®, or RID (permethrin); alternative is to vacuum carefully to pick up living lice and nits.
   B. Specific treatment
      1. Pediculosis capitis (infestation with head lice)
         a. Thoroughly wet hair with Permethrin 1% cream rinse applied to affected areas and washed off after 10 minutes or Triplex Kit (pyrethrins + piperonyl butoxide); Pronto (piperonyl), RID (permethrin) shampoo or R&C shampoo (pyrethrins and piperonyl butoxide), or End Lice (pyrethrins and piperonyl); work up lather, adding water as necessary; shampoo thoroughly leaving shampoo on head for 5 minutes; rinse, or use Pronto shampoo/conditioner (piperonyl butoxide); or Clear® lice killing shampoo (pyrethrin-based) and lice egg remover (permethrin-based) per directions on product or Klout® (nonpesticide ingredients include isopropanol, methylparaben, propylparaben) per directions on product.
         b. Rinse thoroughly, towel dry.
         c. Remove remaining nits with fine-tooth metal comb or tweezers (use of vinegar solution and hair conditioner or olive oil make combing easier).
      2. Pediculosis corporis (infestation with body lice)
         a. Bathe with soap and water if no lice are found.
         b. Wash with hot water and dry in dryer all clothing, bedclothes, towels, etc.
         c. Dry clean items that cannot be washed; for items that cannot be washed or dry cleaned, seal in a plastic bag

for 1 week: lice will suffocate (in cold climates put bags outside for 10 days; temperature change kills lice).

    d. If evidence of lice is found or patient is not relieved by a. and b., Malathion 0.5% lotion applied for 8–12 hours, and thoroughly rinsed off.

  3. Pediculosis pubis (infestation with pubic lice)

    a. Permethrin 1% cream (NIX) rinse applied to affected area and washed off after 10 minutes; OR

    b. Pyrethrins with piperonyl butoxide (RID, Clear, A-200, Pronto, generics) applied to affected area and washed off after 10 minutes; OR

    c. Malathion 0.5% lotion applied for 8–12 hours, and thoroughly rinsed off; OR

    d. Ivermectin 250 µg/kg repeated in 2 weeks

    e. Pregnancy, lactation: use permethrin or pyrethrins with piperonyl butoxide, not lindane

    f. Lindane is not recommended as first-line therapy due to toxicity; it should only be used as an alternative when other therapies fail and only in adults; not in pregnancy or lactation

    g. Treat sexual partners within past month

    h. Wash in hot water and thoroughly dry on heat cycle or dry clean all clothing, bed linen, towels, etc. or remove from body contact for at least 72 hours

C. Stress importance of careful checking of family and household members and close contacts; no treatment is needed unless there is evidence of contamination.

D. Put nonwashable items in hot dryer; or spray with permethrin (RID, NIX)—check safety with children and pets.

E. Screen patients with pediculosis pubis for other STDs.

VIII. Complications

  A. Secondary infection

  B. Sensitivity reactions to treatment

  C. Excoriations

  D. Resistance of lice to pediculicides

IX. Consultation/Referral

  A. Lice found in eyelashes: because shampoo cannot be used, occlusive ophthalmic ointment is applied to the eyelid margins

  B. Treatment failures

  C. Coexisting dermatologic conditions

X. Follow-up

   A. Evaluate in 1 week if symptoms persist.
   B. Instruct patient to return for repeat treatment if symptoms or
       parasites recur.
   C. Treat with alternative regimen if patient's infestation is nonre-
       sponsive.
   See Appendix A and Bibliography.
   Website: http://www.health.state.ny.us/diseases/communicable/
pediculosis/fact_sheet.htm.

NOTE

1. The authors are indebted to Luisa Fertitta, MS, RNC and Mimi Secor, RNC, MS, FNP
   for their expertise on vulvar conditions.

CHAPTER FIVE

Breast Conditions

BREAST MASS

I. Definition

A breast mass is a thickening or lump that is felt in a woman's breast, which may or may not have the following characteristics:
A. Nipple retraction
B. Discharge from nipple
C. Skin dimpling
D. Inflammation or discoloration
E. Skin thickening
F. Palpable axillary or supraclavicular nodes
G. Tenderness

II. Etiology

A. "Fibrocystic disease"—catch-all term for nonmalignant conditions
B. Fibroadenoma
C. Carcinoma
D. Mammary duct ectasia
E. Intraductal papilloma
F. Normal premenstrual breast tissue, i.e., with tenderness and prominent breast tissue secondary to hormone levels—physiologic nodularity, mastoplasia
G. Mastalgia (mastodynia) chronic or cyclic
H. Mastitis: cellulitis, skin boils, abscess
I. Cysts

    J. Fat necrosis
    K. Superficial phlebitis
    L. Phyllodes tumors—painless, solid, smooth, lobular, bulky, stromal hyperplasia
    M. Paget's disease

III. History

    A. What woman may present with
      1. Lump
      2. Pain
      3. Swelling
      4. Redness; bruised area that doesn't resolve
      5. Discharge from nipple
      6. Nipple retraction
      7. Change in appearance of skin and areola
      8. Dimpling, scaliness
    B. Additional information to be considered
      1. Family history of breast disease
      2. History of previous breast lumps or breast disease, biopsy (type) or aspiration; breast surgery including reduction, enlargement, implants, and type
      3. Last menstrual period (has patient noticed a relationship to menses?)
      4. Birth control method(s) used; hormone therapy (type, dose, duration) and how soon after menopause
      5. Diet
      6. Adolescents' most common complaint
        a. Trauma (sports or sexual activity)
      7. Recent pregnancy, lactation
      8. Risk factors
        a. Genetic (70% of breast cancer = no known family history)
          1) Risk increases with 1st or 2nd degree relatives—maternal or paternal—with breast cancer—mother, daughter, sister, aunt, grandmother—and number of these relatives, age at diagnosis
          2) BRCA 1 or BRCA 2 gene mutation; in some ethnic/cultural groups
        b. Hormonal
          1) Early menarche (11 or younger) or late menopause (55 or older)
          2) First full-term pregnancy after 30; nullipara

3) Obesity in postmenopausal women (produce more estrogen); high levels of abdominal fat
4) Breast feeding—may be protective, but data are not conclusive

c. External
1) Other: Previous diagnosis of breast malignancy or atypical hyperplasia
2) Radiation to chest—risk in moderate doses (10–500 rads) (level of radiation in an up-to-date mammogram = 1/4 rad)
3) Exogenous hormones
a) DES exposure in utero or as a DES mother
b) Postmenopausal hormone therapy: possible increased risk with progestin plus estrogen versus estrogen relative risk
c) possibility that organochlorines (pesticides) can act like estrogen in the body
4) Diet (areas under investigation): fat—low fat diet may be beneficial; increased risk with high animal fat diet
5) Alcohol even in moderate amounts (3–9 drinks a week) may increase risk, esp. if on hormone therapy
6) Low vitamin A intake may increase breast cancer risk
7) Exercise—strenuous exercise in adolescence and continued exercise in adulthood may have a protective effect

IV. Physical Examination

A. Breast Physical Examination
1. Examine in both upright and supine positions
2. Measurement, location, consistency of any lesion
3. Note any skin changes such as dimpling, retraction, erythema, nipple scaling, or excoriation
4. Examine for spontaneous breast discharge
5. Examine regional lymph nodes (axillary and suprainfraclavicular)
B. Palpation for the following:
1. Accurate location of any detected lesion
2. Solitary or multiple lesion(s)
3. Consistency and extent of any mass
4. Tenderness of mass

    5. Movable or fixed on chest wall
    6. Displacement or retraction of nipple
    7. Retraction or dimpling of skin overlying mass
    8. Palpability of regional lymph nodes (axillary or supra/infra-clavicular)
    9. Discharge expressed; color, amount, uni- or bilateral, consistency
  C. Express breast for any discharge if none noted on palpation

V. Laboratory Examination

  A. If discharge is present
    1. Microscopic examination to identify fat globules
    2. Guiac all discharge for occult blood

VI. Differential

See Etiology.

VII. Treatment

  A. Medication
    1. Appropriate antibiotic for mastitis, abscess
  B. General measures
    1. If mass does not fit criteria for physician referral, have patient return 1 week after next menses for reevaluation and possible referral.
    2. Dietary; discuss use of caffeine, chocolate, and salt; low-fat diet.
    3. Consider homeopathic remedies; herbals such as evening primrose oil, ginseng tea; vitamins A and B for cyclical mastalgia; vitamin E; green tea; antioxidants.

VIII. Complications

May be grave and extensive if misdiagnosed.

IX. Consultation/Referral

  A. Any of the following lesions should be referred immediately to physician or breast center
    1. Fixed mass
    2. Discrete mass, ultrasound to distinguish cyst from solid mass
    3. Mass associated with nipple retraction

     4. Dimpling of skin; orange peel appearance to skin
     5. Inflammation, swelling, scaling, or excoriation
     6. Palpable axillary or supra/infraclavicular nodes
     7. Nipple discharge
     8. Cystic mass; for possible aspiration
  B. Refer to physician/breast center
     1. Women who do not fit above criteria but in whom mass is still found 1 week past next menses
     2. Women in whom mass is palpable despite negative mammogram
     3. Consider referral to breast center, specialist for evaluation with digital mammography, MRI, galactography; consideration of prophylaxis for high-risk women with a selective estrogen receptor modulator (SERM)
     4. Genetic counseling and testing for women with strong family history of breast or ovarian cancer
     5. When in doubt always refer!

X. Follow-up

  A. Appropriate to VII. B. 1. and VII. B. 2.
  B. Preventive measures to reduce breast cancer risk

XI. Mammogram Screening

  A. All women with a breast mass (although ultrasound may be more useful for women under 35)
  B. Baseline between 35 and 40
  C. Earlier if family history of breast cancer in mother, sister, daughter, aunt, or grandmother
  D. Annually 40 and older

See Appendix A and Bibliography. Web sites: Breast Cancer and Environmental Risk Factors Program (BCERF), www.cfe.cornell.edu/bcerf/.www.cfe.cornell.edu/bcerf/; http://www.mayoclinic.com/health/breast-lumps/BR00013

ABNORMAL BREAST DISCHARGE

I. Definition

Under certain conditions an abnormal fluid may be expressed from the breast(s) or flow spontaneously.

II. Etiology

    A. Physiological cause
        1. Pregnancy, puerperium
        2. Intercourse
        3. Stimulation of the breast
        4. Chest wall surgery or trauma
        5. Exercise
        6. Emotional stress
        7. Sleep (affects measurable amounts of prolactin)
    B. Pharmacological causes
        1. Numerous psychotropic drugs
        2. Cimetidine
        3. Some antihypertensives
        4. Opiates
        5. Estrogens/oral contraceptives/progestins
        6. Antiemetics
        7. Alcohol (chronic abuse)
        8. Marijuana
        9. Danazol
      10. Isoniazid (INH)
    C. Pathological causes
        1. Breast tumor
        2. Pituitary tumor
        3. Hypothalamic tumor
        4. Infections
        5. Empty sella syndrome
        6. Hypothyroidism
        7. Polycystic ovaries (PCOS)
        8. Benign intraductal papilloma
        9. Ductal ectasia

III. History

    A. What the patient may present with
        1. Breast discharge
        2. Amenorrhea
        3. Possibly pain
        4. Possibly localized heat and swelling
        5. Possibly no symptoms (discharge can be an incidental finding
           of breast exam)
    B. Additional information to be considered
        1. Last menstrual period
        2. Sexual activity

3. Birth control method; hormone therapy
4. Medications or illegal drugs currently being used
5. Medications recently taken
6. Recent pregnancy (within 1 year), regardless of outcome
7. Exercise program, e.g., jogging
8. Nipple stimulation, e.g., fondling, sucking
9. Recent trauma to chest or surgery
10. Description of discharge; unilateral or bilateral; only with stimulation? Spontaneous?
11. Chronic illness, e.g., thyroid disease, psychiatric illness
12. Lifestyle changes, e.g., increased stress
13. Alcohol consumption (chronic abuse)
14. Family history of breast disease
15. Breast pain or tenderness
16. Breast surgery: biopsy, reduction, augmentation, implants
17. Duration of discharge

IV. Physical Examination[1]

A. Complete examination
   1. Palpate nipple by compressing nipple areola with thumb and index finger, gently milking the subareolar ducts from just outside the apex of the papilla. Repeat in 3 or 4 different directions, noting number of droplets that appear.
   2. If discharge is expressed, note whether it is unilateral, bilateral, clear, cloudy, dark, light, milky, bloody, thick, thin; note color.
B. Thyroid: palpate for nodes, size
C. Bimanual examination
   1. Ovarian irregularity or enlargement
   2. Uterine enlargement

V. Laboratory Examination

A. Initially on all patients
   1. Guaiac all discharge for occult blood
   2. Microscopic examination for fat globules
   3. Prolactin level; sample should be drawn between 8 and 10 A.M. (literature indicates prolactin level is lowest between 8 and 10 A.M. but not directly after gynecological examination, intercourse, exercise, or breast stimulation including breast examination)
   4. Thyroid panel
   5. Consider mammogram, ultrasound, MRI with consultation

6. Serum pregnancy test if indicated

VI. Differential Diagnosis

See Etiology.

VII. Treatment

As needed according to laboratory report and etiology.

VIII. Complications

Vary by individual, according to diagnosis.

IX. Consultation/Referral

    A. Abnormal lab results
    B. Lack of definitive diagnosis
    C. When in doubt consider referral to breast center, specialist

X. Follow-up

    A. If first visit was a consult visit, encourage complete physical.
    B. Repeat laboratory work as indicated in V.
    Website: http:www.mayoclinic.com/health/nipple-discharge/WO00093
    See Bibliography.

NOTE

1. Per breast mass guidelines.

CHAPTER SIX

Cervical Aberrations

PAPANICOLAOU (PAP) SMEAR AND COLPOSCOPY

I. Definition

The Papanicolaou (Pap) test examines exfoliated cells from the endocervix to detect preinvasive lesions (e.g., dysplasia, carcinoma-in-situ) as well as invasive lesions.

II. Screening

    A. History
1. DES exposure in utero
2. Smoking: exposure to passive smoke
3. Previous abnormal Papanicolaou smear; cervical treatment
4. HPV, other sexually transmitted diseases
5. Sexual practices, partners (number, partner(s) had previous partner(s) with abnormal Paps, partner's sexual history)
6. Family history of cervical cancer; personal history of cancer
7. Age of beginning sexual activity
8. Immunosuppressive therapy; immunosuppression
9. HIV/AIDS or risk
10. Hormone use
11. Per ACOG, American Cancer Society, or guidelines for practice setting

III. Technique

    A. Cytologic specimens may be obtained prior to the bimanual pelvic exam; a nonlubricated speculum must be used (speculum can be warmed with water).

B. May do a palpation of the vagina and cervix to locate the cervix and identify the position of the os.

C. The cervix and vagina must be fully visible when the smear is obtained in order to see entire squamo columnar junction.

D. Vaginal discharge, when present in large amounts, should be carefully removed with a large swab prior to obtaining the smear. The presence of small amount of blood should not preclude cytologic sampling.

E. The spatula is applied to the entire cervix to include the entire squamocolumnar junction. In some settings, the handle of the spatula is used to sample the vaginal pool prior to sampling the cervix. A cytobrush is inserted into the endocervix, rotated ½ turn, removed, and the material is rolled on a slide. If woman is pregnant, do not use cytobrush. Uniform application of the material to the slide, without clumping, both sides of spatula, roll brush on slide and with immediate fixation (within 10 seconds) to prevent drying, is required (spray from 9" to 12" away).

F. For DES-exposed women, additional slides are prepared using smear taken from the upper two-thirds of the vagina at its circumferences. Gentle wiping of the vaginal wall mucosa initially to remove discharge increases the diagnostic accuracy.

G. With the liquid-based technology (Thin Prep Pap Test™, CytoRich®, SurePath™) the sample is collected on a broom-type cervical sampling device. This device then is rinsed in a vial of preserving solution and discarded. The vial is capped, labeled, and sent to the lab. A plastic spatula to sample the portio and cytobrush for the endocervix can be substituted for the broom.

IV. Bethesda 2001 Terminology for Papanicolaou Smears

Specimen Adequacy

Satisfactory for evaluation (note presence/absence of endocervical/transformation zone component)
Unsatisfactory for evaluation (specify reason)
Specimen rejected/not processed (specify reason)
Specimen processed and examined, but unsatisfactory for evaluation of epithelial abnormality because of (specify reason)

General Categorization

Negative for intraepithelial lesion or malignancy
Epithelial cell abnormality
Other

Interpretation/Result

Negative for intraepithelial lesion or malignancy
Organisms

    Trichomonas vaginalis

    Fungal organisms morphologically consistent with Candida species
    Shift in flora suggestive of bacterial vaginosis
    Bacteria morphologically consistent with *Actinomyces* species
    Cellular changes consistent with herpes simplex virus
    Other nonneoplastic findings
    Reactive cellular changes associate with inflammation (includes typical
        repair)
    radiation
    intrauterine contraceptive device
    Glandular cells status posthysterectomy
    Atrophy
Epithelial cell abnormalities
    Squamous cell
    Atypical squamous cells (ASC) of undetermined significance (ASC-US)
    cannot exclude HSIL (ASC-H)
Low-grade squamous intraepithelial lesion (LSIL)
    Encompassing: human papillomavirus/mild dysplasia/cervical in-
    traepithelial neoplasia (CIN) 1
High-grade squamous intraepithelial lesion (HSIL)
        Encompassing: moderate and severe dysplasia, carcinoma in
        situ; CIN 2 and CIN 3
        Squamous cell carcinoma

Glandular cell
    Atypical glandular cells (AGC) (specify endocervical, endometrial, or
        not otherwise specified)
    Atypical glandular cells, favor neoplastic (specify endocervical or not
        otherwise specified)
    Endocervical adenocarcinoma in situ (AIS)
    Adenocarcinoma
Other (list not comprehensive)
    Endometrial cells in a woman ≥ 40 years of age

Automated review and ancilllary testing (include as appropriate)

Educational notes and suggestions:
    The 2001 Bethesda system, *Journal of the American Medical Association, 287* (2114–2119). Available online http://bethesda2001.cancer.gov/terminology/html.

V. Terminology

  A. AutoPap® computer driven cytosmear evaluation technique approved by FDA for selection of 10% of Pap smears to be manually rescreened; selects 10% most likely to exhibit abnormalities

    1. Consider offering to patients when available in lab used; can increase cost

  B. PAPNET® computerized system programmed to recognize cellular abnormalities on Pap slides prepared in the conventional way

    1. Consider offering to patients when available; can add to cost of Pap smear

  C. Adjunctive screening

    1. Speculoscopy; combines with conventional Pap smear

      a. Pap smear is obtained

      b. Cervix is washed with vinegar solution and then illuminated with a chemiluminescent light attached to the upper blade of the speculum (Speculite®) assists clinician in visualizing aceto-white areas of cervix

VI.

At the time of this printing, the 2006 Consensus Guidelines had not yet been published.†The authors are aware of the importance of these new guidelines but agreed with the publisher not to hold up this new edition any longer. The following are the websites to check for the new guidelines.

The Consensus Guidelines for the Management of Women with Cytological Abnormalities 2006 are available at: http://www.asccp.org/consensus.shtml

The guidelines will also appear in the *American Journal of Obstetrics and Gynecology*

www.AJOG.org

The American Society for Colposcopy and Cervical Pathology (ASCCP) held a Consensus Conference to revise the 2001 Guidelines for the Management of Cytological Abnormalities and Cervical Intraepithelial Neoplasia on September 18-19, 2006, at the National Cancer Institute.

Participating national and international medical organizations and Federal agencies include:

American Academy of Family Physicians (AAFP)
American Cancer Society
American College Health Association

American College of Obstetricians and Gynecologists (ACOG)
American Social Health Association
American Society for Clinical Pathology
American Society for Colposcopy and Cervical Pathology
American Society of Cytopathology
Association of Reproductive Health Professionals (ARHP)
Centers for Disease Control's Human Papillomavirus Laboratory, National Center for Infectious Diseases and Division of Viral and Rickettsial Diseases
Centers for Disease Control and Prevention: Division of Cancer Prevention and Control
Centers for Disease Control and Prevention: Division of Laboratory Systems
Centers for Medicare & Medicaid Services (CMS)
College of American Pathologists
Food and Drug Administration
International Academy of Cytology
International Federation for Cervical Pathology and Colposcopy
International Federation of Gynecology and Obstetrics (FIGO)
International Gynecologic Cancer Society
International Society of Gynecologic Pathologists
National Cancer Institute
Nurse Practitioners in Women's Health
Pan American Health Organization
Papanicolaou Society
Planned Parenthood Federation of America
Society of Canadian Colposcopists
Society of Gynecologic Oncologists
Society of Obstetricians & Gynaecologists of Canada

VII. Follow-up for Any Abnormal Papanicolaou Test Finding

    A. Follow-up as indicated in VI
    B. Procedures for follow-up (one example)
        1. If report recommends repeat test or treatment, the patient is notified by letter and perhaps by telephone as well; also it may be useful to have a stamp with "Pap letter sent" on it to stamp the lab result sheet, and the clinician can also sign and date this sheet.
        2. A file card is filled out with the patient's name and ID number, the clinician's initials, and the date and results of the test. (File the card under the months of requested repeat.) In some

settings, a Papanicolaou book is also kept cross-referenced to the card file.[1]

3. At the end of each month, the cards are pulled, attached to the patient's chart, and given to the clinician who performed the Papanicolaou smear originally and who is responsible for sending a letter to the patient reminding her of the need to repeat the test. (The card should be refiled for the next month.) If the patient still has not had a repeat test by the end of the second month, another letter is sent. If the results are less than LSIL, the clinician's responsibility ends. If results are LSIL or greater at this time, a registered letter with this information is sent to the patient. All letters and visits should be documented on charts and file cards.

4. If test results show no abnormal cells but indicate reactive and reparative changes: inflammation, a letter should be sent to the patient stating that the laboratory findings for malignancy were negative but that there is evidence of a possible infection, and that an infection check is recommended if no check was done at the time of the Pap. No follow-up letters are necessary; no entries on cards are necessary.

5. Some settings mark the record in some way and indicate that an annual Papanicolaou was done.

VIII. Indications for Colposcopy

A. As indicated by Papanicolaou test; algorithm with ASCCP guidelines for ASCUS
B. History of physical examination that revealed possible diethylstilbestrol exposure
C. Any obvious lesions of the cervix
D. Lesions in vagina or vulva that are a diagnostic problem
E. If deemed necessary by physician or nurse practitioner

IX. Colposcopy Referral Procedure

A. Refer woman to physician of her choice or one available at same setting or to nurse practitioner or nurse midwife (increasingly being trained in colposcopy).
B. Instruct woman that she will probably be billed for procedure, which is generally covered by insurance; make any arrangements possible if she has no insurance.

C. When patient chooses an outside clinician, a signed release form will be sent with referral sheet so a copy of the referral visit report can be returned to the original facility.

X. Use of Colposcope by Nurse Practitioners

    A. Use of colposcopy examination with HPV treatment

        1. A colposcopy examination of vulva, vagina, and cervix done on all women found to have vulvar HPV lesions prior to beginning treatment

            a. Vulvar warts: treat according to protocol

            b. Cervical warts: refer to gynecologist or treat per clinician preparation

        2. Colposcopy examination may be done at each visit. If warts are still present after 8–12 treatments, consult with gynecologist

        3. Colposcopy examination when warts appear to have resolved to verify treatment

    B. Use of colposcope as diagnostic tool

        1. Used at discretion of clinician for closer inspection of vulva, vagina, and/or cervix

    C. Procedure for colposcopy examination

        1. Explain procedure to patient.

        2. Complete all necessary lab work.

        3. Prepare area

            a. Swab entire vulva and vagina with acetic acid (white vinegar), applying generously.

        4. Examine with colposcope.

        5. Perform any biopsies indicated based on Pap findings.

XI. Follow-up

Per guidelines of setting, based on Papanicolaou findings, colposcopy follow-up protocol; follow-up guidelines for other evaluation methods.

AHCPR report on cervical cytology: www.ahcpr.gov/clinic/

Appendix A contains information about colposcopy that you may wish to photocopy or adapt for your patients. See Bibliography. Web sites: http://cancernet.nci.nih.gov; Bethesda System Web Atlas, http://www.cytopathology.org/NIH/; http://www.cancer.gov/newscenter/bethesda2001, ACS guidelines for screening at, http://www.cancer.org/docroot/CRI/content/CRI_2_4_2X_Can_cervical_cancer_be_prevented_8.asp?sitearea=; ACOG guidelines for Pap smears: http://www.acog. org/acog_districts/dist_notice.cfm?recno=1&bulletin=1698.

CERVICITIS

I. Definition

    A. Chronic or acute inflammation of the cervix that is visible to the clinician. Causes symptoms observed by the woman and/or by cytologic examination.

    B. Mucopurulent cervicitis: characterized by mucopurulent exudate and easily induced cervical bleeding. CDC criteria 2006 for diagnosing indicated by an asterisk(*).

II. Etiology

    A. Bacterial
        1. Neisseria gonorrhoea
        2. Mycoplasmas such as M. genitalium
        3. Ureaplasmas
        4. Chlamydia trachomatis
        5. Bacterial vaginosis

    B. Viral
        1. Herpes simplex
        2. Human papilloma virus (HPV)

    C. Parasitic
        1. Trichomonas vaginalis

    D. Nonmicrobiologic
        1. Inflammation in zone of ectopy
        2. DES exposure
        3. Chemical irritants
        4. Frequent douching

III. History

    A. What the patient may present with
        1. No symptoms
        2. Friable cervix
        3. Postcoital bleeding
        4. Erythema of cervix (*if friable with first pass of swab)
        5. Edematous cervix
        6. Ulcerated or eroded cervix
        7. Hypertrophied cervix
        8. Ectropion

    9. Cervical discharge; may be purulent or mucopurulent endocervical exudate on exam*
  10. Vaginal discharge
  11. Leukoplakia on cervix
  12. Endocervical bleeding
B. Additional information to be considered
    1. Onset of symptoms
    2. Partner with symptoms
    3. History of sexually transmitted diseases
    4. Sexual lifestyle; use of sex toys
    5. Last Papanicolaou smear and results; any history of abnormal Papanicolaou
    6. Contraception past and present
    7. Colposcopy, cone biopsy, cauterization of cervix, cryo, LEEP
    8. Laceration of cervix: childbirth, abortion, D&C, biopsy, sex toys, partner with genital jewelry
    9. Pregnancy history, infertility
  10. Dyspareunia, pelvic pain
  11. Urinary symptoms: frequency, urgency, dysuria
  12. Menstrual history: last menstrual period
  13. DES exposure

IV. Physical Examination

A. Cervix
    1. Color
    2. Character of any discharge: green, yellow, opaque, white, clear, cloudy, purulent, mucopurulent, serous, pH
    3. Size
    4. Lesions
    5. Friability
    6. Hood
    7. Any polyps noted
B. Vagina
    1. Color
    2. Erythema
    3. Lesions
    4. Discharge
C. Bimanual exam
    1. Masses
    2. Tenderness
    3. Cervical motion tenderness
    4. Uterine enlargement
    5. Position of organs
D. Adenopathy

V. Laboratory Examination

    A. As indicated by findings
1. Gonorrhea culture
2. Chlamydia smear
3. Wet prep: saline, KOH: > 10 WBCs/high power field associated wth GC, Chlamydia
4. Papanicolaou smear
5. Culture for bacteria
6. Gram stain > 30 polymorphonuclear (PMN) leukocytes
7. Serology test for syphilis
8. Herpes culture, antibodies
9. Viratyping

VI. Differential Diagnosis

    A. Condyloma acuminata
    B. Chlamydia
    C. Gonorrhea
    D. Cervical cancer
    E. Cervical infection: bacterial including mycoplasma, ureaplasma
    F. Ectropion
    G. Leukoplakia
    H. Herpetic exocervicitis
    I. Trichomonas
    J. Cervical ulceration (erosion) due to trauma: fingernail, cervical biopsy, postpartum, sex toys
    K. Pelvic inflammatory disease (PID)
    L. Infection secondary to trauma with sex toy
    M. Cervical polyp

VII. Treatment

    A. Medication
1. As indicated by organism (see guidelines for gonorrhea, Chlamydia, herpes, condyloma, trichomonas, PID)
2. Bacterial (mycoplasma, urea plasma): see PID guideline
3. Mucopurulent cervicitis (women meeting CDC criteria) without confirmed organism can be treated empirically for gonorrhea and Chlamydia if
    a. prevalance of these is high in patient population such as women less than or equal to 25 years of age
    b. patient might be difficult to locate for treatment
4. Presumptive treatment: Azithromycin 1 gram orally in single dose OR Doxycycline 100 mg orally twice a day for 7 days

B. Other measures
1. Ectropion: evaluate Papanicolaou results and follow-up as indicated; document with diagram and description for later follow-up; with persistent friability: refer or evaluate with colposcopy and biopsy
2. Leukoplakia: refer or evaluate with colposcopy and biopsy
3. Cervical cancer: refer for medical evaluation and intervention; in suspected cases in spite of negative Papanicolaou smear, refer or evaluate with colposcopy and biopsy
4. Cervical ulceration, erosion: follow-up as indicated by extent and nature of trauma; consider referral for medical evaluation and intervention
5. Consider colposcopy for all women who do not meet CDC guidelines for mucopurulent cervicitis, have a negative STD screen, and negative Papanicolaou smear
6. Manage sex partners appropriate for identified or suspected STD
7. Patients and sex partners abstain from sexual intercourse for course of treatment

VIII. Complications

Progression of condition to secondary or systemic infection (depending on organism) or PID; to metastatic disease; infertility; cervical stenosis

IX. Consultation/Referral

A. Unable to evaluate and diagnose
B. No response to treatment
C. For colposcopy, biopsy

X. Follow-up

A. As indicated by condition and treatment
B. Return for reevaluation if symptoms persist
See Bibliography. Web site: http://www.mayoclinic.com/health/cervicitis/DS00518.

NOTE

1. Increasingly, computers are being used for this function. We recommend that a card system be continued for back-up.

CHAPTER SEVEN

Menstrual Disorders

DYSMENORRHEA

I. Definition

    A. Primary dysmenorrhea is the occurrence of painful menses usually beginning within several years of menarche and in the absence of any pelvic pathology but may occur at any time during childbearing years.

    B. Secondary dysmenorrhea is painful menstruation due to an identifiable pathologic or iatrogenic condition, which may be readily identifiable on the basis of the history and the findings in a physical examination.

II. Etiology

    A. Primary dysmenorrhea

        1. Caused by prostaglandins produced in the uterine lining and released into the bloodstream as the lining is shed, causing smooth muscle contraction, nausea, and/or diarrhea

    B. Secondary dysmenorrhea

        1. Extrauterine causes

            a. Endometriosis

            b. Tumors

                1) Subserosal leiomyomata

                2) Malignancies

                3) Pelvic tumors

            c. Ovarian cysts

        d. Pelvic inflammatory disease
2. Intrauterine causes
    a. Adenomyosis
    b. Endometriosis
    c. Intramural leiomyomata
    d. Polyps
       1) Endometrial
       2) Cervical
    e. Presence of an intrauterine device
    f. Cervical stenosis
    g. Endometritis

III. History

  A. What the patient may present with
    1. Regular, recurrent pain may occur monthly, prior to menses, or with menses
      a. Abdominal pain
      b. Pelvic pain
      c. Severe backache
    2. Nausea, diarrhea, or constipation
    3. Weakness
    4. Dizziness
    5. Weight gain
    6. Breast tenderness
    7. Backache
  B. Additional information to be elicited by asking the following questions:
    1. Relationship to menarche
    2. When does pain begin?
    3. How long does it last?
    4. Does anything make it feel better?
    5. Last menstrual period
    6. Birth control method(s) used
    7. Any relationship to intercourse?
    8. Any vaginal discharge?
    9. Any fever related to pain?
   10. What is menstrual flow like?
   11. Is this new; is this a change in pattern?
   12. Sensitivity to aspirin; nonsteroidal anti-inflammatories
   13. History of chronic illness (kidney disease)
   14. Current medications (prescription and over-the-counter)
   15. Postcoital bleeding

16. Home remedies and/or folk remedies tried; use of complementary and alternative therapies
17. STD history, vaginitis/vaginosis

IV. Physical Examination

A. Vital signs
   1. Blood pressure
   2. Pulse
   3. Temperature, if symptoms are present at time of visit
   4. Weight
B. Vaginal examination (speculum): cervix, cervical pathology
C. Bimanual examination

V. Laboratory Examination

A. Chlamydia (if not done within 1 year or woman has a new sexual partner), or cervical picture indicates, or if severity of symptoms has increased
B. Gonorrhea culture (same as Chlamydia)
C. Wet mount

VI. Differential Diagnosis

See Etiology.

VII. Treatment

A. Medication
   1. Ibuprofen (Motrin®) 400 mg 4 times a day, 200–400 mg every 4–6 hours (max. 1.2 grams/day)
   2. Mefenamic acid (Ponstel®) 250 mg, 2 tablets immediately and one every 6 hours
   3. Naproxen (Anaprox®) 275 mg, 2 immediately and 1 every 6–8 hours (no more than 5 tabs 1.375 grams per day); Aleve® 200 mg every 8–12 hours
   4. Naprosyn 500 mg every 12 hours or 250 mg every 6–8 hrs. (max. 1.25 grams 1st day then 1.0 grams/day)
   5. Anaprox DS® 550 mg = one every 12 hours
   6. Aspirin with codeine 1–2 tablets every 4 hours as needed
   7. Ibuprofen (Advil®) 200 mg, 2 tablets every 4–6 hours (max. 1.2 grams/day) (OTC),
   8. Flurbiprofen (Ansaid®) 100 mg orally twice or three times a day

      9. Meclofenamate (Meclomen®) 1 tab (100 mg) every 6 hours prn

    10. Other OTC analogues

    11. Oral or possibly other hormonal contraceptive (to produce anovulatory state)

  B. Other measures

    1. Reassurance

    2. Refer to premenstrual syndrome guidelines for diet, exercise, and vitamin recommendations

    3. Heating pad; microwave pad (filled with nonpopping corn or buckwheat)

VIII. Complications

May occur with failure to recognize presence of entity as described in differential diagnosis that results in lack of appropriate treatment.

IX. Consultation/Referral

  A. Diagnosis of secondary dysmenorrhea

  B. Failure to improve after treatment as in VII

X. Follow-up

  A. Yearly health examination and Papanicolaou smear per guidelines

  B. Secondary dysmenorrhea follow-up as indicated by physician or with consult

See Bibliography.

AMENORRHEA

I. Definition

  A. Primary amenorrhea: failure of the menses to occur by age 15

  B. Secondary amenorrhea: cessation of the menses for longer than 6 months in a woman who has established menses at least 1 year after menarche

II. Etiology

  A. Primary Amenorrhea

    1. Gonadal failure

    2. Congenital absence of uterus & vagina

    3. Constitutional delay

B. Secondary Amenorrhea
   1. Pregnancy; breastfeeding
   2. Pituitary disease or tumor; disruption of hypothalamic-pituitary axis
   3. Menopause
   4. Too little body fat (about 22% required for menses)
   5. Excessive exercise (e.g., long-distance running, ballet dancing, gymnastics, figure skating)
   6. Rapid weight loss
   7. Cessation of menstruation following use of hormonal contraception
   8. Recent change in lifestyle (e.g., increase in stress, travel)
   9. Thyroid disease
   10. Polycystic ovary syndrome
   11. Anorexia nervosa or other eating disorders
   12. Premature ovarian failure, ovarian dysgenesis, infection, hemorrhage, necrosis, neoplasm
   13. Asherman's syndrome
   14. Cervical stenosis—outflow tract anomaly
   15. Medications including psychotropics
   16. Chronic illness
   17. Tuberculosis

III. History

A. What the patient presents with
   1. Absence of menstruation
   2. Possible breast discharge
   3. Other symptoms secondary to underlying etiology
B. Additional information to be considered
   1. Careful menstrual history; pregnancy history
   2. Sexual history
   3. Contraceptive history
   4. Medications—OTC, prescription, homeopathic, herbal
   5. Sources of emotional stress
   6. Symptoms of climacteric
   7. Any current acute illness
   8. History of chronic illness
   9. Present weight, weight 1 year ago
   10. Amount of daily exercise
   11. Recent D&C or abortion
   12. History of tuberculosis
   13. Eating disorder—current or history of

IV. Physical Examination

    A. Weigh patient

    B. Neck: thyroid gland (look for nodes: palpable, enlarged)

    C. Breast: discharge

       1. Breast examination

       2. Milky, clear, dark, light, bloody, thick, thin, color

    D. Vaginal examination (speculum): vagina may be atrophic and there may be no cervical mucus

    E. Bimanual examination

       1. Uterus: may be enlarged

       2. Cervix—scarring, stenosis

       3. Adnexa: ovaries may be enlarged—cystic

       4. Recto-vaginal examination

    F. Measure ratio of body fat to lean mass; BMI

V. Laboratory Examination

    A. Human chorionic gonadotropin (HCG) qualitative, quantitative

    B. Prolactin level

    C. Thyroid stimulating hormone

    D. Follicle stimulating hormone, luteinizing hormone, Dehydroepiandrosterone sulfate (DHEAS), and serum testosterone (if patient is hirsute); hemoglobin, erythrocyte sedimentation rate

    E. Papanicolaou smear

    F. Microscopic examination of cervical mucus

    G. TB test if no history

    H. Consider pituitary function assessment, ultrasound, CAT scan, MRI, hysterosalpingography, hysteroscopy after consultation with a physician

    I. GnRH stimulation test

VI. Differential Diagnosis

See Etiology.

VII. Treatment

    A. If breast discharge is present, do not wait: do work-up as per breast discharge protocol.

    B. If human chorionic gonadotropin (HCG) and prolactin levels are within normal limits, pregnancy test is negative, the nurse practitioner may give Medroxyprogesterone acetate (Provera®) 5–10 mg per day × 5–10 days.

1. If no withdrawal bleed in 3–7 days after progestin, consider follicle stimulating hormone and luteinizing hormone assays 2 weeks after Provera. Try oral estrogen 1.25–2.5 mg to prime the endometrium (estropipate) daily for 21–25 days; if no bleeding, add progestin during last 5–10 days of estrogen. If no withdrawal bleed, refer to physician.
2. If woman wishes to start oral or other hormonal contraceptive and has no withdrawal bleed from Provera, repeat HCG if indicated and start oral contraceptives or other hormonal method the following Sunday regardless of brand of hormonal contraceptive used. If no withdrawal bleed after first cycle, consult with physician.
3. If woman wishes to start oral or other hormonal contraceptives and has withdrawal bleed from Provera, start contraceptive after start of bleed; if Provera is not completed by that time, discontinue and discard remainder (some clinicians have woman complete Provera).
4. If withdrawal bleed occurs with Provera, then no menses for 2 months following the bleed, possible consult with physician, then give Provera 10 mg × 10 days every 2 months. If sexually active, an HCG must be run prior to taking medication each time.
5. If woman has a history of uterine infection or trauma to the uterus through multiple curettages (postpartum or postabortion), or if the work-up is negative and there is no response to Provera, referral for further evaluation (hysterosalpingography; hysteroscopy to lyse adhesions; estrogen to restore endometrium).
6. Instruct woman to complete 10 days of Provera even if withdrawal bleed begins, unless starting oral or other hormonal contraceptive as indicated prior in 3.

VIII. Complications

    A. Inability to conceive
    B. Sequelae of underlying cause

IX. Consultation/Referral

    A. As outlined under Treatment VII.B.5
    B. After work-up for hirsutism is completed (see V.D.)
    C. For all primary amenorrhea cases

X. Follow-up

    A. As deemed necessary with physician consult

B. Yearly

C. PRN if unsatisfactory response to treatment

See Bibliography.

ABNORMAL VAGINAL BLEEDING

I. Definition

Any variation from a woman's usual menstrual pattern; bleeding post-menopause.

II. Etiology

    A. Systemic illnesses, i.e., thyroid disease, blood dyscrasias, adrenal imbalance

    B. Submucous leiomyomata in uterus; polyps, liver disease, clotting disorders, kidney disease, leukemia

    C. Tumor in vagina, uterus

    D. Trauma to vagina, cervix; scar tissue

    E. Cervical lesions

        1. Polyps

        2. Carcinoma

    F. Abnormal hormone secretion (with anovulatory bleeding)

    G. Change in ovarian function (perimenopause)

    H. Endometrial polyps or leiomyomata in cervix, uterus

    I. Pelvic malignancy—nodes, uterus, bladder, rectum, vagina, ovary

    J. Ectopic pregnancy

    K. Abortion

    L. Placental accidents

    M. Hyperplasia

    N. Stress

    O. Postmenopausal bleed

    P. Pharmacotherapeutics

    Q. STDs, PID

    R. Endometriosis/adenomyosis

    S. Hemorrhoids, polyps in colon, colon carcinoma mistaken for vaginal bleeding

III. History

    A. What the patient may present with

        1. Midcycle bleeding

        2. Spotting

        3. Pain

4. Sudden onset of heavy bleeding
5. Postmenopausal bleeding
B. Additional information to be considered
1. Is bleeding recent or since menarche?
2. Onset of bleeding
3. Amount of flow (pads or tampons per hour); clots and size of clots
4. Normal bleeding pattern: how does this episode differ from normal menstruation?
5. Current or recent use of medication; complementary therapies (herbals, homeopathics)
6. Last menstrual period; previous menstrual period
7. Last sexual contact, if sexually active
8. Birth control method(s)
9. Recent trauma to pelvic area or any other part of body (screen for abuse)
10. Characteristics of present bleeding: clots, tissue
11. Any related pain
12. Any fever
13. Any dizziness; syncope
14. Symptoms of changing ovarian function (perimenopause)
15. Recent pelvic surgery including tubal ligation

IV. Physical Examination

A. Vital signs
1. Blood pressure
2. Pulse
3. Temperature
B. Skin: examine for evidence of bleeding disorder, e.g., petechiae or ecchymosis; pallor; fine, thinning hair
C. Neck—thyroid: examine for enlargement, palpate nodes
D. Breasts
1. Development
2. Masses
3. Tenderness, appearance of skin, nipples
4. Discharge
5. Axillary nodes
E. Abdomen
1. Tenderness
2. Guarding
3. Bowel sounds
4. Distension
5. Hepatosplenomegaly

F. Genital examination: Observe perineum for trauma
G. Vaginal examination (speculum)
1. Observe vaginal walls for lesions or evidence of trauma
2. Observe cervix for
a. Polyps
b. Lesions (evidence of trauma)
c. Erosion or ectropion
d. Whether os is closed or dilated; discharge in os
3. Evaluate amount and type of bleeding
H. Bimanual examination
1. Uterus: evaluate size, shape, position, any pain
2. Adnexa: evaluate for possible mass, pain
3. Recto-vaginal exam
a. Fullness (fluid)
b. Pain
c. Bleeding

V. Laboratory Examination (will depend on history and assessment of bleeding)

A. Complete blood count, differential with hematocrit or hemoglobin; platelet count; bleeding and clotting time if indicated
B. Serum pregnancy test
C. Gonococcal culture
D. Chlamydia smear
E. Thyroid studies
F. Hormone levels—LH, FSH, prolactin, GnRh, serum estradiol
G. Urinalysis
H. STD screen including HIV status
I. Wet mount

VI. Differential Diagnosis

See Etiology.

VII. Treatment

A. For light flow/regular/irregular bleeding (e.g., mid-cycle)
1. Lab work as history demands.
2. May observe 2–3 months as indicated by history and physical findings. Woman should be instructed to keep record of days that bleeding occurs.
3. After 2–3 cycles, after normal physical exam and Papanicolaou smear with appropriate lab work, consider
a. Provera 5–10 mg daily × 10 days; or
b. Monophasic OC × 1–3 months or 6–12 months

B. For heavy bleeding
1. Consult/refer to physician after appropriate work-up.
C. For bleeding with IUD in place, see IUD see guideline
D. For heavy bleeding with Depo-Provera,[1] consider addition of low dose contraceptive × 3 cycles or supplemental estrogen until bleeding stops
E. If bleeding persists with a positive HCG
1. Physician consultation
2. Referral as indicated
F. If bleeding postmenopausal will need an endometrial biopsy (see Endometrial Biopsy guideline)

VIII. Complications

A. Severe hemorrhage
B. Shock
C. Of underlying systemic illnesses

IX. Consultation/Referral

A. After completion of all laboratory work and physical examination, nurse practitioner may:
1. Consult with physician for possible Mirena insertion
2. Refer to physician for treatment, i.e., endometrial ablation or D&C
B. Immediate referral to physician if excessive bleeding after laboratory work and work-up by clinician

X. Follow-up

As indicated by diagnosis and treatment.
See Bibliography. Web site: http://www.womenshealth.about.com/cs/ menstrualdisorder/index.htm.

ENDOMETRIAL BIOPSY

I. Definition

Endometrial biopsy is a method of obtaining a sample of the nonpregnant uterine lining for purposes of cytologic and histologic examination. The procedure can be done in an ambulatory setting with or without local anesthesia. The specimen obtained is glandular epithelium.

II. Etiology

A. Reasons for performing this diagnostic procedure may include:

1. Unexplained abnormal vaginal bleeding in the premenopausal, perimenopausal, or postmenopausal woman
2. Rule out endometrial pathology prior to initiation of hormone therapy (HT) in the postmenopausal woman and periodically monitor endometrial status with unopposed estrogen use if indicated
3. Determine response of the endometrium to hormonal intervention in women experiencing infertility
4. Evaluate endometrial response during tamoxifen therapy to rule out pathologic response

III. History

   A. What the patient may present with
      1. Postmenopausal bleeding
      2. Unexplained abnormal vaginal bleeding in a premenopausal woman
      3. Desire for hormone therapy
      4. Currently taking hormone therapy with intact uterus
      5. Unsuccessful attempts at pregnancy
      6. Current tamoxifen therapy for breast disease
   B. Additional information to be considered
      1. Hormone therapy: type, purpose, duration, dosage, side effects, bleeding history; use of hormonal contraception, IUD
      2. Gynecologic and pregnancy including STD and PID episodes; elective abortions
      3. Gynecologic surgery including previous endometrial biopsies and results, tubal ligation, cesarean section
      4. Medical conditions: cardiac, bleeding disorders, hypoglycemia
      5. Current medications including over-the-counter and botanical preparations
      6. Allergies to pharmacologics including local anesthetic agents and povidone-iodine (Betadine®, similar products)
      7. Vasovagal episodes especially with pelvic examinations, uterine sounding, IUD insertion, elective abortion
      8. Symptoms of vaginitis, cervicitis, STD, PID
      9. Contraceptive methods including current method and consistency of use; any recent exposure to pregnancy risk and date
      10. Menstrual cycles, peri- and postmenopausal bleeding; LMP, PMP

IV. Physical Examination

   A. Bimanual examination: uterine position, pain, flexion, size, shape; adnexal or uterine masses, cervical motion tenderness, adnexal exam; any pelvic pain, determine involution if woman is postpartum, postabortion

B. Speculum exam, presence of vaginal discharge

C. Cervical inspection, position, presence of polyps, nebothian cysts, IUD string, mucopurulent discharge

D. Recto-vaginal examination to determine uterine size, position, rule out pregnancy

E. Vital signs: blood pressure, temperature (rule out fever)

F. General status: last meal or snack, fluids (rule out hypoglycemia); offer juice, snack

G. Administer mild prostaglandin inhibitor 20 minutes before biopsy

H. Teach woman about the procedure and possible complications, and obtain her consent to proceed

V. Reasons to Defer Procedure

A. Pregnancy or possible pregnancy

B. PID, STD with PID as complication, cervicitis

C. Poor involution of uterus postpartum or postabortion

D. Fever

E. Blood dyscrasias, especially bleeding disorders, severe anemia

F. Extremely anteflexed or retroflexed uterus or cervical stenosis—may need to do biopsy under general anesthesia

G. Vaginitis—defer procedure until diagnosis and treatment regimen completed

VI. Laboratory

A. Pregnancy test

B. Hematocrit as indicated

C. Vaginal and cervical cultures as indicated

D. Postprocedure biopsy specimen(s) for histologic screening

E. Other per work-up for abnormal uterine bleeding

VII. Biopsy Technique

A. Cleanse cervix and vagina with antiseptic, considering any sensitivities, allergies.

B. Administer local anesthetic agent to the cervix (lidocaine gels, other topical gel or spray products, or paracervical block) if necessary/desired depending on sampling technique and equipment to be used.

C. Sound the uterus (if using curette for sampling); prior to this, grasping the cervix with a fine tenaculum is necessary (using local anesthetic gel at the site for tenaculum placement reduces pain for the woman). Having the patient cough when applying and removing the tenaculum often reduces discomfort.

   D. Insert the sampling device in the os, taking care not to force the device through a resistant os; if the os is stenotic, cervical dilators may be used. Use one of the following techniques:

      1. Pipelle device (flexible sampler with a piston to create suction for sampling): insert up to fundus, pull back completely on the piston to create suction and rotate the pipelle continuously moving it from the fundus and back again several times to collect the sample completely filling the plastic tube; withdraw the pipelle and push in the piston to deposit sample into the preservative. Some devices require cutting off the tip to expel the specimen.

      2. Pipelle device attached to suction pump: insert as above and collect specimen by connecting the external pump, continuing suction until the device is filled.

      3. Suction curette that is steel and reusable or plastic and disposable: sound the uterus stabilizing the cervix with a tenaculum and then insert the curette and gently sample in a manner similar to using the pipelle devices (some are attached to a 10 cc syringe to provide the suction and some to an external pump); withdraw the curette, deposit the specimen in the preservative.

   E. Monitor patient's condition during and after the procedure to assess for vasovagal response, signs and symptoms of uterine perforation.

   F. Allow patient to rest briefly with her legs flat before getting off the examination table. Assure that she is not feeling faint and is able to get dressed safely.

   G. Instruct patient about postprocedure care.

      1. Signs and symptoms of complications: severe cramping or pelvic pain; bright red bleeding with or without clots; fever, chills, foul-smelling vaginal discharge—call provider and/or go to urgent care setting.

      2. Expect spotting for 1–2 days after the biopsy; define spotting and the difference between spotting and bleeding.

      3. Patient may resume vaginal intercourse in 3 days or whenever she desires.

      4. Prostaglandin inhibitor for mild cramping.

      5. Resumption of menses if premenopausal and having menstrual cycles.

VIII. Referral//Consultation for Procedure

   A. Patients with severe cervical stenosis to consider procedure under general anesthesia

B. Patients with contraindications for procedure

IX. Follow-up

A. Arrange for an opportunity to review laboratory findings
B. Care based on reason for endometrial biopsy and laboratory results
C. Treatment of any positive culture results

X. Referral/Consultation for Results

A. Endometrial carcinoma—referral for treatment or co-management
B. Hyperplasia without atypia—usually means atrophic changes
    1. Secretory: follow but no need for treatment unless bleeding persists and consider Provera
    2. Proliferative may benefit from Provera
C. Complex hyperplasia without atypia
    1. Desires pregnancy: consider risks and co-manage with physician
    2. Does not desire pregnancy: to remove unopposed estrogen, cycle with progestins and repeat endometrial biopsy in 3–6 months
D. Complex hyperplasia with atypia—referral for D&C
    1. Co-management for pregnancy if desired and no malignancy or for surgical high risk
    2. Surgery and/or treatment per staging if malignant
    3. Hysterectomy if nonmalignant and no pregnancy desired

See Bibliography. Web sites: http://www.mayoclinic.com/health/vaginal-bleeding/HO000159; http://www.medicinenet.com/endometrial_biopsy/article.htm; http://www.webmd.com/hw/healthy-women/hw4583.asp.

PREMENSTRUAL SYNDROME (PMS)

I. Definition

PMS (premenstrual syndrome) is a cluster of physical, emotional, and behavioral symptoms related to the menstrual cycle, developing or worsening during the luteal phase and clearing with the onset of the menstrual flow.

PMDD (premenstrual dysphoric disorder) is a severe form of PMS sharing symptoms but set apart by the exaggeration and severity.

II. Etiology

No single etiology explains the various symptoms associated with PMS. A multifactorial cause is probable, involving psychosocial, genetic, hormonal, and neurotransmitter components (serotonergic dysfunction).

III. History

    A. What the patient presents with (may include some or all of the following symptoms, in varying degrees)
1. Headache, backache, migraine, syncope
2. Edema
3. Breast tenderness, engorgement, enlargement, heaviness
4. Hot flashes
5. Paresthesia of hands and feet, aggravation of epilepsy, joint or muscle pain
6. Weight gain
7. Fluid retention
8. Abdominal bloating
9. Increase in appetite and/or impulsive eating; craving for sweets and/or salt; food cravings in general
10. Nausea, vomiting, constipation
11. Decreased urine output, cystitis, urethritis, enuresis
12. Exacerbation or recurrence of acne, boils, urticaria, easy bruising, herpes, rhinitis, colds, hoarseness, increased asthma, sore throat, sinusitis
13. Emotional lability (anxiety, depression, crying, fatigue, persistent & marked anger, aggression, irritability), difficulty in concentrating; decreased interest in usual activities
14. Changes in libido
15. Lethargy, fatigue, depression in mood, feeling hopeless
16. Sleep disturbances—hypersomnia, insomnia
17. Palpitations
18. Any symptoms, physical or emotional, that cluster during the same phase of menstrual cycle

    B. Additional information to be considered
1. When did these symptoms first occur in relationship to menarche?
2. When do they begin and end in relationship to menses?
3. Has there been a recent change in symptoms?
4. Do you have cramps with your period?
5. Has there been any change in your lifestyle (work, personal, family)?
6. What is your diet like?
7. How much exercise do you get?
8. Are you or have you ever been in counseling?

9. What medications are you taking?
10. Do you have a history of chronic illness; if so, which, including depression?
11. When was your last menstrual period?
12. What birth control method do you use if any?
13. Have you had tubal ligation and if so, when?
14. Have you ever thought about suicide or harm to others?
15. Have you experienced depression or agitation at other times in your life?

IV. Physical Examination

A. Vital signs
B. Complete physical and gynecologic exam within past year examination
C. Mental status examination

V. Laboratory Examination

A. Only as indicated medically

VI. Treatment

A. Treatment is multifaceted and diverse, aimed at symptoms that patient finds most debilitating. To aid in diagnosis and treatment, 2 months of retrospective daily logs or symptom calendars help to confirm diagnosis and guide selection of appropriate treatment.
   1. Vitamin B6 (pyridoxine). Begin with 50 mg to 100 mg total daily dose. Do not exceed recommended dosage. This vitamin has been shown to be toxic in large doses.
   2. Vitamin E 400 mg daily or twice a day.
   3. Evening Primrose Oil. Begin with 2 capsules twice a day. May increase to 4 capsules twice a day. Improvement will occur slowly over 3–9 months. Contains vitamin E, so patient should not take both.
   4. Prostaglandin inhibitors may provide relief taken during the second half of the menstrual cycle.
   5. May consider
      a. Diuretics
      b. Antidepressants
      c. Antianxiety drugs
      d. Birth control pills (Yaz® has been approved for PMDD), contraceptive patch, ring
   6. Calcium 1000–1200 mg daily; magnesium 300–400 mg daily.

B. General measures
 1. Lifestyle changes including stress reduction, i.e., meditation, yoga, or other relaxation techniques
 2. Diet recommendations (These dietary changes should be on-going. It is not enough to modify one's diet only on the days prior to menstruation.)
    a. Limit consumption of refined sugar (e.g., cookies, cakes, jelly, honey) to 5 tablespoons/day.
    b. Limit salt intake to 3 gm or less per day (e.g., avoid using saltshaker).
    c. Limit intake of alcohol and nicotine.
    d. Avoid caffeine (e.g., coffee, tea, chocolate, soft drinks).
    e. Increase intake of complex carbohydrates (e.g., fresh fruits, vegetables, whole grains, pasta, rice, potatoes).
    f. Consume moderate amounts of protein and fat (decrease animal fats and increase vegetable oils).
    g. Limit red meat consumption to 2 × weekly or less.
 3. Exercise plan recommendations: exercise three times per week for 30–40 minutes (brisk walking, jogging, aerobic dancing, swimming)
 4. Consider other complementary therapies including botanicals, aroma and music therapy, acupuncture, and energy healing
 5. Keep a diary of daily symptoms, diet, body temperature

VII. Differential Diagnosis

A. Sexual dysfunction
B. Chronic pelvic pain
C. Endometriosis
D. Primary dysmenorrhea
E. Post-tubal ligation syndrome
F. Prolactin-producing tumors
G. Perimenopausal symptoms
H. Fibrocystic breast disease
I. Depression
J. Psychopathology
K. Somatization of stress
L. Life stressors
M. Systemic lupus erythematosus
N. Hypertension
O. Meningioma
P. Attention-deficit disorder (residual type)
Q. Thyroid disorders

VIII. Complications

    A. Serious psychological problem misdiagnosed as PMS
    B. Systemic disease misdiagnosed as premenstrual syndrome

IX. Consultation/Referral

    A. Referral at discretion of the nurse practitioner, after review of history and physical examination
    B. Mental health referral if appropriate
    C. Referral to nutritionist if needed/desired by patient
    D. Support group referral if desired

X. Follow-up

    A. Monthly × 3 checks
    B. Yearly if improvement in relief of symptoms
    C. If symptoms increase or change

See Complementary and Alternative therapies guideline, and Bibliography. Web site: http://www.womenshealth.gov/faq/pms.htm.

NOTE

1. Approach this regime with caution remembering that menstrual changes are recognized as an early phenomenon with progestin-only contraception, decreasing with prolonged use. If patient is a long time user, the onset of new bleeding may indicate underlying pathology.

CHAPTER EIGHT

Medical Abortion

I. Definition

To terminate a pregnancy between 6 and 9 weeks with use of Misoprostol and Mifepristone.

Mifepristone (Cytotec): derivative of norethindrone with strong affinity for progesterone receptors. The progestin antagonist effect of mifepristone interferes with the maintenance of early pregnancy. Mifepristone acts on the decidua to break down the capillary epithelial cells, causing the trophoblast to separate from the decidua. This leads to the disruption of the integrity of the pregnancy, bleeding and a decrease in the maternal human chorionic gonadotrophin (hCG).

Misoprostol (Mifeprex): synthetic prostaglandin analogue. Misoprostol efficiently ripens the cervix and induces uterine contractility.

II. Etiology

Therapeutic abortion—Patient presents with desire to terminate early pregnancy by nonsurgical means.

III. History

A. Medical Guidelines for Eligibility
1. Amenorrhea with positive pregnancy test
2. Pelvic or transvaginal ultrasound documenting intrauterine pregnancy between 6 and 9 weeks gestation (gestational age cut off depending on office protocol)
3. Fetal cardiac activity identified on ultrasound
4. Full medical and surgical including but not limited to:
   a. Diabetes

    b. Cardiovascular
    c. Infectious disease (including STIs, hepatitis, HIV, TB)
    d. Thyroid
    e. Lung
    f. Autoimmune
    g. Eating disorders (especially if currently active)
    h. Metabolic conditions
    i. Psychiatric illness
    j. Epilepsy
    k. Allergies
    l. Kidney
    m. Surgeries, especially gynecologic

5. Full psychosocial history including but not limited to:
    a. Drug and alcohol use/abuse (including prescriptives, non-prescriptive, street drugs, and herbal preparations) that contain Misoprostol (i.e., Cytotec, Arthrotec), or any component of the product
    b. Tobacco use
    c. Domestic violence (with regard to safety)
    d. High-risk behaviors
    e. Patient's social network—including support systems, especially with her knowledge of pregnancy and decision to terminate
    f. Cultural beliefs—especially with regard to pregnancy and abortion

6. Full gynecologic/obstetrical history including but not limited to:
    a. Menstrual history
    b. Gynecologic history
    c. Pap smear history
    d. High-risk behaviors (especially STDs and number of sexual partners)
    e. Pregnancy history including number of pregnancies, deliveries, miscarriages, previous abortions (medical and surgical), ectopic pregnancies, stillbirths, and other neonatal losses or infant/child deaths (e.g., SIDS)
    f. Contraceptive history and desire for contraception after abortion is complete
    g. History of attempt to end current pregnancy with prescriptive, nonprescriptive, or herbal preparations or street drugs

IV. Contraindications and Ineligibility

    A. Greater than 50 days amenorrhea or beyond last menstrual period (depending on office protocol for gestational cut-off)

B. Intrauterine device in-situ; IUD must be removed prior to taking Mifeprex®

C. Inconclusive pelvic or transvaginal ultrasound for intrauterine pregnancy or documented/suspected extrauterine pregnancy

D. History of adrenal failure

E. History of current anticoagulant therapy

F. History of any bleeding disorder

G. History of specific current steroidal medication therapy

H. Documented allergy to mifepristone, misoprostol, or other medications

I. History of severe asthma uncontrolled by therapy

J. History of long-term glucocorticoid therapy

K. History of complicated diabetes mellitus

L. History of severe anemia without documented normal lab values

M. Inherited porphyria

N. Contraindication to prostaglandin analogue selected

O. Undiagnosed adnexal mass

P. Additional information to be considered
    1. Must be absolutely certain in decision to terminate pregnancy
    2. Must agree to participate in their own abortion and take responsibility for their own care
    3. Must agree to return for follow-up visit(s)
    4. Must be able to understand and follow instructions for medical abortion as well as the risks, benefits, and side effects of medications used
    5. Must not have comprehension or language barriers
    6. Must agree to have a surgical abortion, should the medical abortion fail
    7. Must have access to telephone in case of emergency
    8. Must have access and transportation to an emergency facility if one is needed
    9. Must agree not to take any herbal medications or supplements or prescription medication without asking the clinician, during the medical abortion
    10. Must agree to not use any of the following medications/foods/herbs during the abortion procedure:
        a. Ketoconazole
        b. Itraconazole
        c. Erythromycin
        d. Grapefruit juice
        e. Klonopin
        f. Rifampin
        g. Dexamethasone

    h. St. John's Wort
    i. Carbamazapine
    j. Corticosteroids

V. Physical Examination

  A. Vital signs: blood pressure, pulse, temperature, respirations
  B. Pelvic exam: unnecessary unless patient has complaints
  C. Pelvic or transvaginal ultrasound (depending upon office protocol)
  D. Urine pregnancy test (if ultrasound is inconclusive for intrauterine pregnancy)
  E. Laboratory values: hemoglobin and Rh testing
  F. Height and weight

VI. Counseling and Consent Signing

  A. Patient should be counseled on options for current pregnancy to include:
    1. delivery, adoption, and abortion
  B. Patient will be required to read material provided by office on medical abortion.
  C. Discussion with patient regarding the FDA approved dosage of medication and evidence-based use of medication.
  D. Patient should be counseled as to risks, benefits, and side effects of Misoprostol® and Mifepristone®.
  E. Patient should be counseled as to instructions for medication use—to include taking Mifepristone® in office and when to insert Misoprostol® at home.
  F. Patient should be counseled as to what she might experience once each medication is taken, to include bleeding and passing tissue, cramping, nausea, vomiting, and fever.
  G. Patient should be counseled as to what to do if abortion does not occur.
  H. Patient should be counseled as to what to do in case of emergency including heavy, uncontrollable bleeding, pain that does not respond to medication, or fever over 101 degrees F.
  I. Patient should be counseled on when to begin contraception.
  J. Patient will be required to read Mifeprex® medication guide and sign a patient agreement.
  K. Patient will be given written instructions and information on aftercare.
  L. Patient will be counseled as to importance of attending follow-up visit to insure completed procedure.
  M. Patient to be counseled as to importance of presenting letter from clinician if seen in an emergency room. Letter explains medical

abortion procedure, medications that interfere with procedure, and phone number of clinician.

N. Patients should be counseled that there were four deaths in California following medical abortion due to sepsis.

O. Patient to be given both verbal and written instructions.

P. Aftercare instructions to be given include: pain medication, heating pad use, anti-emetics and comfort care; discussion about diet, exercise, heavy lifting, and other restrictions post AB.

Q. Educate patient on how to identify complications.

VII. Medication Regimen (Based on office protocol)

A. Mifepristone® 200 mg orally and 400–800 mcg Misoprostol® intravaginally between 24–72 hours after taking Mifepristone® (Evidence based protocol)

B. Mifepristone® 600 mg orally and 400 mcg Misoprostol® orally 36–40 hours later (FDA approved protocol)

C. Mifepristone® 200 mg orally and 800 mcg Misoprostol® intravaginally in simultaneous dosing (Creinin®)

VIII. Other Medications to Consider

A. Rhogam (D) 1 cc must be given after oral dose of Mifepristone to all women who test Rh negative

B. Anti-emetic (i.e., Zofran ODT, Compazine, ginger, B6)—per office guidelines

C. Pain medication (i.e., Ibuprofen 800 mg every 8 hours, Vicodin 1 orally every 4–6 hrs; Percocet every 4–6 hrs)—per office guidelines

IX. Complications With Medical Abortion

A. Patient to be instructed to seek emergency treatment if:
  1. Bleeding (soaking through two thick full-sized sanitary pads per hour for two consecutive hours
  2. Pelvic pain uncontrolled with medication regimens recommended
  3. Fever greater than 100.4 degrees F or higher that lasts for more than 4 hours
  4. Severe abdominal pain
  5. Weakness, nausea, vomiting, or diarrhea more than 24 hours after taking Misoprostol®

X. Consultation/Referral for Signs of Incomplete Abortion or Infection

A. Uncontrolled bleeding

B. Continued pregnancy symptoms (i.e, nausea/vomiting or breast tenderness) 1 week after medical abortion

C. Unexplained fever

D. Failure to return to pre-pregnancy baseline

XI. Follow-up

A. Follow-up visit should occur 2–3 weeks post abortion and should include:

1. Vital signs

2. Urine pregnancy test

3. Medical and psychosocial history since medical abortion including bleeding pattern, pain or cramping, fever, pregnancy symptoms, support network, signs and symptoms of depression or anxiety due to decision to terminate

4. Pelvic exam to assess:

   a. Involution of uterus

   b. Vulvo-vaginal infection post abortion

   c. Resolution of bleeding

   d. Pelvic pain or PID

5. Review of birth control management or plan to include:

   a. Current method used, evaluate:

      1) effective vs. ineffective

      2) user friendly

      3) side effect profile

      4) need for sample, refill, or new prescription

   b. If no current method used, evaluate:

      1) need for method—review options

      2) review risks, benefits, side effects, and instructions for use

      3) give sample, refill, or new prescription

See Bibliography. Web site: http://www.fwhc.org/abortion/medical-ab.htm.

Guideline developed by Amy Kassirer, RNC, MS, MSW, Women's Health Nurse Practitioner at the Ob/Gyn Office of Dr. Marie Lemoier and at Four Women.

POSTABORTION CARE, MEDICAL AND SURGICAL

Examination after Medical or Surgical Abortion

I. Definition

An examination usually 2 weeks after uncomplicated therapeutic abortion to assess the patient's physical and mental status.

II. Etiology

> Therapeutic or elective abortion.

III. History

> A. What patient may present with
> > 1. Surgical
> > > a. No unusual complaints
> > > b. Rare complications may include:
> > > > 1) Excessive blood loss (typical length of light to moderate flow is 9 days)
> > > > 2) Pelvic infection
> > > > 3) Pelvic perforation
> > > > 4) Acute hematometra
> > 2. Medical
> > > a. Nausea
> > > b. Vomiting
> > > c. Headaches
> > > d. Fever
> > > e. Chills
> > > f. Bleeding: average length of bleeding is 10 to 13 days; however, heavy bleeding may occur
> B. Additional information to be considered
> > 1. Date of abortion; type of procedure
> > 2. Date of last menstrual period
> > 3. Are pregnancy symptoms gone; if not what symptoms continue?
> > 4. How long after procedure did bleeding continue; any pain associated with bleeding; how much bleeding; any clots, character of bleeding, odor to discharge; fever?
> > 5. Results of pathological examination of products of conception (if available)
> > 6. Any change in relationship with partner?
> > 7. Present emotional status
> > 8. Birth control method
> > 9. Intercourse since procedure
> > 10. Medications taken including antibiotics, oxytocins, herbals, vitamins, homeopathics

IV. Physical Examination

> A. Vital signs: blood pressure, pulse
> B. Abdominal examination: suprapubic tenderness, guarding, rigidity

    C. Vaginal examination (speculum)
1. Observe for bleeding or other discharge
2. Cervix
    a. Os closed
    b. Any lesions
    c. Any discharge
    D. Bimanual exam
1. Uterus
    a. Size
    b. Consistency
    c. Tenderness
    b. Cervix: positive cervical motion tenderness (CMT)
2. Adnexa
    a. Tenderness
    b. Masses
3. Rectovaginal: any abnormal findings

V. Treatment

    A. Birth control
1. Hormonal contraception: birth control pills, Depo-Provera®, contraceptive ring, patch, implant
2. Diaphragm, FemCap, Lea's Shield
3. Intrauterine device
4. Other methods (OTC): condoms, spermicides, sponge, film
5. Sterilization (if desired)
    B. General measures: review use and sign informed consent form for birth control method (See Appendix B)

VI. Laboratory Examination

    A. Pregnancy test as indicated
    B. Wet mount as indicated

VII. Differential Diagnosis

None

VIII. Complications

See Postabortion with Complications, pages 203 to 205

IX. Consultation/Referral

    A. See Postabortion with Complications, pages 203 to 205
    B. If unresolved issues are apparent, follow-up counseling will be recommended.

X. Follow-up

    A. Yearly for health examination, Papanicolaou smear, reevaluation of family planning needs

    B. As per guideline for contraceptive of woman's choice

See Appendix A and Bibliography. Web site: http://www.nlm.nih.gov/medlineplus/ency/article/001512.htm.

POSTABORTION WITH COMPLICATIONS

I. Definition

Any sequelae or unexpected/untoward events or conditions following a therapeutic/elective abortion either medical or surgical.

II. Etiology

Therapeutic/elective abortion: medical or surgical.

III. History

    A. What the patient may present with
        1. Fever, body aches, chills
        2. Pelvic pain, severe cramps
        3. Bleeding; more than one pad an hour
        4. Passing clots larger than a quarter
        5. Abdominal pain: R or L side or bilateral; onset, duration, how relieved
        6. Nausea, vomiting, diarrhea
        7. Breast tenderness, discharge
        8. Foul odor to vaginal discharge
        9. Vertigo, headache
    B. Additional information to be considered
        1. Where and when was the procedure done; has the woman spoken to that facility regarding her symptoms or follow-up care; type of procedure (medical or surgical)
        2. How much physical activity since procedure, type of activity
        3. Any intercourse since procedure
        4. Anything used in vagina since procedure: contraceptive device, tampons, sex toy, douche product
        5. Any exposure to flu or anyone with similar symptoms
        6. Any medications taken such as analgesics, ergotrate, antibiotics, over-the-counter or prescription drugs, including herbals, vitamins
        7. Urinary tract symptoms

8. Bowel symptoms
9. Still feels pregnant; symptoms of pregnancy

IV. Physical Examination

A. Vital signs
   1. Temperature
   2. Pulse
   3. Blood pressure
   4. Respirations
B. Breast examination: tender/more/less/same as before procedure (if indicated); discharge
C. Abdomen
   1. Bowel signs
   2. Guarding
   3. Rebound tenderness
   4. Referred pain (shoulder pain)
D. Vaginal examination (sterile if within 1 week after procedure):
   1. Os dilated
   2. Any tissue in os
   3. Amount of bleeding; character
   4. Any discharge present; odor
E. Bimanual examination
   1. Cervical motion tenderness: positive Chandelier's sign
   2. Uterine tenderness, enlargement; note consistency
   3. Adnexa
      a. Tenderness
      b. Mass
      c. Fullness
   4. Rectovaginal examination: tenderness; if present, describe location

V. Laboratory Examination

A. Serum pregnancy test: quantitative
B. Gonococcal culture
C. Chlamydia smear
D. Cervical culture
E. Complete blood count with differential, sedimentation rate
F. Urinalysis and urine culture
G. Call laboratory of referring facility to get results of pathology report

VI. Differential Diagnosis

A. Retained secundae; continuation of pregnancy

  B. Uterine infection, endometritis
  C. Delayed involution
  D. Pelvic inflammatory disease
  E. Urinary tract infection
  F. Uterine perforation, bowel perforation
  G. Ectopic pregnancy
  H. See Acute Pelvic Pain and Abdominal Pain guidelines

VII. Treatment

As indicated by symptoms and diagnosis; may include appropriate antibiotics, treatment of any urinary infection, ergotrate product to promote involution; re-evacuation or evacuation if failure of medical abortion; referral for evaluation of possible ectopic pregnancy (see Pelvic Inflammatory Disease guideline and Genitourinary Tract [Urinary Tract Infection] guideline).

VIII. Complications

  A. Sepsis
  B. Ruptured ectopic pregnancy
  C. Hemorrhage
  D. Uterine perforation, bowel perforation
  E. Ascherman's syndrome

IX. Consultation/Referral

Call facility or clinician who performed the abortion for a consult and arrangement for return visit and further evaluation.

X. Follow-up

Follow routine postabortion guideline.
    See Appendix A and Bibliography.

CHAPTER NINE

Abuse and Violence

ASSESSMENT FOR ABUSE AND/OR VIOLENCE

I. Definition

Abuse and/or violence in a relationship is said to occur when one person physically, sexually, verbally, and/or emotionally abuses or economically abuses/controls another person and/or destroys the property of the person. Experiencing fear for one's person in a relationship is characteristic of an abusive situation, regardless of whether or not there is physical violence. Fearing physical harm is enough to consider the relationship abusive. Power or control by one person over another in a relationship can constitute abuse; power and control in a relationship are hallmarks of abuse. Constant degradation damages ego, self-esteem, and confidence. Dating violence affects an estimated 1:8 adolescents and domestic violence, 1:4 to 1:10 women.

II. History

Consider each woman in any setting abused until proven otherwise.
A. What the patient may present with
1. Description of abuse or violence in the relationship
2. Unexplained symptoms or injuries such as bruises or fractures inconsistent with any disease pathology
3. Numerous psychosomatic complaints with no physical evidence
4. Vague physical complaints
5. The woman's partner gives history and answers questions directed toward woman

    6. Delay between presenting injury or problem and seeking care
    7. Woman seems embarrassed or evasive in giving history
    8. Woman seems fearful, withdrawn, does not name friends, family members as resources

B. Additional information to be considered (see questions on the Abuse Assessment Screen and the Danger Assessment in the Appendices C and D)
    1. Psychiatric, alcohol, and/or drug abuse by patient and/or partner
    2. Suicide gestures or attempts; suicidal ideation
    3. Many accidents in medical record, visits to emergency department
    4. Any gynecologic or gastrointestinal complaints
    5. Level of anxiety the woman demonstrates over the visit or the physical exam

III. Physical Examination

A. Unexplained bruises; whiplike injuries consistent with shaking; erythematous areas consistent with slapping; lacerations, burn marks, fractures, and/or multiple injuries in various stages of healing

B. Injuries on body hidden by clothing and injuries inconsistent with common accidents such as on the genitals, breasts, chest, head, face, and abdomen

C. Evidence of sexual abuse such as lacerations on breasts, labia, urethra, perineum, anal area

D. Healed fractures or scars

E. Fractures inconsistent with story of accident

F. Apprehensive during examination and injuries and other findings are inappropriate to her story or inexplicable

G. Abuse can have no symptoms; well woman without visible injuries

IV. Laboratory Examination

A. As indicated by physical findings

B. May include x-rays for evidence of new, healing, or old fractures

V. Interviewing the Woman

A. Provide a safe place alone and private where partner/spouse/abuser cannot hear.

B. Assure her of confidentiality and safety.

C. Phrase questions in a nonthreatening way conveying empathy such as: "I notice you have some bruises. Can you tell me how they happened? Have you been hit by someone? Has anyone hurt you in any way? When was the last time you cried?" (see also questions on Abuse Assessment Screen (AAS) in Appendix C).

D. Assess for current danger and for emotional and/or physical injuries (see Danger Assessment tool in Appendix D).

VI. Documenting Evidence

A. Collect data from medical records and those of other health care providers.

B. Record most recent, as well as past incidents.

C. Record any witnesses to abuse.

D. Quote the woman's statements of abuse with, "Patient states . . ."

E. Protect patient by deleting any statements such as, "He hurt me so much I wanted to kill him."

F. If woman denies any abuse, record your assessment and suspicions for possible future use.

G. Record any injuries or symptoms in detail as to size, location, duration, onset, age, pattern. Make a body map and locate injuries in as much detail as you can. Indicate any evidence of sexual abuse or restraint marks on skin.

H. Collect physical evidence of injuries and label after obtaining with the woman's written permission to do so.

I. Photograph all evidence of injuries with the woman's written permission.

VII. Treatment

A. Assure the woman she is not alone.

B. Assure the woman of confidentiality and that only she can authorize the release of evidence to the police, the release of her records, and your verbal testimony.

C. Provide support that she does not deserve abuse and that no person should perpetrate any kind of abuse or violence on her.

D. Show her the documentation in her record and indicate that its purpose is to protect her.

E. Provide resources for her safety and for escape if she decides to do so; empower her to make her own plans and choices.

F. Teach her about the patterns of violence and the laws in your state concerning abuse and violence in relationships; have copies of the state laws available.

G. If she chooses to remain in the relationship, you can offer her emergency numbers of police, any domestic violence units or special forces, local emergency room(s) and shelters; help make a safety plan (money, car keys, important documents, where to go); for undocumented immigrant women who need counseling, give phone numbers of culturally sensitive programs.

VIII. Referrals/Consultation

A. Medical consultation as appropriate for treatment of injuries
B. Police, if woman chooses to file a complaint or police report
C. Shelters, special services for women in abusing/violent relationships
D. Mental health consultation if you believe woman is suicidal
E. Substance abuse, alcohol abuse treatment programs as appropriate and desired by the woman

IX. Follow-up

A. Plan return visit so woman has another opportunity for contact with you. Women may seem fine but may be degraded, depressed, afraid, or subjugated by a powerful partner who may control finances, children's money and welfare, and may be occasionally rewarding and caring.
B. As appropriate for care of injuries, presenting concerns, contraceptive needs, treatment of STDs, vaginitis, gynecologic conditions.

Appendix C abuse assessment screen and Appendix D on danger assessment may be photocopied or adapted for your patients.

See Bibliography on abuse and violence. Web site: http://www.nnvawi.org.

CHAPTER TEN

Sexual Dysfunction

I. Definition

Diminished libido or lack of libido, diminished sexual response or lack of response to sexual stimulation. Vaginismus, involuntary spasm or constriction of the distal third of the vaginal musculature around the introitus on one or more occasions.

II. Etiology

A. Organic and physiologic disorders
   1. Hormonal imbalance
   2. Injuries or anomalies of the genital tract
   3. Infection of the genitalia
   4. Lesions
   5. Nerve impairment
   6. Substance abuse: alcohol, recreational drugs
   7. Recent pregnancy
   8. Effects of medications—prescription or over-the-counter
   9. Chronic illness
B. Relationship disorders
   1. Partner's and/or patient's lack of desire for sex
   2. Medical conditions
   3. Lack of privacy
   4. Fear of failure in the sexual act; lack of knowledge about sexual response(s)
   5. Shame, guilt
   6. Expectations different from those of partner; miscommunication

    7. Rape trauma; sexual assault, or abuse at any age; domestic violence

    8. Improper use of barrier or chemical contraceptives

    9. Recent gynecological event affecting sexuality, such as sterilization, pregnancy, tubal ligation, abortion, hysterectomy, mastectomy

   10. Difficulties in sexual orientation; or confusion over gender identity

   11. Clinical depression of patient and/or partner

III. History

  A. What the patient may present with
1. Lack of sexual desire
2. Lack of response to stimulation
3. Inability to have an orgasm
4. Vaginal or vulvar irritation, bleeding, soreness
5. Lack of vaginal lubrication
6. Inability to have vaginal intercourse
7. Dyspareunia

  B. Other signs and symptoms
1. Rectal or perineal pain
2. Perineal lesions
3. Abdominal pain, pelvic pain
4. Fever
5. Bladder, urethral pain

  C. Additional information to be considered
1. Sexual history: ever had intercourse; ever experienced orgasm; partners—men, women, both
2. Contraceptive history and method presently using
3. Any gynecological/obstetrical history, diethylstilbestrol exposure, perimenopausal problems, pelvic surgery, tubal ligation, carcinomas
4. Any recent contributing events: change of partner or new relationship, marriage, divorce, separation, sterilization, pregnancy, infection, surgery, or sexual assault, incest, domestic violence
5. Any cultural or religious beliefs that relate to sexual activity
6. Alcohol, drug use; any changes
7. Expectations of self and partner, health of sexual partner
8. Any problems with privacy, time together, living arrangements
9. Use of sex toys
10. Pattern of sexual expression; availability of sexual partner

11. You might ask, "What do you do, how do you do it, and how does it make you feel?"
12. Sexual fantasies, preoccupations
13. Difficulties focusing on tactile or other sensations previously erotic

IV. Physical Examination

  A. Vital signs
    1. Blood pressure
    2. Weight
  B. General physical examination including thyroid, breasts, CVA tenderness, neurological
  C. Abdominal examination with special attention to
    1. Guarding
    2. Pain
    3. Masses
  D. External examination
    1. Anomalies
    2. Skene's glands
    3. Clitoris
    4. Status of hymen
    5. Perineum
    6. Bartholin's glands
    7. Urethra
    8. Lesions, signs of infection, injury
  E. Vaginal examination (speculum)
    1. Vaginal walls: infection, anomalies, atrophy, injuries
    2. Discharge, lesions
    3. Cervix: lesions, signs of infection, anomalies, scarring
    4. Tolerance of speculum and size accommodated, length of vagina
  F. Bimanual examination
    1. Pain on cervical manipulation
    2. Uterus: tenderness, position
    3. Adnexa: mass, tenderness
    4. Vaginal lesions

V. Laboratory Examination

  A. Appropriate cultures when evidence of infection; wet mount; urinalysis
  B. Consider thyroid panel, FBS, liver, renal function tests, serum corticosteroids if history and/or clinical findings warrant
  C. Hormone assays as indicated

VI. Differential Diagnosis

  A. Hormonal imbalance: estrogen, androgens
  B. Anomaly, injury
  C. Infection
  D. Substance abuse: drugs, alcohol, smoking
  E. Nerve impairment: spinal cord injury, neurologic diseases
  F. Changes due to aging: slower responses
  G. Adrenal, thyroid, liver, kidney problems
  H. Diabetes, diabetic neuropathy
  I. Medication side effects
  J. Depression
  K. Psychosocial problems, eating disorders
  L. Posttraumatic stress disorder (PTSD) secondary to incest, rape, sexual assault, domestic violence
  M. Vestibulitis, vulvodynia
  N. Physical and/or intellectual disabilities

VII. Treatment

  A. Medications: treat any infection present (see specific guideline); consider hormones especially if peri or postmenopausal; new drugs for women—analogues to Sildennafil citrate (Viagra®) when available. Nonprescription dietary supplement-Avilimil® (salvia rubis)
  B. General measures
    1. Education about changes in sexual response that accompany aging; need for privacy, making time for intimacy
    2. Education about a woman's sexual response, how it differs from that of a man; teach Kegel (pelvic floor) exercises; positions
    3. Explore partner relationship: changes, previous responsiveness, sexual preference, communication, expectations, guilt; screen for abuse
    4. Education on techniques for stretching hymen, vagina
    5. Education and techniques for learning about sexual response and excitation, self and partner
    6. Emphasize role of self-care: diet, exercise, vitamins, hygiene, stress reduction
    7. Education about lubricants, nonhormonal agents to restore/maintain vaginal mucosa and moisture, other sexual aids

VIII. Complications

  A. Long-term disruption of relationships
  B. Exploitation in relationships: abuse, violence, infidelity

IX. Consultation/Referral

    A. Physician for possible hormonal imbalance, genital anomaly, nerve impairment, medical conditions underlying problem

    B. Counselor for rape trauma, PTSD, exploitative relationships, abuse, depression, gender identity, sexual preferences

    C. Sex therapist—single or couples

    D. Support group

X. Follow-up

    A. Check if infection is present; reevaluate for further treatment.

    B. Arrange repeat visit as appropriate for discussion of relationship problems.

    C. Assess success of vaginal, hymenal stretching; stimulation techniques.

    D. For medical/medication problems, laboratory results as appropriate.

See Bibliography. Web site: http://familydoctor.org/612.xml.

Peri- and Postmenopause

GENERAL CARE MEASURES

I. Definition

The menopause is the landmark event of the climacteric, the 10-to-15-year period, beginning at about age 35 to 40, when women's bodies are changing and preparing for cessation of menses. A woman cannot say that she has gone through menopause until at least 1 year has passed without any menstrual period (uterine bleeding). The postmenopausal time begins when menopause is complete and menses no longer occur. For women today, the postmenopausal years may comprise as much as three-eighths of their lives or more, the age for menopause being about 50 in the United States (mean 50.4 years). A woman who has had a hysterectomy (removal of uterus only) is not considered menopausal with cessation of menses.

II. Etiology

    A. Physiologic: The gradual diminution of estrogens, resulting in cessation of ovulation and thus of menstruation.

    B. Anatomic: Surgical removal of the uterus and ovaries resulting in surgical menopause, an abrupt end to ovulation and menstruation.

III. History

    A. What the patient presents with
        1. Changes in character of the menstrual cycle
            a. Menstrual periods that are more frequent, less frequent, of longer duration or shorter duration
            b. Scanty flow
            c. Flooding at onset of flow
            d. Gradual or abrupt cessation of menses for 1 or more months
            e. Irregular periods over a period of time or abrupt cessation of menstruation
        2. Changes related to menopause and/or the aging process (these changes are the presenting complaint of women with previous surgical removal of the uterus and intact ovaries)
            a. Hot flashes, hot flushes
            b. Vaginal dryness, atrophy of vaginal tissues
            c. Night sweats
            d. Dry skin and hair; skeletal pain or stiffness
            e. Graying of hair
            f. Loss of skin elasticity
            g. Alterations in sleep patterns
            h. Developmental occurrences of aging: empty nest, caring for aging parents, grandchildren, changing roles, retirement
                1) Alterations in sexual response: longer time needed for arousal, lessened vaginal lubrication
            j. Mons and vulva flatten, less fatty tissue padding, thinning of pubic hair
        3. Recent history of gynecologic surgery: hysterectomy, oophorectomy, salpingectomy, dilatation, and curettage
    B. Additional information to be considered
        1. Menstrual history, past year; previous year
        2. Contraceptive use to present
        3. Obstetrical history: pregnancies, abortions, stillbirths
        4. Gynecologic history: surgery, endometriosis, infertility, anomalies, last Papanicolaou smear, any breast problems, last mammogram, sexually transmitted disease, infections; does she do SBE; any stress or urge incontinence
        5. Sexual history: dysfunction, unresponsiveness, recent changes, use of sex toys (see sexual dysfunction guideline); high risk sexual behaviors
        6. Life event changes: resumption of career, retirement, caring for older family members, adult children in or out of home,

divorce, separation, marriage, new sexual relationship, caring for grandchildren, loss of a child
   7. Lifestyle: exercise, diet, smoking, recreation, stressors, recreational drugs
   8. Medical history: chronic disease, medications (OTC, prescription); depression, anxiety
   9. Family medical history
   10. Use of complementary therapies (botanicals, homeopathics, massage, Tai Chi, acupuncture, Chinese medicine, aromatherapy, etc.)
   11. Beliefs about menopause and expectations
   12. Domestic violence, elder abuse

IV. Physical Examination

   A. Vital signs
      1. Blood pressure
      2. Pulse
      3. Height
      4. Weight, BMI
   B. General health examination
      1. Head
      2. Neck
      3. Heart
      4. Lungs
      5. Abdomen
      6. Extremities, joints, spine
   C. External examination for lesions, infection, atrophy, anomaly
      1. Urethral orifice
      2. Clitoris
      3. Labia
      4. Perineum
   D. Vaginal examination (speculum)
      1. Walls
      2. Discharge
      3. Lesions in the vaginal vault, noting if posthysterectomy
      4. Cervix
      5. Careful inspection of entire vagina
   E. Bimanual examination
      1. Adnexa
         a. Tenderness
         b. Masses
         c. Palpable tubes or ovaries, if present

2. Uterus
   a. Size
   b. Mobility
   c. Tenderness
   d. Masses
3. Cystocle, rectocele, urethrocele
F. Rectal examination: fecal occult blood

V. Laboratory Examination

A. Appropriate cultures, smears if suspicion of infection
B. Papanicolaou smear if none done in past year
C. Mammogram per American Cancer Society guidelines: (baseline at 35, annually at 40 and after); may be altered with family history or personal risk factors for breast cancer and new recommendations from ACS or NCI
D. Consider serum FSH level to assess for menopause if no menses for 12 months or on hormonal contraception age 50 or > and/or desire to consider HT [FSH equal to or > 2–40 mIU/ml]; discontinue hormones for the 2 weeks prior to serum assay of FSH
E. Blood glucose and lipid levels, TSH

VI. Differential Diagnosis

A. Carcinoma of genital tract
B. Pregnancy
C. Endocrine disorders
D. Decreased nutritional state; obesity
E. Marked increase in exercise regimen

VII. Treatment

A. Medication
   1. Perimenopausal: consider low dose oral contraceptive or other hormonal contraception after assessment for risks, desire for contraceptive protection; consider cycling with Provera 10 mg x 10 days monthly if intermenstrual time decreases and/or heavy bleeding/flooding characterize menses.
   2. Postmenopausal: consider nonhormonal or hormone (see hormone therapy guideline) interventions per clinical picture and patient's wishes.
B. General measures
   1. Teaching about normal menopausal symptoms, changes with aging, need for more time for arousal, use of supplemental lubrication (saliva, water-soluble jelly, water soluble

lubricants—these come as creams, jellies, and as vaginal inserts), nonhormonal agents to restore/maintain vaginal mucosa and vaginal moisture such as Replens®, Comfrey ointment, vitamin E supplement + 100–600 mg/day, or evening primrose oil 2–4 capsules/day[1] (also helpful for hot flashes), Calendula, black cohosh (20–40 mg twice a day), changes in sexual response that accompany removal of the uterus/ovaries.

2. Teaching about self-care: diet, exercise—aerobic, weight bearing, and strengthening—prevention of osteoporosis (calcium intake 1200–1500 grams/day and 400–800 IU [20 mg] vitamin D/day in foods or supplement); breast self-examination, need for Papanicolaou smear as indicated by history and past Paps and pelvic examination yearly; regular mammograms; contraception until 1 year without menses (some say 2 years); signs and symptoms of problems: postmenopausal bleeding; prevention of vaginal infections.

3. Teaching re: urinary health: 6–8 glasses of water a day, decrease caffeine, Kegel exercises; quit smoking.

4. Teaching re: triggers for hot flashes—electric blanket, alcohol, spicy foods, overheating, constrictive clothing; symptom management with evening primrose oil, licorice root, phytoestrogens, sage or sarsaparilla, black cohash (see complimentary therapies).

5. Consider nonhormonal synthetic medication and bioflavonoid alternatives for symptom management; other botanicals, homeopathic medicines (e.g., for sleep disorders: hops, valerian tea or tincture, melatonin, exercise, relaxation techniques; for memory: ginkgo biloba (120–240 mg/day); for irritability: anise, chasteberry, dongquai, flaxseed, ginseng, kava kava (60–120 mg), red raspberry leaf).

6. Diet: low fat, avoid or decrease caffeine, zinc 15 mg/day in foods and/or in supplements; vitamin C and B complex vitamins, fiber; phytoestrogens (soy protein isoflavone 40–160 mg/day; lignans such as flax seed, cereal bran; other isoflavones chick peas, legumes, bluegrass, clover).

VIII. Complications/Risks

  A. Pregnancy

  B. Carcinoma of reproductive tract

  C. Breast cancer (risk is higher after menopausal years)

  D. Incapacitating menopausal symptoms: hot flashes that disrupt normal life, night sweats, sleep disturbances

E. Osteoporosis

F. Possible increased risk for heart attacks, coronary heart disease (see Women and Heart Disease: Risk Factor Assessment in Appendix F)

G. Interactions, adverse effects of herbals, vitamins; negative interactions with prescription medications

IX. Consultation/Referral

A. To physician or other clinician as appropriate for complications listed above

B. Sex therapist for prolonged or severe disruption in sexual relationship

C. Counseling: stresses of the middle years, depression

D. Mammogram, sigmoidoscopy, or colonoscopy per protocol and risk

E. Bone mineral density

F. Consider consultation with homeopath, herbalist, naturopath, Ayurvedic practitioner

X. Follow-up

A. Annual examination, Papanicolaou smear as recommended, pelvic exam

B. Mammograms and bone mineral density testing as recommended

C. As needed if problems continue or become exacerbated

See Bibliography. Web sites: http://www.menopause.org; www.herbalgram.org; http://womenshealth.med.ucla.edu/community/newsletter.

HORMONE THERAPY[2]

I. Definition

Hormone therapy is the use of exogenous natural or synthetic estrogen or estrogen and progestin in combination by the postmenopausal woman (whether natural or surgical menopause has occurred) to alleviate the symptoms of lower amounts of natural estrogen.

II. Etiology

A. The theca intema and granulosa cells of the ovarian follicles and the corpus luteum produce three naturally occurring estrogens: estradiol, estrone, and estriol, in concert with precursors LH and FSH from the anterior pituitary and androstenedione from the adrenals. The corpus luteum and ovarian follicle produce

progesterone. The stromal tissues of the ovaries produce insignif-
icant amounts of androgens; the major sources of androgens in
women are the adrenals. During the perimenopausal years, there
is a gradual decrease of the production of these hormones.

III. History (see also Perimenopause Guideline)

A. What the patient may present with
   1. Irregular menstrual cycles: longer than 35 days, shorter than 21 days
   2. Changes in character of cycles: scanty, brief duration, begin with flooding, clots, dysmenorrhea
   3. Sleep disturbances, night sweats
   4. Experiencing hot flashes and hot flushes
   5. Dyspareunia
   6. Changes in vaginal tissue: dryness, itching, burning of vulva
   7. Urinary urgency or frequency; urethral pain; irritation at meatus
   8. No vaginal bleeding for prior 12 months or more
   9. Surgical menopause: hysterectomy with bilateral oophorectomy and salpingectomy

B. Additional information to be considered
   1. Age of patient and of her biological mother at menopause
   2. Last Papanicolaou smear, breast self-examination, mammo-gram, bone density testing
   3. Medical, surgical, and gynecologic/obstetric history; history of pelvic surgery
   4. Family medical history, especially osteoporosis, heart disease, carcinoma, Alzheimer disease
   5. Signs, symptoms of possible vaginitis, vaginosis, STD, cystitis
   6. Lifestyle: diet, exercise, smoking, alcohol
   7. Change in mood or sense of well-being
   8. All medications including OTC, herbals, homeopathics

IV. Physical Examination

A. Vital signs
B. Complete physical examination
C. Pelvic examination
   1. Vulva and perineum, noting any signs of infection, atrophy, irritation; hair distribution and signs of thinning; loss of adipose tissue
   2. Vagina: color, rugae, signs of atrophy, infection, or irritation, length
   3. Cervix: color, any lesions, ectropion

4. Urethral os: signs of irritation, atrophy, urethrocele
5. Pelvic floor integrity: cystocele, rectocele, uterine prolapse
6. Uterus: size, shape, position, contour, mobility, presence of masses, tenderness
7. Adnexa: masses, tenderness
8. Rectal exam: masses, rectocele, uterine anomalies, occult blood

V. Laboratory

A. Papanicolaou smear with maturation index
B. Mammogram
C. May consider endometrial biopsy with intact uterus
D. Vaginal and/or urine cultures: HIV, STD screen as appropriate
E. Serum FSH or testosterone assay as indicated
F. Lipid profiles, thyroid function test, serum glucose
G. Hematocrit or hemoglobin as indicated
H. Bone density assays if indicated and feasible
I. Pelvic ultrasound if pelvic examination is positive for masses (vaginal probe)
J. May consider baseline EKG
K. Per findings of physical examination and from history

VI. Considering HT[3]

A. Contraindications[4]
   1. Undiagnosed vaginal bleeding
   2. Known or suspected pregnancy
   3. History of nontraumatic pulmonary embolism (PE) or deep vein thrombosis (DVT), or PE or DVT in past 6 months
   4. Known or suspected cancer of the breast or reproductive tract (estrogen-dependent carcinomas); malignant melanoma at any stage
   5. Currently on anticoagulants or tamoxifen
B. Precautions: consider clinical data, risk, and benefits
   1. Active gallbladder disease
   2. Family history of breast cancer
   3. Migraine headaches
   4. Elevated triglycerides, high LDL, low HDL
C. Weighing risks and benefits
   1. Osteoporosis in family or personal history; risk factors for osteoporosis (see osteoporosis handout in Appendix A)
   2. Personal and family medical history including heart and Alzheimer disease, breast cancer, ovarian, endometrial, colon cancer

3. Presence of indicators for benefits in absence of absolute contraindications and weighing of relative risks; emerging data from the Women's Health Initiative
4. Consideration of risks with smoking, hypertension, epilepsy, migraines, benign breast or uterine disease, endometriosis
5. Consideration of benefits to genitourinary tract, feelings of well-being
6. The use of hormone therapy remains a highly individualized decision and controversial issues remain
7. Access to health care for follow-up: endometrial biopsy, mammography, monitoring for side effects, danger signs
8. Alternatives to HT: diet, exercise, calcium from exogenous source in addition to foods, botanicals, vitamins, nonhormonal vaginal lubricants (such as Astroglide®), naturalistic interventions, homeopathic preparations (see peri- and postmenopausal general care guideline and complementary therapies guideline)

VII. Hormone Regimens

A. Absence of uterus: estrogen only or estrogen and androgen
1. Conjugated equine estrogen (Premarin®) 0.3–2.5 mg/day orally daily (or days 1–25).
2. Enjuvia estrogens conjugated 0.3–1.25 mg/day.
3. Modified estrone from plant compounds (Estratab®/Menest®) 0.3–2.5 mg/day orally daily (or days 1–25).
4. Micronized plant estrogen, estradiol (Estrace®) 0.5–2 mg/day (or days 1–25), Gynodiol (estradiol) 1 mg, 1.5 mg, 2 mg/day.
5. Estropipate (synthesized from estrone) (Ogen®, Ortho-Est®) 0.625–2.5 mg/day orally daily (or days 1–25); Cenestin® synthesized conjugated estrogens 0.3–1.25 mg one tab/day.
6. Estro Gel, estradiol topical 0.06% gel, apply 1.5 gm once daily.
7. Estrasorb, estradiol topical 1.74 gm/pkg/emulsion, apply 3.48 gm to skin once daily.
8. Estradiol natural plant compound transdermal patch
   a. Alora® 0.025–0.1 mg/day—apply patch twice/week
   b. Climara® 0.025–0.1 mg day—apply patch once/week
   c. Estraderm® 0.05–0.1 mg/day—apply patch twice/week
   d. FemPatch® 0.025 mg/day—apply patch once/week
   e. Vivelle® 0.025 mg–0.1 mg/day—apply patch twice/week
   f. Vivelle-Dot® 0.025–0.1 mg estradiol/day—apply patch twice/week

   g. Esclim® 0.025–0.1 mg estradiol apply patch twice/week
   h. Menostar ®0.014 mg/day estradiol—apply patch once/ week

9. Estrogen vaginal cream or suppository for dryness, atrophy: Dienestol 0.7 mg (DV) or diethylstilbestrol 0.1 mg or 0.2 mg suppositories 1 or 2 daily; conjugated estrogens (Premarin) 0.625 mg/gram or dienestrol 0.01% (OrthoDienestrol), or dienestrol 0.01% with lactose (DV, Estrogard), or estropipate 1.5 mg/gm (Ogen) cream 1–2 applicators full per day; estradiol cream 0.1 mg/gram (Estrace) 2–4 gm daily for 1–2 weeks, then 1–2 gm daily for 1–2 weeks; maintenance 1 gram 1–3 times a week 3 weeks on, one off.

10. Vagifem® estradiol vaginal tablet 25 mg one tab/day for 2 weeks then maintenance one tab vaginally 2x/week.

11. Estradiol (Estring®) (2 mg) vaginal ring (rapid release for first 24 hours, then continuous low dose of 7.5 mg/24 hours). Replaced every 90 days. May be used by postmenopausal women both with and without a uterus who desire symptomatic relief from local symptoms of urogenital atrophy. Addition of progestin not necessary for woman with a uterus since adverse effects on endometrium unlikely with consistent low daily dose.

12. Estradiol acetate (Femring®) available in 2 dosages, 0.05 mg/day and 0.1 mg/day. Replace every 90 days.

13. Estratab/methyltestosterone (Estratest®) 1.25 mg esterified estrogen/2.5 mg testosterone, or Estratest HS® 1/2 strength 0.625 mg esterified estrogen, 1.25 mg methyl-testosterone

B. Presence of uterus: add progestin

1. Medroxyprogesterone acetate (MPA) synthetic progesterone (Provera®) 2.5–10 orally
   a. 10 mg MPA orally taken in combination with estrogen for last 12 days (days 14–25)
   b. 2.5–5 mg MPA orally taken in combination with estrogen on days 1–5 or daily

2. Norethindrone or norethindrone acetate synthetic progesterone (Micronor®, Aygestin®) 5 mg/day orally taken as in B.1a.,b.

3. Micronized progesterone from plant sources (Prometrium®) 100–200 mg/day orally taken as in B.1a.,b (capsules contain peanut oil; avoid for patients with peanut allergies); Promensil® natural plant estrogens 40 mg/day (1 tablet).

4. Micronized progesterone from plant sources time-release intrauterine device (IUD) Mirena® (levonorgestrel-releasing

intrauterine system) 20 μg/day provides continuous source of progestin for combination therapy.

5. Combination products
   a. Conjugated estrogens 0.62 mg/2.5–5 mg, 0.45 mg/1.5 mg daily orally (Prempro®)
   b. Conjugated estrogens 0.625 mg p.o. alone for 14 days (Premphase®); conjugated estrogens 0.625 mg MPA orally for 14 days
   c. Estradiol/norethindrone acetate transdermal system (CombiPatch®). Two systems available: Continuous combined regimen 0.05 mg estradiol/0.14 or 0.25 mg norethindrone acetate continuously, changed × 2/week; continuous sequential regimen 0.05 mg estradiol patch × 14 days (Vivelle®) (replaced × 2 weekly) then 0.05 mg estradiol/0. 14 mg norethinrone acetate (CombiPatch®) (replaced × 2 weekly) Climara Pro® 0.045/0.015 mg weekly (estradiol/levonorgestrel)
   d. Activella® 1 mg estradiol/0.5 mg norethindrone once daily
   e. Femhrt® norethindrone acetate and ethinyl estradiol 2.5 mcg/0.5 mg and 5 mcg/1 mg
   f. Orthoprefest estradiol 1.0 mg = norgestimate 0.09 mg in alternating 3-day cycles. 3 days of estradiol alone, 3 days of estradiol and norgestimate, repeating pattern continuously

C. Other
   1. Raloxifene hydrochloride (Evista®) synthetic selective estrogen-receptor modulator 60 mg orally daily. Use daily for osteoporosis protection.
   2. Custom compounded hormone therapy, oral, topical, and pellet implant (estrogen, progesterone, and testosterone) may be compounded by many pharmacists and mail order pharmacies specializing in natural hormones such as:
      a. College Pharmacy, Colorado Springs, Colorado 1-800-888 9358
      b. Women's International Pharmacy, Madison, WI 608-221-7800 and Sun City, AZ 623-214-7700, http://www.womensinternational.com
      c. Referral to compounding pharmacists at http://www.iacprx.org (International Academy of Compounding Pharmacists)

D. Withdrawal bleeding
   1. Will occur with sequential use of progestin
   2. No bleeding should occur with continuous use

VIII. Clinical Management
  A. Side effects
    1. Bleeding with hormone use
      a. with sequential use
      b. with continuous use
        1) Consider change in dosage or medication
        2) If not effective, do endometrial biopsy
      c. Unopposed estrogen use (still prescribed by some providers)
        1) Encourage combination therapy; prior to changing therapy, consider using Provera® 10 mg for 10 days. If no bleeding, begin new regimen. If bleeding does occur, do endometrial biopsy or do an ultrasound to measure lining.
    2. Breast tenderness
    3. Fluid retention
    4. Weight gain (increased appetite)
    5. Dysmenorrhea with withdrawal bleed
    6. Depression
    7. Irritability or emotional lability
    8. Possible increase in size of uterine leiomyomata
    9. Allergic response to patch
    10. Virilization with androgens (rare)
  B. Other clinical management strategies
    1. Short-term topical estrogen for vaginal dryness; discontinue after 6 months or when no longer necessary
    2. Alternative nonhormonal vaginal lubricants such as Astroglide® or Replens®
    3. Complementary/alternative modalities to be considered, including many botanicals as well as acupuncture, massage, and relaxation; can increase a woman's feeling of well-being
    4. Careful teaching about modalities utilized
  C. Follow-up and lifestyle on HT
    1. Reinforce need for calcium intake both from food and supplementary sources. Will also need a consistent source of vitamin D + magnesium in appropriate dose for adequate absorption.
    2. Regular program of exercise, strength training.
    3. Reinforce knowledge of risks and benefits.
    4. Preventive health care: annual examination, Papanicolaou smear as indicated, mammography, breast, and vulvar self-examination.
    5. Consider periodic monitoring for bone density, lipid profile.

6. Vaginal lubricants, signs of vaginal infection or cystitis versus dryness, Kegel exercises, sexuality.
7. Careful use of herbals, vitamins, and isoflavones with HT.
See Appendix A and Bibliography.

OSTEOPOROSIS

I. Definition

Osteoporosis, a largely preventable skeletal disease, is characterized by low bone mass and microarchitectual deterioration of bone tissue, leading to enhanced bone fragility and a consequent increase in fracture risk.

II. Etiology

  A. Two main factors are responsible for the fragility of bone:
    1. Reduced bone mass
    2. Impaired repair of microdamage caused by normal wear and tear of bone, with disruption in continuity of the plates in cancellous (trabecular) bone

III. Clinical Types

  A. Primary or idiopathic osteoporosis
    1. Type I bone loss occurs primarily in the trabecular compartment and is closely related to postmenopausal loss of ovarian function
    2. Type II bone loss involves cortical bone and is thought to be an exaggeration of the physiologic aging process
  B. Secondary osteoporosis
    1. Medical conditions
      a. Chronic renal failure
      b. Gastrectomy and intestinal bypass
      c. Malabsorption syndrome
      d. Metastic cancer
      e. Fractures
      f. Alcoholism
      g. Celiac disease
      h. Vitamin B12 deficiency
      i. Vitamin D deficiency
    2. Endocrinopathies
      a. Hyperprolactinemia
      b. Hyperthyroidism
      c. Hyperparathyroidism

    d. Adrenocortical
    e. Diabetes
    f. Turners syndrome
    g. Premature ovarian failure
    h. Hypogonadism over-activity
    i. Hypercalciuria
3. Connective tissue disorder
    a. Osteogenesis imperfecta
    b. Ehlers-Danlos syndrome
    c. Homocystinuria
    d. Rheumatoid arthritis
4. Medications
    a. Anticonvulsants
    b. Antacids (with aluminum)
    c. Thyroid hormone therapy
    d. Glucocorticoids-oral, inhaled
    e. Luteinizing hormone-releasing hormone
    f. Lithium
    g. Long-term Depo Provera use
    h. Aromatase inhibitors
    i. Immunosuppressants
    j. Insulin
    k. Phenothiazines
    l. Butyrophenones
    m. Methotrexate
    n. Heparin
    o. Sodium Fluoride

IV. History

  A. Woman's medical history, including but not limited to: refer to III.B
  B. Medication history
    1. Current prescription medication
    2. Current over-the-counter medication
    3. Current vitamin and botanical use
  C. Ob-gyn history
    1. Age at menarche
    2. Age at menopause
    3. Months (years) of oral or other hormonal contraceptive, Depo-Provera use
    4. Parity
    5. Estrogen use

6. History of menstrual dysfunction
   a. Late menarche
   b. Oligohypomenorrhea
   c. Exercise-induced amenorrhea
   d. Previous hysterectomy with oophorectomy
7. History of extended breastfeeding
D. Nutritional status
   1. Height and weight
   2. Eating habits
   3. Consumption of caffeine and alcoholic beverages
   4. History of an eating disorder
   5. Current and past exercise habits
   6. Smoker
E. Lifestyle
   1. Excessive use of alcohol
   2. Smoking
   3. Caffeine ingestion
   4. Inactivity
F. Family history
   1. Maternal history of osteoporosis or fractures

V. Physical Examination

A. Height (compare to previous measurement), (loss of 1 ½")
B. Weight; body mass index
C. Observe back for dorsal kyphosis and cervical lordosis
D. Assess for physical abnormalities that interfere with mobility
E. Assess for bone pain
F. Assess for change of stature

VI. Laboratory

A. Consider one of the following screening tests
   1. X-ray densitometry (DEXA) gold standard
   2. Bone ultrasound
   3. Genotyping
   4. Bone turnover markers (Urinary N-Tetopeptide) (NTX)
   5. Single Energy X-ray absorptrometry (measures the bones of the wrist or heel)
   6. Quantitative Computed Tomography (measures the bone density of the spine); this test is expensive and exposes the woman to a higher dose of radiation than other screening tests
   7. Consider calcium and albumin (hyperparathyroidism)
   8. Consider 25 hydroxy, vitamin D (vitamin D deficiency)

    9. Consider Thyroid Stimulating Hormone (TSH) (hyperthyroidism)
   10. Consider CBC with sedimentation rate
   11. Consider liver function test
   12. Immunoglobulin A (IgA)
   13. Antitissue Transglutaminase (+TGA)
   14. IgA Antiendomysial Antibodies (AEA)
   15. Serum protein electrophoresis

VII. Treatment

  A. Medication
    1. Estrogen (see Hormone Therapy guideline)
    2. Bisphosphonates regime should include Fosamax®, Actonel®, and Boniva®; an Alendronate regimen should include:
      a. 5 mg/10 mg a day or 35–70 mg once a week with 6–8 ounces of water on arising, at least a half hour before breakfast or 150 mg monthly with 6–8 ounces of water on arising, at least 1 hour before breakfast
      b. Calcium supplements and antacids interfere with absorption of Alendronate; these should be taken at least a half hour later
      c. To prevent GI complications, the woman must remain in an upright position for 1 half hour after taking medication
    3. Calcitonin-Salmon—Fortical
      a. Injection treatment: 100 IU subcutaneously or intramuscularly every other day
      b. Nasal spray treatment: 200 IU intranasally once a day (Miacalcin® or Fortical)
    4. Selective estrogen receptor modulators: Raloxifene (Evista®) 60 mg daily
    5. Calcium, 1200–1500 mg with vitamin D, 400–800 IU daily (20 mg), and a multivitamin with magnesium 600 mg daily
    6. Fortio (parathyroid hormone) 20 mcg subcutaneously daily (may treat up to 2 years)
    7. Phytoestrogens
  B. General measures
    1. Increase exercise
      a. Muscle strengthening exercises concentrating on large muscle groups
      b. Aerobic exercise: walking, walking on a treadmill, climbing a Stairmaster, riding a bicycle, using a cross-country ski-type apparatus

2. Increase dietary intake of calcium, vitamin D, magnesium
3. Decrease dietary intake of caffeine and alcohol, red meat
4. Decrease or stop smoking (see smoking cessation guideline)

VIII. Differential Diagnosis

A. Osteopenia—reduced bone mass due to inadequate osteoid synthesis
B. Arthritis
C. Paget's disease
D. Fracture

IX. Complications

A. Fracture with associated complications
B. Physical deformity

X. Referral/Consultation

A. Lack of response to treatment
B. Fractures
C. Nutritional guidance
D. Exercise program (organizations providing moderate to low cost for physical fitness)
E. Smoking cessation

See Appendix A and Bibliography. Web sites: for menopause, http://www.menopause-online.com, http://www.mayoclinic.com/health/menopause, http://www.fbhc.org/patients/betterhealth/menpause; for hormone therapy, http://www.nih.gov/PHTindex.htm, http://www.nim.nih.gov/medlineplus/hormonereplacementtherapy.html, http://www.mayoclinic.com/health/hormone-therapy/WO00046, http://www.osteo.org, http://www.4woman.gov/faq/oseopor.htm.

NOTES

1. See complementary alternative therapies guidelines.
2. The use of HT continues to be controversial. The decision about the use of HT requires evaluation of the risks and benefits for each individual woman. Clinicians should keep up to date with AGOG guidelines to assist them with decision making.
3. The decision about use of HT requires evaluation of the risks and benefits for each individual woman. For women currently using HT, it is important to assess their reasons for use and to evaluate potential risks, benefits, and alternatives. See ACOG Web site www.acog.org and keep up to date with results from the Women's Health Initiative, the HERS study—heart and estrogen replacement study; the PEPI Trial—Post menopausal estrogen/progestin intervention and the Nurses' Health Study.
4. From the Women's Health Initiative Criteria, NIH.

CHAPTER TWELVE

Smoking Cessation

I. Definition

Smoking is the leading cause of preventable illness and premature death in the United States causing approximately 440,000 deaths annually. An estimated 40 million Americans smoke, and it is estimated that of this number 70 percent want to quit. Quitting involves the process of fighting both the physical and psychological dependence of smoking. It is believed that nicotine is as addictive as cocaine, opiates, amphetamines, and alcohol. Nicotine dependence is classified as a substance use disorder in *DSM-IV*.

II. Etiology

A. The nicotine contained in inhaled cigarette smoke reaches the brain in approximately 10 seconds. Once received in the brain, nicotine causes the brain to release dopamine and norepinephrine. When nicotine is inhaled in a regular fashion, the brain accepts the chemicals by increasing the number of nicotine receptor sites. This mechanism is believed to underlie nicotine dependence. When inhaled nicotine binds to these receptor sites, it causes arousal, stimulation, increased heart rate, and increased blood pressure. These physical reactions cause the smoker to experience mood elevation, reduced anxiety, and stimulation within seconds of inhalation. Signs and symptoms of withdrawal may begin within a few hours of the last cigarette, peak at 48–72 hours and return to baseline 3–4 weeks after quitting.

B. Problems associated with smoking
   1. Pregnancy complications (low birthweight, miscarriage, preterm delivery), increased asthma risk in children, other respiratory problems
   2. Cervical dysplasia
   3. Increased risk for cancer (esophageal, bladder, kidney, pancreatic, leukemia, breast, gynecologic)
   4. Gastric and duodenal ulcers
   5. Premature wrinkling of the skin
   6. Decreased bone density, osteoporosis, fractures
   7. Impotence and fertility problems
   8. Lung disease
   9. Decreased HDL
   10. Peripheral vascular disease
   11. Periodontal and dental diseases; oral cancers
   12. Depression
   13. Early menopause

III. Barriers to Smoking Cessation

A. Physical dependence
   1. Withdrawal symptoms
      a. Depressed mood
      b. Insomnia
      c. Irritability
      d. Difficulty concentrating
      e. Increased appetite—weight gain
      f. Anger
      g. Restlessness
      h. Frustration
      i. Increased heart rate
B. Psychological dependence
   1. Behaviors associated with smoking become integrated into a person's routine
   2. Smoking once integrated into routine becomes associated with pleasure and enjoyment
   3. Smoking may also be used to cope with stress or lessen negative emotions

IV. History

A. Risk assessment
   1. Do you smoke? Ask all patients at annual visit.
   2. How many cigarettes a day? For how long?
   3. How soon after awakening do you smoke your first cigarette?

    4. Do you waken at night to smoke?

    5. Is it difficult for you to observe "no smoking" rules?

    6. Which cigarette would be hardest to give up?

    7. Do you smoke more cigarettes in the first hours of your days than at other times?

    8. Have you ever attempted to stop smoking?

    9. If yes, what got in your way?

B. What the patient may present with

    1. Nagging, chronic cough

    2. Sinus congestion

    3. Shortness of breath

    4. Fatigue

    5. Elevated blood pressure

    6. Inability to meet physical challenges (run for a bus, play with young children)

    7. Decreased fertility

    8. Osteoporosis, decreased bone density

    9. Premature wrinkling

   10. Gum disease

C. Additional questions to be asked

    1. Pregnancy complications

    2. History of abnormal Pap smears

    3. History of, or presently existing, cancer

    4. Fractures

    5. Cataracts/glaucoma

    6. Problems with cold hands or feet or leg pain

    7. Diabetes

    8. Gastric or duodenal ulcer

    9. Current medicines including herbals, homeopathics, vitamins

V. Physical Examination

A. Vital signs

    1. Temperature

    2. Pulse, respirations

    3. Blood pressure

B. Skin

    1. Observe for color, tone, and premature wrinkling

C. ENT

    1. Thorough examination of oral cavity. Observe for dental cavities, stained teeth, tongue or buccal lesions, gum disease, foul breath

D. Lungs

    1. Listen for adventitious sounds (wheezes, rales, crackles)

    E. Breast examination

    F. Abdominal examination

    G. Gynecologic examination (Pap, cultures, bimanual)

    H. Extremities

       1. Observe extremities for signs of circulatory, peripheral vessel involvement, pulses, pedal edema

V. Laboratory Examination

    A. CBC (elevated hematocrit, WBC, platelets, decreased leukocytes)

    B. Lipid level (decreased HDL)

    C. Consider

       1. Vitamin C level (decreased)

       2. Serum uric acid (decreased)

       3. Serum albumin (decreased)

       4. Pulmonary function tests

VI. Differential Diagnosis

    A. Per physical findings

    B. Depression

    C. Anxiety

VII. Treatment

    A. Intervention needs to be multifaceted and tailored to each patient's needs—multiple nicotine medication interventions may be used simultaneously without adverse effect.

    B. Any approach needs to include information regarding the following:

       1. A clear, strong stop smoking message

       2. Risks associated with smoking

       3. Benefits of cessation, advise all users to stop

       4. Addictive components of smoking

       5. What to expect during withdrawal period

       6. Potential risk of relapse

    C. Personalize the risks to each individual. Relate her current health problems or findings on physical examination to the effects of smoking.

    D. Emphasize how smoking cessation can reward the individual.

    E. If the patient indicates a willingness to quit, form a contract for a quit date. This date should be within a short time frame (1–2 weeks). A notation of this date should be made and the clinician should reinforce the contract with a phone call.

F. Factors involved in successful cessation efforts include:
   1. Timely intervention and motivation by clinician
   2. Individual's desire and motivation
   3. Multifaceted program
   4. Individualization of program to patient's situation
G. Methods (may be used individually or in conjunction with each other)
   1. Behavioral
      a. Draft a list of reasons to quit smoking and the rewards of quitting. This list should be kept with the person and reviewed when the urge to smoke "hits" and he or she is in need of reinforcement.
      b. Inform family and friends and ask for their support and encouragement.
      c. Smoker should keep a journal. In precessation stage the smoker can use the journal to record each cigarette smoked, the social cues experienced, the setting, the intensity of the craving, and the time of day. This can help identify the individual's triggers and assist smoker to adapt strategies and coping skills to get past the triggers. Keeping a journal during cessation is helpful for expressing feelings and recording the steps of the journey.
      d. Patient should avoid alcohol, which weakens resolve.
      e. Patient should throw out all cigarettes, ashtrays, etc.
      f. Patient should avoid being around smokers.
      g. If possible, patient should establish a "no smoking" living space.
      h. Patient should increase exercise level (walking, weight lifting, yoga). Exercise assists in weight management, stress reduction, and sense of well-being.
      i. Consider use of meditation or relaxation tapes.
   2. Nicotine replacement. The theory behind nicotine replacement is that by replacing the nicotine, the smoker can deal with the emotional factors and utilize behavioral changes without having to deal with the full impact of physical withdrawal at the same time.
      a. Gum—offers episodic satisfaction for nicotine craving as it arises
         1) Nicotine Polacrilex (Nicorette™) 2 mg per piece (maximum 30 pieces per day)
         2) Nicotine Polacrilex (Nicorette D.S.™) 4 mg per piece—maximum 20 pieces per day
         3) Adverse effects:

    a) Mouth sores
    b) Dyspepsia
    c) Hiccup
    d) Jaw ache
    e) 10% of those who use gum may become
       dependent requiring long-term use (1–2 years)
       to remain abstinent
  b. Transdermal patches. If a patient chooses to use the
     patch, there should be a contract not to smoke during
     its use.
     1) Nicotine transdermal therapeutic system (Habitrol™)
        21 mg/day (24 hours) for 4–6 weeks, then 14 mg/day
        for 2–4 weeks, then 7 mg/day for 2–4 weeks
     2) Nicotine transdermal system (Nicoderm CQ™) 21
        mg/day (24 hours) for 4–6 weeks, then 14 mg/day for
        2–4 weeks, then 7 mg/day for 4–6 weeks
     3) Nicotine transdermal system (Nicotrol™) 15 mg/day
        (16 hours) for 4–6 weeks
     4) Nicotine transdermal system (ProStep™) 22 mg/day
        (24 hours) for 4–8 weeks, then 11 mg/day for 2–4
        weeks
     5) Adverse effects:
        a) Skin reactions
        b) Insomnia
        c) Vivid dreams
        d) Myalgia
     6) If vivid dreams and/or insomnia are a problem, the
        patient may remove the patch prior to retiring and
        apply new patch on arising. NOTE: If waking during
        the night is a problem, the 24-hour patches may
        provide more relief.
  c. Nasal spray—has the advantage of being an accelerated
     delivery system, delivering nicotine on demand (within
     10 seconds) as a cigarette does
     1) Nicotine nasal spray (Nicotrol NS™) 1 spray (0. 5
        mg) in each nostril (8–40 mg/day) to a maximum of
        5 times per hour or 40 times per 24 hours. Max: 3
        months treatment
     2) Adverse effects:
        a) Higher incidence of dependence
        b) Nasal irritation
        c) Throat irritation
        d) Rhinitis

e) Sneezing

f) Watering eyes

g) Coughing

d. Nicotrol inhaler 10 mg/cartridge (4 mg delivered) 6–16 cartridges/day for up to 12 weeks, reduce gradually over 12 more weeks then discontinue. Max: 6 months treatment

e. Oral medication

1) Bupropion Hydrochloride (Zyban™ or Wellbutrin™ SR) 150 mg every day for 2 days then 150 mg twice a day for 7–12 weeks. Initiate medication 1 week prior to start date. This week allows the patient to initiate behavioral interventions and prepare psychologically for quitting. Bupropion Hydrochloride is an antidepressant that acts as an inhibitor of the neuronal uptake of norepinephrine, serotonin, and dopamine. The mechanism of action in smoking cessation is unknown, but it may serve to mimic the neurochemical effects of nicotine that serve as the pathway to addiction.

a) Contraindications

i) History of seizure disorder

ii) Prior diagnosis of eating disorder

iii) Concurrent use of monoamine oxidase inhibitor

b) Possible adverse reactions:

i) Rash

ii) Nausea

iii) Agitation

iv) Migraine

NOTE: If a prescription is written for Zyban Advantage Plan™ the patient receives material providing a toll-free 800 number. A phone call will enroll the patient in an individualized program providing behavioral modification and patient support materials as well as information on smoking cessation and 3 months of personal support at no additional cost.

2) Chantix (varencline) acts on receptor sites by activating them and blocking nicotine from attaching to them. Dosage days—3 white tablets (0.5 mg) 1 orally every day for days 4–7; one white tablet (0.5 mg) orally twice a day (morning and evening) days 8 to end of treatment; blue tablet 1 mg orally twice a day (morning and evening)

a) Important facts
   i) Patients with kidney problem or dialysis may need lower dose (see package insert)
   ii) Should be taken after meals with full glass of water
   iii) If a dose is missed, it should be taken as soon as remembered. If it is close to time of next dose, skip missed dose, take regular dose on time.
   iv) Patients taking other medications such as blood thinner, insulin and asthma medication may need to have dosages altered after cessation of smoking.
b) How to start
   i) Choose quit date
   ii) Begin taking Chantix 7 days before quit date. This allows Chantix to build up in the body. Patients can continue to smoke during this time.
   iii) Most patients will take Chantix for up to 12 weeks. If medication has been successful another 12 weeks may be prescribed to help patient remain cigarette free.
c) Patients may join Get Quit by calling (877) 242-6849.
3) Nortriptyline (Pamelor™) (tricyclic antidepressant) 25 mg daily x 4 days, 50 mg daily x 4 days then 75 mg daily x 12 wks. For best results start medication 14 days prior to quit date
4) Citrol™ (dietary citric acid supplement). Spray 2–4 times directly on back of throat to reduce desire to smoke for approximately 1 hr. Use as needed.
   f. Hypnosis
   g. Plastic "cigarettes"

VII. Complications

A. Relapse—most people who return to smoking do so within a month of quitting. The longer persons have abstained, the more likely they are to continue to do so.
   1. Patient may be doing well when a situation or stressor makes smoking too enticing to resist
   2. Patient may experience side effects from product used and lose resolve

VIII. Consultation

    A. Question regarding possible medical contraindication to use of nicotine replacement or Bupropion Hydrochloride

    B. Referral to intensive group sessions such as those offered by Nicotine Anonymous, American Cancer Society, American Lung Association, or a local hospital

IX. Follow-up

    A. Telephone call to patient within 1–2 weeks of quit date

    B. Office follow-up at 1 and 3 months

    C. If relapse occurs

        1. Discuss and review problems and stressors that contributed to relapse

        2. Review and reinforce strategies that smoker can utilize to meet future challenges

        3. Renew smoker's commitment to total abstinence

        4. Review why patient wishes to quit; contract with patient to set another quit date

        5. Reassure patient that success is often achieved only after 5 to 6 repeated attempts; success may take several years

See Appendix A for a patient information sheet for photocopying or adapting. See Bibliography. Web sites: http://www.smoking-cessation.org; http://www.surgeongeneral.go/tobacco; http://www.cdc.gov/tobacco/how2quit.htm

CHAPTER THIRTEEN

Loss of Integrity of Pelvic Floor Structures

I. Definition

Loss of tone of pelvic floor soft tissues can be attributed to a wide variety of causes including childbirth, increased BMI, exercise, chronic constipation, and/or the general effects of aging, and may result in cystocele, rectocele, urethrocele, incontinence, and/or uterine prolapse. It can also result from sexual assault or abuse including incest.

Urinary incontinence is one of the most common results, categorized as stress or urge incontinence, as well as leaking of urine.

II. Etiology

A. Childbirth trauma resulting in nerve or muscle damage: precipitous delivery, especially of a very large baby, grand multigravida, inadequate repair of episiotomy or of lacerations
B. Aging: loss of muscle tone, relaxation of muscles, ligaments; atrophic vaginitis
C. Trauma due to sexual assault, incest, abuse
D. Secondary to surgery, infection especially STDs with scarring
E. Medication side effects; bladder irritants—smoking, caffeine, artificial sweeteners, alcohol
F. Obesity; increase in BMI
G. Diseases: multiple sclerosis, diabetic neuropathy, chronic cough, dementia, stroke, impaired mobility, Parkinson's, tumor, congestive heart failure
H. Behavioral: excessive caffeine and alcohol intake, psychological conditions, poor bowel/toilet habits

III. History

    A. What the patient may present with
1. Stress incontinence; urge incontinence; mixed incontinence; leaking of urine
2. Feeling of pressure in pelvic area—heaviness, fullness
3. Pain on defecation, fecal incontinence
4. Inability to empty bladder completely; frequency, urgency; overactive bladder characterized by sudden urge to urinate with/without urine loss, frequency, nocturia
5. Dyspareunia
6. Lower abdominal, groin, or lower back pulling or aching
7. Bulging of organs against vaginal wall, prolapse through vagina

    B. Additional information to be considered
1. Menstrual and reproductive history; pregnancies, route of delivery, any laceration, episiotomy, pelvic surgery or repair, reproductive tract cancers
2. Symptoms: type, onset, frequency, severity, conditions under which they occur, relief measures and results; precipitating factors
3. Contraceptive history: methods used, present method
4. History of sexual assault, abuse, incest
5. STDs, especially with tissue destruction and scarring
6. History of ritual circumcision, genital cutting
7. Caffeine intake, diet, alcohol, smoking
8. Medications use and timing: OTC and herbals, vitamins, homeopathics
9. Weight gain

IV. Physical Examination

    A. Abdominal examination
1. Masses, fullness
2. Tenderness—suprapubic

    B. External examination
1. Urethra
2. Perineum
3. Vulva
    a. Cystocele; cystourethrocele
    b. Rectocele, enterocele
    c. Urethrocele
    d. Prolapsed uterus
    e. Ritual circumcision, genital cutting

     f. Atrophy

     g. Skin excoriation

     h. Evidence of urine leakage

C. Vaginal examination

  1. Speculum

     a. Condition of vagina: lax, good tone, any lesions, rugae

     b. Presence of cervix

     c. Integrity of vaginal walls

     d. Visible cystocele, urethrocele, and/or rectocele; uterine prolapse

  2. Digital

     a. Palpate cystocele, urethrocele

     b. Palpate rectocele both vaginally and rectally

D. Biannual examination

  1. Uterus

     a. Position

     b. Tenderness

     c. Masses

  2. Adnexa

     a. Masses

     b. Tenderness

  3. Palpable cystocele, urethrocele, scars; palpate bladder and urethra for tenderness

  4. Assess strength and duration of levator muscle contraction—with fingers in vagina ask patient to try to squeeze as if stopping urine stream

  5. Rectal exam: rectocele; occult blood; masses, anal tone, have patient squeeze

E. Standing evaluation: cough stress test to confirm urine loss from urethra

F. Use perineometer to measure strength of pelvic floor contractions

G. Sterile cotton swab (Q-tip) test—lubricate with lidocaine gel and place through urethra into bladder (using sterile technique) and withdraw until meeting resistance; ask woman to bear down and observe angle of Q-tip > 30 degrees urethral hypermobility; < 30 degrees with history of stress incontinence, sphincter deficiency

V. Laboratory Examination

A. Urinalysis with culture for stress or urge incontinence, to rule out infection

B. Postvoid residual volume test: catheterization or pelvic ultrasound

VI. Differential Diagnosis

   A. Urinary tract infection
   B. Genital tract mass/carcinoma
   C. Undiagnosed underlying disease (see II. G)

VII. Treatment

   A. Medication
      1. Prescription for urinary tract infection if indicated (see urinary tract infection guideline in Appendix A)
      2. Consider hormone therapy—oral, patch, vaginal ring, or topical
      3. Treat any vaginitis, vaginosis, STD
      4. Nonhormonal vaginal moisturizers such as Replens®
      5. Detrol® (Tolterodine tartrate) 2 mg twice a day or Detrol® LA 4 mg/day can reduce to 2 mg/day for overactive bladder, urinary frequency, urgency, or urge incontinence
      6. Ditropan® XL (oxybutynin chloride) 5 mg/day; or Ditropan® 5 mg twice or 3 times a day; Oxytrol™ (oxybutynin transdermal system) 3.9 mg/day applied twice a week
   B. General measures
      1. Teach Kegel (pelvic floor muscle training) exercises for stress incontinence (if there is no prolapse, cystocele, or urethrocele). (A commercial product of graduated weighted cones is available to assist in Kegel exercises; a cone is inserted in the vagina and Kegels are performed using the cone's feedback; when weight of cone can be maintained 15 minutes when walking or standing, move to next cone.) Biofeedback devices are available, or electrical stimulation for passive exercise; intravaginal device (sphere) Colpexin™ to strengthen pelvic organ support.
      2. Keep diary of occurrence of incontinence (see Appendix A for teaching materials and diaries; bladder retraining techniques).
      3. Suggestions for hygiene measures.
      4. Eliminate bladder irritants including milk products, sugar, chocolate, many cough medications, caffeine, nicotine, alcohol, artificial sweeteners, spicy and acidic foods.
      5. Improve hydration.
      6. Relaxation training.
      7. Pessary for uterine prolapse (continence ring, Mar-Land, Eva Care®, Milex® pessaries).

8. Stress incontinence devices: bladder neck support prosthesis (Introl®), the Reliance urethral insert, the Softpatch®, FemAssist®, Impress® soft patch, FemSoft® insert, Viva® plug.

VIII. Consultation/Referral

A. To physician or incontinence specialty practice for:
1. Possible surgical repair, hysterectomy
2. Possible reconstruction secondary to prior surgery, scarring
3. Videodynamic evaluation with anterior wall relaxation

See Appendix A, which can be photocopied or adapted for your patients. See Bibliography. Web sites: http://kidney.niddk.nih.gov/kudiseases/pubs/uiwomen/index.htm; http://kidney.niddk.nih.gov/kudiseases/pubs/bladdercontrol/index.htm.

CHAPTER FOURTEEN

Genitourinary Tract

URINARY TRACT INFECTION

I. Definition

An infection of the urethra, bladder (cystitis), ureters, or kidneys.

II. Etiology

  A. Specific causes
    1. Bacteria
      a. Escherichia coli (E. coli) 75–90% of all acute uncomplicated infections
      b. Staphylococcus saprophyticus, second most commonly isolated organism; formerly thought to be a contaminant; now thought to be of causative significance, especially in women aged 16–25
      c. Others in descending order of implication: Staphylococcus saprophyticus, Klebsiella, Proteus mirabilis, Enterobacteriaceae, Citrobacter, Enterococcus, and other including Serratia, Providencia, Pseudomonas, Group B Streptococcus, Staphylococcus aureus, Staphylococcus epidermidis, Mycoplasma, and Chlamydia
    2. Fungi: especially in diabetes and patients with catheters; immunocompromised persons
    3. Viruses that cause viruria: measles, mumps, herpes simplex, cytomegalo-virus, adenovirus varicella zoster leading to hemorrhage in bladder, and cystitis
  B. Mechanism: most commonly ascending infection

    1. In females: gastrointestinal flora (E. coli)

    2. In males: prostate plays a role in harboring infection, constricting urethra causing urine retention

C. Other predisposing factors

    1. Size of inoculum

    2. Virulence of organism

    3. Incomplete or infrequent bladder emptying

    4. Urinary tract abnormalities: obstruction, calculi, congenital defects, prostatic hypertrophy

    5. Use of catheters

    6. Newly sexually active (honeymoon cystitis)

    7. Chemical contamination secondary to spermicidal, barrier methods of contraception

    8. Possibly being postmenopausal with estrogen deficiency

    9. Family history of UTIs

III. History

A. What the patient may present with

    1. Dysuria

    2. Frequency, urgency

    3. Suprapubic pain, ache, pressure, scorched feeling after urination

    4. Back pain; ache or pressure in genitals

    5. No systemic symptoms except occasionally a low grade fever, < 101 degrees F.

    6. Gross hematuria

    7. Vague abdominal discomfort

B. Additional information to consider

    1. Any previous cystitis or pyelonephritis: when, how treated, response to treatment

    2. Previous urologic work-up

    3. Any vaginal discharge, character, onset

    4. Any chronic condition, diabetes, paraplegia, quadriplegia, cerebral palsy, meningomyelocele, spina bifida

    5. Duration of symptoms

    6. Possible pregnancy with high-risk complications or use of contraindicated drugs

    7. Sexual activity, especially 24–48 hours post vaginal intercourse

    8. Method of contraception

IV. Physical Examination

A. Vital signs: temperature

B. Abdomen: any tenderness, masses

C. Back: any costovertebral angle (CVA) tenderness or pain
D. Pelvic examination essential to rule out pelvic inflammatory disease, vaginitis, vaginosis, or sexually transmitted disease

V. Laboratory Examination

A. U/A: clean catch midstream urine; pyuria = > 5 WBC/high power field
B. Culture alone is sufficient on first time ever with urinary tract infection with no risk factor; all others should have culture and sensitivities
    1. Culture and sensitivities typically > 100,000 organisms felt to be diagnostic
    2. If between 10,000 and 100,000, probably significant if clinical symptoms support diagnosis
C. Note: Urine may be stored at room temperature for 1 hour or refrigerated up to 72 hours
D. Acute uncomplicated cystitis (nonpregnant woman) dipstick if + for nitrates and + for leukocyte esterase, or microscopic examination of urine shows increased WBCs (10 in high powered field) consider treating presumptively

VI. Differential Diagnosis

A. Upper tract disease: pyelonephritis
B. Urethritis due to
    1. Chlamydia
    2. Bacteria from urethral manipulation causing irritation; thought to be early cystitis
C. Vaginitis
D. Pelvic inflammatory disease
E. Sexually transmitted disease
F. Interstitial cystitis
G. No recognized pathology, honeymoon cystitis
H. Pregnancy
I. Hormonal urethral changes
J. Urologic cancer

VII. Treatment

A. Antibiotics
    1. For first episode of urinary tract infection in women without risk factors: institute treatment with any of the following, provided the woman is not allergic to the drug
        a. Nitrofurantoin (Macrodantin®) 50 mg 4 times a day x 7 days and, depending on repeat culture results, possibly

25 mg 4 times a day x 7 more days or Macrobid® 100 mg twice a day x 7 days

b. Trimethoprim (160 mg) sulfamethoxazole (800 mg) (Septra DS), Bactrim DS twice a day x 10–14 days or Septra or Bactrim (80 mg trimethoprim and 400 mg sulfamethoxazole) 2 tabs twice a day x 10–14 days

c. For uncomplicated first or second episodes, Trimethoprim (160 mg) and sulfamethoxazole (800 mg) 2 (Septra DS®) or Bactrim DS® STAT or twice a day for 3 days or Trimethoprim 100 mg twice a day x 3 days

d. Cipro® (ciprofloxacin HCL) 100–250 mg twice a day x 3 days OR Ciprofloxacin estended release 500 mg once a day x 3 days OR Floxin® (ofloxacin) 200 mg twice a day x 3 days OR Gatifloxacin 400 mg once a day for 3 days or a single 400 mg dose OR Augmentum® (amoxicillin 400 mg/clavulantic acid 125 mg) one twice a day x 3 days OR Noroxin® (norfloxacin) 400 mg twice a day x 3 days OR Maxaquin® (lomefloxacin) 400 mg once a day x 3 days (these drugs should be reserved for complicated UTIs and in areas where local resistance rates to trimethoprim-sulfamethoxazole are high)

e. Monurol® (fosfomycin) 3 grams in a single dose mixed in 3–4 ounces of cold water (not recommended under age 18)

2. For reinfection or urinary tract infection in women without risk factors, same as for the first episode. Important to distinguish reinfection from relapse. Reinfection occurs within weeks to months of preceding episode, and is often caused by a new organism. Relapse is a recurrence of symptoms and infection after finishing a medication course, and is caused by the same organism as the original infection.

3. For relapse in women
   a. Consider retreatment with same medication, with a test of cure 24–48 hours after completion of medication.
   b. Consider change of medication with test of cure 24–48 hours after completion of medication.
   c. For second relapse, consult with physician.

4. For patients with risk factors (past history of pyelonephritis, known urinary tract abnormality, use of catheter, diabetes), consider referral to physician

B. For pregnant women
   1. The causative pathogen in pregnant women is usually E. coli. Do culture before treatment; sensitivity only if no improvement from medication

    a. First choice: Ampicillin 250 mg one 4 times a day for 10 days (caution of increasing resistance of antibacterial resistance among urinary E. Coli)

    b. Second choice: Nitrofurantoin (Macrodantin®) or Macrobid® (pregnancy category B); note caution of use near time of labor and delivery

    c. In areas with high resistance of E. Coli consider Fosfomycin (pregnancy category B)

    d. Do not use Sulfa, Septra®, or Bactrim® (Trimethoprim), or Ciprofloxacin (category C) in pregnancy

C. Pain relief: Phenazopyridine hydrochloride (Pyridium®, Azo-Standard, Baridium, Di-Azo, Phenazo, Urodine) 200 mg 3 times a day x 24 hours; Uristat (phenazopyridine HCL 95 mg) 2 tabs 3 times a day for no more than 2 days (available OTC) (not recommended in pregnancy)

D. General measures
1. Advise voiding before and after sex
2. Advise adequate lubrication for sex
3. Teaching re: hygiene, contamination
4. Treat as above (A.) if bacteria present
5. Consider treatment with Pyridium® Azo®Standard (Phenazopyridine hydrochloride), Uristat® or other such product only if patient symptomatic in absence of pathogenic organism
6. Cranberry juice; 6–8 glasses of water a day; cranberry juice capsules Azo-cranberry 450 mg cranberry juice concentrate 1–4 capsules per day with meals; CranXact® urinary formula (tannins in cranberries prevent E. Coli from attaching to urinary tract)
7. Decrease bladder irritants such as caffeine, smoking, artificial sweeteners
8. Cotton underwear, avoid tight-fitting garments
9. Consider topical or vaginal estrogen in postmenopausal woman with recurrent cystitis as adjunct

VIII. Complications

A. Pyelonephritis

IX. Consultation/Referral

A. Consider physician consult on
1. Women with relapsed infections
2. Women who are symptomatic after 3 days of treatment
3. Women who have more than 3 episodes in a year

4. Complicated UTIs
5. Pregnant women especially close to term

X. Follow-up

A. Follow-up culture if symptoms do not resolve after treatment.
B. Consider test of cure up to 1 week after completion of medication.

Appendix A, on cystitis, may be photocopied or adapted for your patients.

See Bibliography.

INTERSTITIAL CYSTITIS

I. Definition

Interstitial cystitis (IC) is a chronic, inflammatory, noninfectious disorder of the bladder with no associated histologic changes affecting both men and women. IC is more common in women than men. Of the 1 million Americans with IC, up to 90 percent are women.

II. Etiology

A. The exact pathogenesis and etiology of IC remain unclear; they are thought to be multifactorial:
1. Abnormal bladder epithelial permeability
2. Neurogenic abnormalities
3. Autoimmune disorders
4. Allergic reactions
5. Infectious etiologies
6. May present as part of a more visceral pain syndrome
B. Genetics

Researchers have found a higher than expected prevalence of IC among first degree relatives of index IC cases.

III. History

A. What a patient may present with:
1. Urinary urgency, A.M. and P.M.
2. Urinary frequency, A.M. and P.M.
3. Dyspareunia
4. Pressure, pain (can be worse during menstruation) and tenderness around bladder, pelvis, and perineum
B. Additional information to consider

1. Treatment of UTI—no response to antibiotics
2. Pain worse with menses
3. Pain influenced by diet
4. Feeling of depression or anxiety
5. Decreased quality of life

IV. Physical Examination

  A. Thorough medical history
  B. Pelvic exam essential to rule out PID, vaginitis, vaginosis, or STD
  C. Abdominal exam, tenderness, mass
  D. Vital signs

V. Laboratory Examination

  A. Urinalysis and culture
  B. Urine cytology
  C. Vaginal and cervical cultures
  D. Bladder diagnosis:
     1. PST—Potassium Sensitivity Test—Test may be done in office as a minimally invasive procedure that involves the instillation of a potassium chloride (KCL) solution into the bladder to determine the degree of the patient's pain or urgency response.
  E. Cystoscopy with biopsy
  F. Patient assessment questionnaire

VI. Differential Diagnosis

  A. Endometriosis
  B. Irritable bowel syndrome
  C. UTI
  D. Vulvodynia
  E. Nonbacterial prostatitis (males)
  F. Fibromyalgia
  G. Co-existing depression and anxiety
  H. Bladder cancer
   I. Kidney Disorders
  J. STDs
  K. Neurological or rheumatologic disorders

VII. Treatment

  A. Bladder distention—researchers are not sure why distention helps, but some believe that it may increase capacity and interfere with pain signals transmitted by nerves in the bladder.

B. Bladder instillation (bladder wash or bath)—the bladder is filled with a solution that is held on average of 10–15 minutes before being emptied.
   1. Dimethylsulfoxide (DMSO, RIMSO-50) treatments are given every week or two for 6–8 weeks and repeated as needed. Most people who respond to DMSO notice improvement 3–4 weeks after the first 6–8 week cycle of treatment.
C. Oral Drugs
   1. Elmiron 100 mg 3 times a day
   2. Analgesic medications
   3. Tricyclic antidepressants
   4. Antihistamines
   5. Antispasmodics
   6. Antichotinergics
D. Transcutaneous Electrical Nerve Simulation (TENS).
E. Diet: There is no scientific evidence linking diet to IC/PBS, but many health care providers and patients find that the following may contribute to bladder irritation and inflammation:
   1. Alcohol
   2. Tomatoes
   3. Spices
   4. Chocolate
   5. Caffeinated beverages
   6. Citrus beverages and fruits
   7. Highly acidic foods
   8. Artificial sweeteners
F. Eliminate smoking: Many patients feel that smoking makes their symptoms worse.
G. Exercise: Gentle stretching exercises may help relieve IC/PBS symptoms.
H. Bladder Training: Methods vary but basically patients void at designated times and use relaxation techniques and distractions to keep to the schedule.
I. Physical therapy and biofeedback.

VII. Complications

A. Missed diagnosis
B. Depression—rare cases—suicidal ideation

VIII. Consultation

A. Consult with physician regarding appropriate testing
B. Refer to physician for appropriate testing
C. Refer to urologist or IC specialist

IX. Follow-up

    A. 1–2 weeks after initial work-up and evaluation

    B. 4–6 weeks after starting any treatment

    C. Initially as needed to adjust treatment measures and symptoms—this may take months

    D. Regular follow up visits to monitor symptoms and progress

Web sites: http://www.ichelp/.org; http://www.ic-network.com; http://www.mayoclinic.com/health/interstitialcystitis/DS00497.

CHAPTER FIFTEEN

Preconception Care

I. Definition

Advanced planning aimed at reducing maternal and perinatal mortality and morbidity.

II. Etiology

    A. Reasons for promoting preconception care (PCC) include:
        1. Maximize healthy life for woman and baby
        2. Identify any medical condition or medications in either prospective parent
        3. Identify genetic disorders
        4. Review past gestational and pregnancy history
        5. Identify high risk exposures, e.g., tobacco, drug, and alcohol use; environmental hazards (toxins, chemicals including pesticides, gases, foods)

III. History

    A. Woman's medical and surgical history including but not limited to:
        1. Diabetes
        2. Phenylketonuria
        3. Cardiovascular including high B/P
        4. Lung
        5. Thyroid
        6. Kidney
        7. Infectious diseases (e.g., HIV, hepatitis B and C, toxoplasmosis, rubella, varicella, TB, STDs, vaginosis, vaginitis)
        8. Autoimmune diseases

   9. Connective tissue disorders
   10. Eating disorders
   11. Metabolic conditions
   12. Psychiatric illness; mental health issues
   13. Epilepsy
   14. Thromboembolic episodes
   15. Any surgery?
   16. DES exposure
   17. Allergies
B. Obstetrical and gynecological history
   1. Contraception
   2. Menstrual history
   3. Gynecological history
   4. Pap smear history
   5. High-risk behaviors (including STDs)
   6. Pregnancy history including SAB, TAB
C. Immune status: need to have documentation
   1. Rubella
   2. TB
   3. Hepatitis A, B, C
   4. Varicella
   5. Tetanus if ≥ 10 years
   6. Polio
   7. Influenza
D. Drug history
   1. Current prescription medications: some medications have different safety periods between cessation and conception
   2. Current over-the-counter medications
   3. Current vitamin and botanical use
   4. "Street" drug use history
E. Nutritional status
   1. Height and weight, body mass index
   2. Eating habits; note especially fad diets, vegan
   3. Food allergies
   4. Caffeine and artificial sweetener intake
   5. History of being over- or underweight: underweight BMI < 19.8; overweight BMI > 26.1–29.0; obese BMI > 29.0
   6. History of an eating disorder
   7. Current exercise habits and other physical activities
F. Genetic history
   1. May use a Genogram, identify couples with a personal or family history of problematic diseases such as:
      a. Tay-Sachs
      b. Thalassemia

        c. Sickle-cell disease or trait
        d. Phenylketonuria
        e. Cystic fibrosis
        f. Hemophilia
        g. Mental retardation
        h. Myotonic dystrophy
        i. Adult polycystic kidney disease
        j. Birth defects
        k. Other anemias
      2. Family background
        a. Related outside marriage
        b. Ethnic background: African American, Mediterranean, Ashkenazi Jew, Asian
  G. Exposure to teratogenic toxins: Areas of concern include:
      1. Exposure to:
        a. Metals (lead)
        b. Organic solvents
        c. Gases
        d. Ionizing radiation
        e. Pollutants (e.g., second hand smoke)
        f. Pesticides, herbicides
        g. Lead paint
        h. Plastics, vinyl monomers
        i. Hyperthermia
      2. Consumption of:
        a. Alcohol
        b. Cigarette smoke
        c. Street drugs
  H. Social history
      1. Age
      2. Marital, partner status
      3. Family structure; household composition
      4. Support systems
      5. Employment/financial status
      6. Cultural beliefs
      7. Child care issues
      8. Safety issues (e.g., spousal/partner abuse)
      9. Work history: exposure to chemicals, radiation, standing at work, occupational risks, such as wearing respirator, mask, special clothing
  I. Partner health history
      1. Thorough health/genetic/social history should be taken on prospective fathers. Little conclusive research has been done on how partner's exposures to chemicals/toxins/drugs may

affect fetal development. Recent studies have indicated that alcohol consumption in the month prior to conception contributes to low spermatogenesis.
2. Findings need to be integrated with maternal health history findings.

IV. Physical Examination

A. Baseline height, weight, BMI, vital signs
B. General physical, including pelvic
C. Comprehensive exam based on medical history

V. Laboratory

A. Papanicolaou smear
B. Baseline studies may be considered, including:
   1. Blood Rh, type
   2. Hemoglobin/hematocrit
   3. Urinalysis
   4. RPR/VDRL
   5. Check status for
      a. Hepatitis B, C
      b. Varicella
      c. Rubella
      d. HIV
      e. TB
   6. Based on history, check:
      a. Toxoplasmosis
      b. CMV
   7. GC, Chlamydia, wet mount, mycoplasma, and ureaplasma

VI. Education

A. Begin at least 1 month prior to planned conception
   1. Avoid environmental toxins.
   2. Cease smoking and alcohol consumption, use of street drugs.
   3. Begin exercise program (e.g., walking, swimming, cycling) heart rate not to exceed 140 beats per second.
   4. Bring immunizations up to date (if live vaccine used, postpone conception at least 3 months).
   5. Eat a balanced diet.
   6. Start vitamin therapy.
      a. 0.4 mg orally of folic acid daily (increase dosage for women who are at increased risk for neural tube defects to 0.8 mg daily; some sources say 5 mg/day)

      b. Increase calcium intake to an equivalent of 1 quart of milk daily (or 1200–1500 mg/day)
7. Avoid or at least decrease caffeine intake.
8. Consult with primary care provider regarding prescription medications (e.g., psychotropics, antihypertensives, anticonvulsants); botanicals, vitamins.
9. If hemoglobin < 12 g/dl add iron to prenatal vitamins.
10. Women with PKU should start a low phenylalanine diet.
11. Avoid hot tubs, saunas (bringing body temperature above 101 degrees F can damage the embryo).
12. Don't empty cat litter box.
13. Don't consume raw meat or raw fish.

VII. Referral/Consultation

A. For genetic consultation if indicated
B. Evaluation of prescriptive medication use with specialists
C. Substance abuse counseling if indicated
D. Nutritional counseling if indicated (e.g., obesity, gestational diabetes with prior pregnancies, vegetarian)
E. Community/federal programs for financial assistance if indicated
F. Domestic violence intervention

VIII. Follow-up

A. Refer for obstetrical care if pregnancy occurs (if setting does not provide care).
B. If conception does not occur within 1 year, return for further evaluation/possible referral. Consider sooner if over age 30.

Appendix A may be photocopied or adapted for your patients. See Bibliography. Web site: http://www.cdc.gov/mmwr/preview/mmwrhtml/rr5506a1.htm.

CHAPTER SIXTEEN

Polycystic Ovary Syndrome (PCOS)

I. Definition

PCOS, known in the past as Stein-Leventhal Syndrome, is an endocrinological condition with complex pathophysiology and a wide variety of clinical presentations. It is one of the most common reproductive tract problems in women under 30 years of age. Typical clinical and biochemical manifestations are anovulatory cycles, infertility, and hyperandrogenicity, but many women do not exhibit these characteristic signs. Some women with PCOS have ovaries with a thickened capsule and multiple follicular cysts (polycystic ovaries—PCO). Women with PCO do not necessarily have PCOS, and those with PCOS do not always have PCO.

II. Etiology (unknown but posited)

A. Genetic factors
B. Possible autosomal transmission of responsible genetic sequences
C. A gene or gene series may render the ovary susceptible to insulin stimulation of androgen secretion and block follicular maturation

III. History

A. What the patient may present with (only 20–30% symptomatic)
   1. Anovulatory cycles
   2. History or presence of infertility
   3. Oligoamenorrhoea

   4. Amenorrhea
   5. Prolonged erratic menstrual bleeding
   6. Signs of hyperandrogenism, including hirsutism, acne, and alopecia (especially crown pattern baldness)
   7. Galactorrhea
   8. Increased waist to hip ratio: > 0.85
   9. Hyperpigmentation: nape of neck, axillae, inguinal areas (acanthosis nigricans)
   B. Additional information to be considered
   1. Menstrual cycle history, patterns (onset, length, duration, amount of bleeding)
   2. Pregnancy history
   3. Contraceptive history
   4. History of weight gain, hirsutism
   5. Voice changes, frontal balding, increased muscle mass, acromegaly
   6. Any chronic diseases, especially diabetes
   7. Family history of PCOS, infertility, diabetes
   8. Medication history

IV. Physical examination

   A. Complete physical examination including height, weight, blood pressure
   B. Pelvic examination—speculum and bimanual to check for enlarged PCO
   C. Breast examination to rule out galactorrhea
   D. Full body scan for hirsutism, acanthosis nigricans, body shape, waist to hip ratio, hair growth patterns

V. Laboratory and Other Diagnostics

   A. FSH
   B. LH
   C. LH/FSH ratio
   D. Prolactin
   E. Androstenedione
   F. Glucose (fasting)
   G. Testosterone (total and free)
   H. 17-ketosteroids
   I. Dehydroepiandrosterone sulfate (DHEAS)
   J. Sex hormone binding globulin
   K. Comprehensive metabolic panel
   L. Transvaginal ultrasound

M. TSH
N. Lipid profile
O. Insulin (fasting)
P. HCG

VI. Differential diagnosis

   A. Late manifestation congenital adrenal hyperplasia
   B. Adrenal adenoma
   C. Adrenal carcinoma
   D. Hyperthecosis
   E. Ovarian carcinoma
   F. Cushing's syndrome
   G. Acromegaly
   H. Idiopathic hirsutism
   I. Hyperprolactinemias
   J. Thyroid disorders
   K. Disorders of adrenal and pituitary glands

VII. Treatment

   A. Weight loss and exercise program
   B. Low dose, low androgenic combination oral contraceptives to restore cyclic menses
   C. Possibly antiandrogens for hirsutism and acne
   D. Insulin-sensitizing agents: metformin, troglitazone
   E. Electrolysis, depilatories
   F. Ovulation induction

VIII. Complications

   A. Insulin resistance and development of type 2 diabetes, metabolic syndrome
   B. Miscarriage
   C. Infertility
   D. Hysterectomy
   E. Endometrial cancer
   F. Ovarian cancer
   G. Cardiovascular disease (atherosclerosis, hypertension, increased triglycerides)

IX. Consultation and Referral

   A. For infertility treatment
   B. For nonpharmacologic treatment of hirsutism

X. Follow-up

    A. Education about PCOS and lifestyle alterations

    B. Education about pharmacologic interventions

    C. Education about fertility

    See Bibliography. Web sites: http://www.pcosupport.org; http://www.familydoctor.org/20.xml; http://www.obgyn.net/pcos/pcos.asp.

CHAPTER SEVENTEEN

Weight Management

I. Definition

Obesity is an excess of body fat. The most commonly utilized method for measuring body composition is the Body Mass Index (BMI) (see Appendix G). BMI is expressed in weight in kilograms divided by height in meters squared (Kg/m^2). Normal weight is defined as a BMI of 18.5–24.9, overweight as a BMI between 25 and 29.9, mild obesity as a BMI between 30 and 34.9, moderate obesity 35–39.9 and morbid obesity, > 40. Health risks begin to surface with a BMI greater than 25, the risk increasing as the BMI increases.

Increasingly a subset of obese patients is being identified with Metabolic Syndrome. This syndrome, also called Syndrome X and Insulin Resistance Syndrome, is a cluster of conditions that can lead to an increased risk to cardiovascular disease and diabetes. Criteria for diagnosis include:

A. Obesity
   1. BMI greater than 30
   2. Increased visceral adipose tissue with a waist circumference of greater than 35 inches in women
   3. A small number of persons not meeting the criteria for obesity but who present with laboratory values that identify them as metabolically obese
B. Dyslipidemia
   1. Hypertriglyceridemia 150 mg/dL or higher
   2. Decreased HDL-C levels less than 50 mg/dL in females
   3. LDL-C levels may be normal

    C. Elevated blood pressure
      1. New Advanced Technology Program III guidelines define elevated blood pressure as 130/85 or greater (see Web site site: www.atp.nist.gov/atp/psag-co.htm)
    D. Impaired glucose function
      1. Fasting blood glucose of greater than 100 mg/dL
    E. Increased fasting insulin levels
    F. Polycystic Ovary Syndrome is not included in the criteria for diagnosis, but is present in a large percentage of women with metabolic syndrome.

II. Epidemiology

Obesity is among the most serious and prevalent health problems in the United States, second only to cigarette smoking. Over 97 million Americans are defined as having a weight problem. Of these, 58 million are obese.

Prevalence continues to rise, in the past decade rising from 25 to 35 percent. Researchers have shown that prevalence varies greatly by sex, age, race, and socioeconomic status. Over 55 percent of the population defined as obese are women. Obesity in women is twice as common in lower socioeconomic groups than in women with higher socioeconomic status. Obesity itself is an independent risk factor for many medical conditions and negatively contributes to many others.

III. Etiology

    A. Obesity is a multifactorial disorder occurring as a result of an imbalance between energy expended and food consumed and with other contributing factors such as:
      1. Metabolic (less than 1% of obese)
        a. Hypothyroidism
        b. Cortisol excess (Cushing's Syndrome)
        c. Stein-Leventhal Syndrome (polycystic ovary disease)
      2. Medication
        a. Antidiabetics
        b. Antipsychotics
        c. Antidepressants
        d. Antiepileptics
        e. Adenergic antagonists
        f. Serotonin and histamine antagonists
        g. Steroids
      3. Food consumption
        a. Portion size

      b. Selection of foods
        1) Foods high in fat
        2) Foods and beverages high in sugar and complex carbohydrates
   4. Lifestyles
      a. Sedentary/lack of physical activity
      b. Lack of calorie burning (aerobic) exercise
      c. Use of food for comfort and to reduce stress
   5. Other
      a. Of lesser contribution
        1) Endocrine
        2) Deviant eating patterns, i.e., binge-eating, night-eating

IV. Risks Associated With Obesity

  A. Obesity is associated with increased morbidity and mortality. It has been associated with over 30 illnesses, among them:
    1. Type 2 diabetes
    2. Hypertension
    3. Coronary artery disease
    4. Dyslipidemia
    5. Gallstone formation
    6. Osteoarthritis
    7. Gastrointestinal disorders
    8. Sleep apnea
    9. Breast inflammation
   10. Respiratory diseases
   11. Some cancers
   12. Gynecologic conditions
   13. Increased risks in pregnancy

V. History

  A. Risk Assessment
    1. Overweight and obese patients may not present with the stated desire to lose weight.
    2. Presenting complaints are most commonly those associated with the risk factors listed in IV. A.
    3. A weight-loss assessment should be part of an annual exam.
    4. Weight-loss assessment
      a. Patient's recognition of need for weight reduction
      b. Patient's readiness to change
      c. Previous attempts at weight loss

    d. Dietary assessment
       1) Type and amounts of food typically consumed
       2) Patterns of eating
       3) Meals
       4) Snacks
       5) Spontaneous eating
    e. Alcohol consumption
       1) Amount
       2) Frequency
    f. Physical activity
       1) Type
       2) How often, for how long
    g. Presence of obesity-related problems
    h. Family history of weight and weight-related problems
    i. Signs and symptoms of depression
    j. Medications: prescribed, over-the-counter including herbals, homeopathics, and nutritional supplements
    k. Smoker/nonsmoker

VI. Physical Exam

A. As indicated by known problem or presenting complaint or to rule out a secondary cause of obesity
B. Regardless of above, exam should include:
    1. Height
    2. Weight
    3. Blood pressure
C. Head and neck examination for presence of:
    1. Moon facies
    2. Hirsutism
    3. Goiter
    4. Buffalo hump
D. Skin
    1. Striae
    2. Hirsutism
    3. Edema
    4. Dryness
E. Calculation of BMI
    1. BMI may be calculated by dividing the weight in pounds, by the square of the height (square inches) and multiplying the result by 703.
    2. BMI may also be assessed by consulting a BMI Table (see Appendix G).

F. Waist circumference measurement
   1. Waist circumference of > 35 on women

VII. Laboratory Exam

   A. As indicated by known history or physical exam
   B. The following should be considered if no underlying physical problem is indicated:
      1. Lipid profile
      2. TSH, free T⁴
      3. Fasting blood sugar; 2-hour postprandial
      4. CBC
      5. Baseline electrocardiogram
      6. Sleep studies if indicated
   C. If metabolic syndrome is to be ruled out
      1. Lipid levels
      2. Fasting blood sugar; 2-hour postprandial
      3. Fasting Insulin level
      4. Laboratory workup specific for PCOS (see Chapter 16)

VIII. Treatment

   A. Intervention needs to be multifaceted and tailored to meet the patient's needs and readiness for change.
   B. The need for weight loss should be presented to the patient in a nonjudgmental, nonconfrontational manner. Approach the problem as a partnership in an endeavor that will help the patient to enjoy a longer, healthier life.
   C. Assessment of patient's willingness to make a change:
      1. Patient may not be interested in making a change despite the identified risk and potential consequences.
      2. Patient may be interested, acknowledge the risk factors, but may not yet be ready to take action.
      3. Patient is ready to take on the challenge of weight loss.
   D. Assessment of the amount of weight to be lost based on physical findings and risk factors.
   E. Plan
      1. Assessment of caloric intake
      2. Assessment of energy expenditure and level of physical activity
      3. Assessment of limitations and/or existing factors
         a. Physical limitation
         b. Medications (alternatives may be considered)
         c. Financial limitations
         d. Cues or stimuli that affect eating

4. Set realistic goals and expectations regarding the amount of weight to be lost
   a. Short-term
      1) 5–10 percent loss in initial weight at 1–2 lb/week rate
   b. Long-term
      1) Realization of ideal weight
      2) Maintaining ideal weight
5. Contract with patient a framework for realization of goals

F. Interventions
   1. Diet/with emphasis on long range behavior changes
      a. Nutritionist for evaluation and plan
      b. Self-help
         1) Weight Watchers
         2) Take Off Pounds Sensibly (TOPS)
         3) Overeaters Anonymous
         4) Community-based programs
         5) Meal replacement programs
         6) Books, magazine articles
         7) Web site weight-loss programs
   2. Education in food selection and change in eating patterns (NHLBI/NIDDK guidelines are a good source of information—see Web site: www.nhlbi.gov)
      a. Low fats, increase omega-3 fatty acids
      b. Moderate use of complex carbohydrates
      c. Decrease consumption of simple carbohydrates, i.e., sugary drinks, candy
      d. Moderate use of low-fat protein
      e. Decrease in portion size
      f. Omit late night eating
      g. Eating more slowly (20 minutes should pass between first and last bites of a meal)
      h. Drinking 8 (8 oz) glasses of water/day
      i. Use of daily food diary to keep track of consumption
   3. Physical Activity
      a. Activity needs to be tailored to the patient's needs and limitation.
      b. A guideline of 30–40 min/day of aerobic exercise, 3–4 x/week for strenuous exercise; 4–5 x/week for moderate exercise. This may be done at divided times (i.e., three 10-minute sessions).
      c. Moderate-intensity physical activity provides significant health benefits, but needs to be done more often.
      d. Aerobic exercise may include (according to patient's ability):

    1) Running/jogging
    2) Brisk walking (3 mph)
    3) Swimming
    4) Bicycling > 10 mph for strenuous exercise; < 10 mph for moderate exercise
    5) Cross-country skiing
    6) Rowing

  e. Flexibility, resistence/strength training are important components of an exercise program and provide additional health benefits. Activities include:
    1) Light weight lifting
    2) Resistance bands
    3) Pilates
    4) Yoga

4. Pharmacotherapeutic options
  a. Pharmaceutic intervention may be helpful in patients with a BMI of > 30 kg/m^2. This may also be helpful in patients who are slightly less obese (i.e., BMI of 27–29.9) but who have a comorbidity.
    1) Sibutramine (Meridia®). A serotonin and norepinephrine—reuptake inhibitor (in the same class that includes Prozac®/Zoloft®/Wellbutrin®).
      a) How sibutramine works
        i) Makes the patient feel full for a longer period of time, thus helping to control appetite
        ii) Reduces food cravings
        iii) Improves the comorbid conditions associated with being overweight, which results in improvements in triglycerides, HDL, cholesterol, uric acid, and glucose
      b) Dosage
        i) 10 mg daily orally
        ii) increasing to 15 mg daily
        iii) May be decreased to 5 mg daily if not tolerated at higher level
      c) Minor side effects include:
        i) Headache
        ii) Dry mouth
      d) More major side effects include:
        i) Increased blood pressure and pulse rate
      e) Contraindications
        i) Hypertension
        ii) CHD

       iii) History of stroke

       iv) Patients on SSRI or SSNRI

2) Orlistat (Xenical®) a pancreatic lipase inhibitor

   a) How it works

      i) Blocks absorption of about 30% of ingested dietary fats

      ii) Not an appetite suppressant

      iii) Improves comorbid conditions related to obesity especially hyperlipidemia and diabetes

   b) Dosage

      i) 120 mg orally three times a day taken just prior to meal containing fat

      ii) In patients with side effects, medication may be started by taking one 120 mg tablet with the largest fat containing meal of the day and gradually titrating up to advised dosage as patient adjusts

   c) Side effects (are directly related to amount of fat in meal consumed)

      i) Soft stools

      ii) Diarrhea (may be explosive and foul smelling)

      iii) Anal leakage

   d) Additional information

      i) A daily multiple vitamin should be recommended as Orlistat® inhibits absorption of fat soluble vitamins

3) Herbal or alternative medications

   a) Currently not recommended as alternative medications

      i) Not under any regulation

      ii) Ingredients i.e., Ma Hung, possess the potential for serious side effects

4) Behavioral

   a) Stimulus control

      i) Identifying factors contributing to overeating and underexercising

      ii) Identify ways in which contributory factors may be eliminated

      iii) Structuring mechanism for elimination of the negative stimuli

   b) Stress management

      i) Meditation, progressive relaxation

      ii) Guided imagery

c) Cognitive restructuring
   i) Identification of inner dialogue, i.e., self-talk, distorted/negative self-image
   ii) Replacement of these negative and self-defeating cognitions with more positive ones

d) Social support
   i) Seek out support/educational groups as noted in VIII. F.1.
   ii) Join and participate in exercise groups, and other recreation programs geared toward physical well-being and body conditioning
   iii) Seek support systems within family or peer group
   iv) Daily journal

5) Surgical
  a) May be considered for patients who have failed trials of diet, lifestyle changes, pharmacotherapy
  b) Most often used for patients under age 55 and in good health with a BMI < 40 kg/m^2 and possessing a significant cofactor
  c) Prior to surgery patient should undergo assessment by multidisciplinary team. Assessment should include:
   i) Medical
   ii) Surgical
   iii) Psychological
   iv) Nutritional
  d) Patient should be well motivated and well informed about potential benefits and risks
  e) Types of procedures
   i) Vertical banding—restricting gastric volume
   ii) Roux-en-y gastric bypass, in addition to restricting volume also alters digestion
  f) Success rates
   i) Regardless of procedure, most patients lose one-half to two-thirds their excess weight within 18 months.
  g) Risks
   i) Postoperative wound infection
   ii) Atelectasis
   iii) Dehiscence
   iv) Deep vein thromboembolism
   v) Anastomotic leaks

          vi) Marginal ulcers
         vii) Pouch and distal esophageal dilation
       viii) Persistent vomiting
         ix) Cholecystitis
          x) Development of dumping syndrome
         xi) Vitamin deficiencies, i.e., B12, folate, iron

6) Other
   a) Preconception counseling
   b) Preconception weight stabilization
   c) Counseling of pregnant women as to micronutrient and vitamin supplementation and close monitoring for appropriate weight maintenance and weight gain

X. Consultation

   A. BMI > 40 (morbidly obese)
   B. Psychiatric disorder (bulimia/depression)
   C. Sleep apnea
   D. Uncontrolled cofactor
      1. Hypertension
      2. Diabetes
      3. Heart disease
   E. Assessment and treatment for metabolic syndrome (consider endocrinologist)

X. Follow-Up

   A. Weight checks on regularly scheduled contracted schedule—4 weeks if no adverse events and weight loss is being achieved.
   B. Measurements as part of above.
   C. Review and reassessment of goals on regular schedule.
   D. Review of food and exercise diaries.
   E. Review and assessment of problems, concerns, and side effects associated with pharmaceutical interventions.

See Bibliography. Web sites: National Heart, Lung and Blood Institute (NHLBI), http://www.nhlbi.gov/; National Institute of Diabetes, Digestive, and Kidney Diseases, http://www.niddk.gov/; http//www.nhlbi.nih.gov/guidelines/ obesity/ob_home.htm; http://www.nhlbi.nih.gov/health/public/heart/ obesity/lose_wt/index.htm; http://www.health.gov/dietary guidelines; http://www.63.73.158.75; http://www.cyberdiet.com; USDA Nutrient Data Laboratory, http://www.nalusda.gov/fnic/foodcomp; North American Association for the Study of Obesity, http://www.naaso.org; American Obesity Association, http://www.obesity.org; Eat Right America Program, http://www.eatright.org; Advanced Technology Program, US Department of Commerce, http://www.atp.nist.gov/atp/psag-co.htm

CHAPTER EIGHTEEN

Complementary/ Alternative Therapies (CAM)

Increasingly, women are using complementary and alternative therapy for preventative and palliative care as alternative or adjunct therapies to their traditional medical care. In the following, we will present an overview of commonly used therapies for peri/menopause, PMS, and depression.

I. Definition

Alternative therapies refer to treatment approaches that, although used for many years, have not been evaluated and tested by conventional methods. The term complementary therapies is utilized to convey the concept that these therapies are often used in conjunction with conventional medically accepted treatments. When looked at in this manner, the term assumes a more holistic view of women's health care needs.

II. Types

    A. The following are therapies commonly utilized by women:
        1. Vitamins
        2. Minerals
        3. Herbals
        4. Phytoestrogens (dietary)
        5. Natural estrogen
        6. Natural progesterones

7. Acupuncture
8. Biofeedback/hypnosis
9. Homeopathy
10. Therapeutic touch, massage, Reiki
11. Traditional medicines
   a. Ayurveda
   b. Traditional Chinese medicines
   c. Tibetan
   d. Wise woman traditional
   e. Herbalism
   f. These traditional methods may have
      1) Complex theoretic structure
      2) Literature-based traditions
      3) Classic gynecologic texts
      4) Materia medica with specific herbs for reproductive and gynecologic problems
12. Therapies based on oral tradition

III. Reasons for Selection/Use of CAM

A. Preference for more "natural" treatment
B. Belief in unconventional (non-Western) medicine
C. Concern about potential side effects of conventional medicines and treatments
D. Dissatisfaction with or lack of confidence in conventional methods
E. Desire to have control over ones own health and health care
F. Being raised in a culture that believes in and uses CAM therapies

IV. Problems and Concerns

A. Lack of systemized research and well-designed studies to measure safety and efficacy
B. Self-medication based on insufficient information
C. Lack of standardization of therapeutics
D. Failure to inform health care practitioner of CAM use; supplements can interact with prescription or over the counter medications

V. Cautions

A. Remember "natural" isn't synonymous with safe.
B. CAM should be used only for minor problems, not for conditions that have potential to be life-altering or life-threatening.
C. CAM should not be used in pregnancy or breast feeding without discussion with health care practitioner.

D. Use should be limited to recommended dosages for recommended time frames.

E. Users need to be knowledgeable about CAM methods. Do not use CAM therapy that has not been personally researched and its use understood. The Internet should not be the only source of research and information.

F. Use should begin with a smaller than recommended dose to observe for adverse reaction.

G. Buy or seek therapies only from reputable manufacturers and practitioners.

VI. Frequently Used/Recommended CAM Therapies

   A. Menopause
      1. B Complex vitamins
        a. Usual dose 50–300 mg daily
        b. Conditions
          1) Stress/depression
          2) Water retention
        c. Toxicity/adverse effects
          1) None known
      2. Vitamin C
        a. Usual dose 500 mg daily
        b. Conditions
          1) Free radical scavenger/antioxidant
          2) Linked with raising levels HDL, lowering LDL
          3) Maintaining bone structures
          4) Maintaining healthy connective tissues
        c. Toxicity/adverse effects
          1) Use with caution and medical supervision if history of compromised kidney function
          2) Increased doses (5,000 mg per day) associated with intestinal gas and loose stool; if history of reflux, take buffered vitamin C
      3. Vitamin D
        a. Usual daily dose 400–800 IU daily
        b. Conditions
          1) Osteoporosis—increase mineral absorption, bone mineralization
        c. Toxicity/adverse effects
          1) Unwise to exceed 1,000 IU per day
          2) Hypervitaminosis (mild), treatable
          3) Hypercalcemia from extended doses of over 1,000 IUs per day may be irreversible

4. Vitamin E
   a. Usual daily dose 400–800 IU may be used up to 1,200 IU safely
   b. Conditions
      1) Hot flashes
      2) Cardiovascular prevention (controversial), poor circulation, atrophic vaginitis
   c. Toxicity/adverse effects
      1) Use with caution if patient is on high blood pressure medication (may decrease blood pressure)
      2) Use with caution or not at all if patient is on anticoagulant therapy
      3) Using more than recommended dose can result in nausea, flatulence, diarrhea, heart palpitations, fainting (all reversible with dose decrease)
5. Calcium
   a. Usual daily dose in divided doses 1,200–2,000 mg— should be used in conjunction with Vitamin D to aid in bone remineralization
   b. Conditions
      1) Osteoporosis (prevention and treatment) provides reintegration of calcium into bones
      2) Hypertension—aids in contraction and expansion of heart muscle
   c. Toxicity/adverse effects
      1) Calcium has no known toxic effects (caution in use of antacids as calcium supplements; in addition to calcium many of these products contain aluminum that interferes with calcium absorption)
6. Essential fatty acids (EFAs)
   a. Usual daily dose Omega 3/Omega 6 (3,000 to 4,000 mg/day)
   b. Conditions
      1) Hot flashes, vaginal atrophy, mood swings and irritability, bloating and fluid retention, decreased libido
      2) Cardiovascular disease osteoporosis: a correct balance of EFAs is essential for the rebuilding and production of new cells and to decrease inflammation and modulate hormone imbalance
      3) EFAs consist of EPA (eicosapentaenoic acid Omega 3), DHCA (docosahexaenoic acid Omega 3), and GLA (gamina linolenic acid Omega 6)

    c. Toxicity/adverse effects
      1) No known adverse effects
  7. Coenzyme Q10 (ubiquinone)
    a. Usual daily dose 30–100 mg
    b. Conditions
      1) The name ubiquinone is appropriate because coenzyme Q10 is found everywhere in the body. A powerful antioxidant, it stimulates the immune system, increases tissue oxygenation, and has vital antiaging effects. Extensive research has been done regarding its impact on heart disease. It is mentioned here because of its preventative effects.
    c. Toxicity/adverse effects
      1) No known adverse effects
  8. Dong Quai (angelica sinensis)
    a. Usual daily dosage—consult preparation instructions
    b. Conditions
      1) Hot flashes, irritability, insomnia, restlessness, night sweats, headaches, toxicity
    c. Toxicity/adverse effects
      1) No known toxicity; may cause minor GI upset (do not use Dong Quai during menses if hypermenorrhea is a problem). Interacts with and increases the activity of the anticoagulant drug Warfarin. This can lead to increased bleeding.
  9. Chasteberry (Vitex-agnus-castus)
    a. Usual daily dosage—consult individual preparation
    b. Conditions
      1) Mood swings, irritability, depression, balances estrogen–progesterone levels in the body
      2) Hot flashes—balances estrogen, progesterone
    c. Toxicity/adverse effects
      1) Usually without adverse effects—rarely causes nausea, diarrhea, weight gain, headaches, allergic rash—spontaneously disappear when discontinued
 10. Black Cohosh (cimicifuga racemosa) does not act like estrogen as previously thought. Has good safety record.
    a. Usual daily dosage—100–600 mg/day
    b. Conditions
      1) Hot flashes
      2) Fatigue
      3) Irritability

      4) Night sweats
      5) Headaches
      6) Insomnia
      7) Heart palpitations
   c. Toxicity/adverse effects
      1) No known adverse effects

11. Licorice (glycyrrhiza glabra)
   a. Usual daily dose varies with type of preparation
   b. Conditions
      1) Hot flashes
      2) Fatigue—appears to estradiol levels while raising progesterone
   c. Toxicity/adverse effects
      1) Should not be used in patients with kidney problems, high blood pressure, patients taking potassium. Not advisable for use in persons who are on low salt diets or persons taking diuretics, corticoid treatments, cardiac glycosides, or medication for hypertension.

12. Ginkgo biloba
   a. Usual daily dosage—consult preparation directions
   b. Conditions
      1) Circulation
      2) Forgetfulness
      3) Cold hands and feet
      4) Antitoxin/anti-inflammatory
   c. Toxicity/adverse effects
      1) Headaches
      2) Nausea
      3) Dizziness
      4) Allergic skin reactions
      5) Do not use if taking anticoagulants or prior to surgery

13. St. John's Wort (hypericum perforatum)
   a. Usual daily dose—300 mg
   b. Conditions
      1) Depression, anxiety, sleep disorders
   c. Toxicity/adverse effects
      1) May alter liver enzyme function in processing some drugs, including HIV medications, digoxin, warfarin, oral contraceptives, antidepressants

14. Ginseng
   a. There are three kinds of Ginseng—Asian (Chinese or Korean), American, and Siberian. The first two are authentic

Ginseng. Siberian Ginseng is not, however it looks similar and has similar effects on the body.
   1) Usual daily dose 200–400 mg/day
   b. Conditions (it is advised to limit use to 3 consecutive months then take a 3 month break before resuming)
      1) Stress
      2) Fatigue
      3) Loss of libido
      4) Depression
      5) Vaginal dryness—Ginseng has a direct estrogenic effect
   c. Toxicity/adverse effects
      1) Headache
      2) Gastrointestinal problems
15. Dietary phytoestrogens are naturally found in foods. These compounds may produce effects similar to estrogen; found in cereal, legumes, and grasses.
   a. There are three main groups of phytoestrogens: isoflavones, lignans, and coumestans.
      1) Isoflavones are found in soy, garbanzo beans, and other legumes. They may be consumed in the form of soy, miso, and tofu.
      2) Lignans are found in seed oils such as flaxseed.
      3) Coumestans are found in red clover, sunflower seeds, and bean sprouts.
   b. Phytoestrogens are thought to be helpful in minimizing hot flashes, maintaining bone density, and lowering cholesterol, LDLs, and triglycerides.
   c. Natural progesterones manufactured from wild yams—patients should be discouraged from using OTC preparations of topical progestins for their progesterone imbalance since there is no standardized compounding. Replacement hormones are usually synthesized.
16. Melatonin is helpful with sleep disturbances—difficulty falling asleep and waking in the middle of the night unable to go back to sleep. Dosage is 1–3 mg and it comes regular and timed release.
17. Other
   a. Relaxation techniques
   b. Biofeedback
   c. Meditation
   d. Tai Chi and Qi Gong
   e. Yoga

These techniques can be helpful in helping the body regain homeo-stasis, thus making it more possible to adapt to change without increasing stress.

      f. Ayurvedic and Chinese herbals may also be used. There are several preparations on the market. They include:

         1) Meno-care® used to alleviate palpitations, insomnia, mood swings, and hot flashes. Usual dose—1 tablets twice a day.

         2) Geriforte® used to address the overall stress of aging. Usual dose—2 tablets twice a day. Source: health food store or through the manufacturer, Himalaya, USA (1-800-869-4640).

         3) Nukeba Zhen Wan (Women's Precious Pills)—an herbal blend, generally used to address low estrogen levels, hot flashes, forgetfulness, confusion, insomnia, and tearfulness. Usual dose—8 small pellets 3 times/day.

         4) Er Xian Tang Wan (Two mortals) helpful in fatigue, hot flashes, night sweats, low libido. Usual daily dose is 8 pills 3 times a day.

These herbals may be found in health food stores or ordered from Ethical Nutrients (1-800-638-2848). Although these preparations are easily available, consultation with a Ayurvedic or Chinese medicine clinician is recommended.

      g. Homeopathic remedies are based on the premise that the body has the capacity to heal itself. Formulas are compounded that use very minute quantities of an agent to trigger the body's innate capacity to heal. Preparations specific to a symptom can be found in health food stores for self-treatment. Homeopathic practitioners are also available to work with a patient to customize preparations to fit the person's symptoms.

VI. PMS

    A. B Complex
        1. Usual dose 50–300 mg/day
        2. Symptoms
            a. Stress/depression
            b. Water retention (Especially B6)
        3. Toxicity/adverse effects
           a. none known
    B. Vitamin B6 usual dose 100–200 mg/day

C. Magnesium usual dose 400 mg/day
D. Vitamin E usual dose 400–600mg/day
E. Chromium usual dose 250 mcg daily or twice a day to reduce sugar cravings
F. Essential Fatty Acids—EFAs (also helpful with dysmenorrhea)
  1. Usual daily dose—as indicated on individual preparation/no daily optimum dose
  2. Conditions
    a. Help to reduce depression, irritability, cramps, nausea, bloating, and headaches. Correct balance of EFAs is essential for the rebuilding and production of new cells— decrease inflammation, moderate hormone imbalance
G. Licorice (Glycyrrhiza glabra)
  1. Usual daily dose varies with preparation
  2. Conditions addressed—estrogen-like activity helps in irritability, mood swings, stimulates adrenal glands
  3. Toxicities—should not be used by women with kidney problems, high blood pressure, patients taking potassium. Not advisable for use in persons who are on low salt diets or persons taking diuretics, corticoid treatments, cardiac glycosides, or medications for hypertention.
H. Black Cohosh (cimicifuga raccmosa)
  1. Usual daily dosage—as indicated on individual preparation
  2. Conditions
    a. Nervousness
    b. Irritability
    c. Sleep disturbances
    d. Depressive moods
    e. Headaches

VII. Depression

Consult guideline on emotional/mental health issues. See Bibliography. Web sites: CAM on PubMed, http://www.ncbi.nlm.nih.gov/pubmed; National Center for Complementary and Alternative Medicine, National Institutes of Health, http://www.nccam. nih.gov; The Nurse Healers— Professional Associates, http://www.therapeutic-touch.org; http://www. herbalgram.org/herbalgram/

CHAPTER NINETEEN

Emotional/Mental Health Issues

APPROPRIATE FOR ASSESSMENT AND TREATMENT IN A WOMEN'S HEALTH CARE SETTING

I. Definition

An alteration in mood or behavior resulting in discomfort to the woman. These changes may place the woman in chronic or acute distress. Attempting to cope with this distress may alter her ability to function, causing family relationship or workplace disturbances, as well as somatic manifestations that may contribute to morbidity and mortality.

II. Psychiatric Conditions Commonly Seen in a Women's Health Care Setting:

A. In this guideline, one asterisk (*) indicates a condition appropriate for assessment by a clinician in an office setting, two (**) indicates a condition appropriate for referral for further assessment and treatment, and three (***) indicates condition appropriate for immediate referral to a hospital emergency room or other immediate care settings.

B. Mood Disorders
1. Bipolar disorder**
2. Dysthymia*
3. Major depression**
4. Postpartum depression* or **
5. Premenstrual dysphoric disorder—PMDD*
6. Seasonal affective disorder (SAD)*

   C. Anxiety Disorders
1. General anxiety disorder*
2. Obsessive compulsive disorder (OCD)* or **
3. Panic disorder**
4. Posttraumatic stress disorder (PTSD)**
5. Social phobia*

   D. Eating Disorders
1. Anorexia**
2. Bulimia**

   E. Personality Disorders
1. Borderline personality disorder**
2. Narcissistic**
3. Avoidant**
4. Dependent**
5. Self-defeating*

   F. Cognitive Disorders
1. Dementia**
2. Delirium***

   G. Psychotic Disorders
1. Schizophrenia** or ***
2. Other psychotic disorders** or ***

   H. Sexual Dysfunction* or **

   I. Sleep Disturbances
1. Insomnia* or **
   a. Difficulty falling asleep
   b. Restless/wakeful sleep
2. Early morning awakening with inability to resume sleep

   J. Substance Abuse Disorders**

   K. Suicidal Threats or Ideation***

   L. Somatoform Disorders
1. Body dysmorphic disorder*
2. Hypochondriasis*
3. Conversion disorder**

III. Responsibilities of Clinicians

   A. Knowledge of signs and symptoms indicating a psychiatric condition or a psychiatric component in a medical condition

   B. Screening and assessment

   C. Intervention
1. Treatment
2. Referral for further assessment
3. Emergency intervention if condition warrants

IV. History

  A. What the patient may present with:
1. Stomach pain
2. Back pain
3. Pain in arms, legs, joints
4. Mood changes associated with menses
5. Loss of libido
6. Headaches
7. Chest pain
8. Dizziness
9. Rapid/pounding heart
10. Shortness of breath
11. Gastrointestinal complaints: pain, diarrhea, constipation, nausea, vomiting
12. Fatigue and/or low energy
13. Sleeping difficulties
14. Feeling edgy or nervous
15. Excessive worry
16. Difficulty swallowing or "lump in throat"
17. Feelings of sadness without known cause

  B. Additional information to be considered
1. Generalized feeling of sadness or hopelessness
2. Weight loss or weight gain; what was patient's weight 6 months ago/1 year ago?
3. Alcohol consumption/use of prescription or illicit drugs
4. Has partner or close associates commented on alcohol consumption?
5. Does patient feel guilty about drinking?
6. Does patient avoid social situations?
7. Change in interest in sex or responsiveness during intimacy
8. History of depression or other psychiatric problem in biological family
9. Number of visits to health care provider in past year
10. Has patient found it difficult to concentrate or been easily distracted, finding it hard to find words, forgetting things?
11. Changes in work or family environment
12. Suicidal thoughts, plan or attempt
13. Seasonal pattern
14. Prescription, OTC, or herbal or other CAM used currently
15. Information on any of the problems listed in II if not spontaneously volunteered

C. Interview Techniques
  1. Nonverbal messages are important in obtaining a reliable psychiatric history
     a. Patient and clinician should be seated at equal height with no furniture between them, i.e., desk
     b. Establish eye contact
     c. Put pen down, give patient your full attention
     d. Ask clear, open-ended questions
     e. Allow patient to talk
     f. Be supportive
     g. Be watchful for important subtexts, i.e., changing the subject, avoidance, careless, or exaggerated responses, inability to maintain eye contact
     h. Maintain a nonjudgmental attitude; however, be open to challenge contradictory statements

V. Physical Exam

  A. Appropriate to physical complaint or symptomatology
  B. In addition to appropriate physical exam, clinician should be alert for the following physical manifestations of emotional distress:
     1. Appearance of sadness
     2. Gross anxiety
     3. Elevated respiratory rate and pulse
     4. Excessive perspiration
     5. Coldness and dampness of hands
     6. Tremor
     7. Inability to make eye contact
     8. Unkempt appearance
  C. If indicated by information and observation of above, a general mental status exam or a mini-mental status exam should be conducted.
     1. Mini-mental status exam
        a. Appearance
           1) Grooming
           2) Clothing; dirty, clean, appropriate to seasonal condition, revealing
        b. Behavior
           1) Are mannerisms and gestures appropriate?
        c. Attitude
           1) Is patient aggressive, angry, guarded, cooperative?
        d. Mood
           1) Anxious
           2) Depressed

        3) Manic or hyperactive
        4) Alternating moods
     e. Speech
        1) Quantity and quality
        2) Speed; pressure
     f. Cognitive functions
        1) Concentration
        2) Memory
     g. Affect
        1) Normal variety of facial expression
        2) Blunted, flat, or immobilization of facial features

VI. Differential Diagnosis

   A. Mental and physical disorders are frequently overlapping; the challenge presented in diagnosis is consideration of both dimensions at the same time and ability to differentiate between the two; by the way in which both entities may be present and contributing to the symptomatology.
     1. Hypothyroidism
     2. Hyperthyroidism
     3. Hypoglycemia
     4. Mitral valve prolapse
     5. Meniere syndrome/vestibular neuronitis
     6. Esophageal tumors or other obstructions
     7. Asthma
     8. Caffeine abuse
     9. Coronary disease
    10. Alzheimer disease or senile dementia
    11. Irritable bowel syndrome
    12. Crohn's disease
    13. Brain tumors
   B. Signs and symptoms of conditions indicated in II as suitable for diagnosis and treatment in a primary women's health care setting.
     1. Dysthymia—milder form of depression, symptoms are not disabling but chronic, typically lasting for many years. These symptoms may be so much a part of an individual's life that they are taken for granted and patient does not complain to provider.
       a. Depressed mood
       b. Poor appetite
       c. Insomnia
       d. Hypersomnia
       e. Low energy/fatigue

    f. Low self-esteem

    g. Poor concentration

    h. Difficulty making decisions

    i. Feelings of hopelessness

2. Postpartum Depression (PPD). A self-limiting period of affective lability occurring within a few days to a week or so after childbirth. Many times PPD goes without diagnosis, which may leave the woman with lifelong feelings of guilt, fear, and inadequacy. The following symptoms (a) through (d) indicate a nonpsychotic PPD and (e) through (i) may indicate a psychotic illness. The psychotic and/or delusional mother may be at risk to herself and/or her child. Evaluation by a mental health professional is indicated. Women who have experienced one episode of PPD are at greater risk for another. Women with inadequately treated psychotic symptoms are at greater risk for future mental health illness.

    a. Sleeplessness

    b. Weeping

    c. Sadness

    d. Guilt

    e. Agitation

    f. Prolonged sleeplessness

    g. Lack of personal hygiene

    h. Anorexia

    i. Preoccupation with concerns or delusions about the infant

    j. Untreated, the above may contribute to lack of bonding and has been implicated in lifelong problems for mother and infant

3. Premenstrual Dysphoric Disorder (PMDD). A cluster of symptoms regularly presenting during the last week of the luteal phase, beginning to remit within a few days of the follicular phase. Symptoms are always absent in the week following the menses. Symptoms are not present prior to the last week of the luteal phase. Symptoms are of comparable severity but not duration to those displayed in a major depressive episode including:

    a. Sadness

    b. Hopelessness

    c. Anxiety/tension/feeling on edge

    d. Mood instability with tearfulness

    e. Persistent irritability

    f. Increased anger

      g. Increased interpersonal conflicts

      h. Binge-eating

      i. Insomnia

      j. It is helpful in making a diagnosis if the patient maintains a daily diary charting symptoms over a 2-month period.

   4. Seasonal Affective Disorder (SAD)

      a. Essential feature is that symptoms of a depressive episode occur seasonally, during fall or winter, remitting during spring

   5. Generalized Anxiety Disorder (GAD). An essential feature is excessive anxiety and worry occurring more days than not during a period of 6 months. Other symptoms include:

      a. Restlessness

      b. Easy fatigue

      c. Difficulty concentrating

      d. Irritability

      e. Muscle tension

      f. Disturbed sleep patterns

      g. Fearfulness

      h. Somatic complaints, i.e., cold hands, lump in throat, etc.

   6. Body Dysmorphic Disorder (BDD). An essential feature of BDD is a preoccupation with a defect in appearance. This preoccupation must cause significant distress or impairment in lifestyle and in other areas of function. Complaints commonly include:

      a. Hair thinning

      b. Acne

      c. Wrinkles

      d. Scars

      e. Vascular markings

      f. Paleness or redness of complexion

      g. Facial asymmetry or disproportion

      h. Excessive hair on face

      i. Preoccupation with a bodily part

VII. Laboratory Examination

   A. The following may be considered according to presenting complaint and symptomatology

      1. CBC

      2. Urinalysis

      3. Electrolytes

      4. Blood glucose levels

5. Thyroid function tests
6. Liver enzymes
7. Hormone levels
8. EKG
9. EEG
10. Drug screen if indicated

VIII. Treatment

A. Medication—All of the conditions listed as suitable for office treatment usually respond well to the use of an antidepressant or antianxiety medication. Most antidepressants are effective in treating anxiety as well as depression. Included below are those medications that can be most effectively and safely used in a general practice setting. When a patient does not respond well to one choice she/he may do better with another. When switching medications, do not stop initial drug abruptly prior to starting a new one, instead cross taper over a few weeks. For pregnant women, only Prozac® is currently approved.

1. Antidepressant/antianxiety medications
   a. Selective Seratonin Reuptake Inhibitors (SSRIs)
      1) Citalopram hydrobromide (Celexa®)—Starting dose: 10–20 mg per day; usual daily dose: 20–60 mg per day.
      2) Fluoxetine hydrochloride (Prozac®/Sarafem®)—Starting dose: 10–20 mg per day; usual daily dose: 20–60 mg/per day. Sarafem® is used for PMDD and is generally given for the 2 weeks prior to menses. Usual dose: 20–40 mg per day.
      3) Fluvoxamine maleate (Luvox®)—Starting dose: 50 mg per day; usual daily dose: 50–300 mg per day.
      4) Paroxetine hydrochloride (Paxil®)—Starting dose: 10–20 mg per day; usual daily dose: 20–60 mg per day.
      5) Sertraline hydrochloride (Zoloft®)—Starting dose: 25–50 mg per day; usual daily dose: 50–200 mg.
      6) Eszitalopram (Lexapro®)—Starting dose: 10 mg per day; usual daily dose: 10 mg.
      7) Major side effects of SSRIs include:
         a) GI disturbances
         b) Sexual side effects
         c) Restlessness
         d) Insomnia
         e) Headaches

      f) Orgasmic dysfunction

      g) Activation of mania in patients with bipolar disorder

b. Dopamine—norepinephrine reuptake inhibitors (DNRIs).

  1) Bupropion hydrochloride (Wellbutrin®)—Starting dose: 100 mg per day; usual daily dose: 100 mg 3 times a day.

  2) Bupropion hydrochloride—sustained release (Wellbutrin SR®)—Starting dose: 100 mg or 150 mg per day; usual daily dose: 300 per day (150 mg twice a day).

  3) Bupropion hydrochloride Wellbutrin XR 150 mg–300 mg. Starting dose: 150 mg daily x 7 days; usual daily dose: 300 mg daily in the am. Useful in SAD—start in autumn, taper and stop in early spring.

  4) Major side effects of DNRIs

      a) Seizures possible with high dose (450 mg/day and history of eating disorder or seizure disorder)

      b) Nausea and vomiting with SR formulation

      c) Headaches

      d) Psychosis (use cautiously in psychotic disorders)

c. Serotonin—norepinephrine reuptake inhibitors (SNRIs)

  1) Venlafaxine (Effexor®)—Starting dose: 37.5 mg daily; usual daily dose: 7.5 mg twice a day.

  2) Venlafaxine extended release (Effexor XR®)—Starting dose: 37.5 mg per day; usual daily dose: 75–225 mg per day.

  3) Duloxetine (as HCI) Cymbalta 20 mg, 30 mg, 60 mg

  4) Major side effects with SNRIs

      a) Hypertension

      b) Nausea

      c) Activation

      d) Sexual dysfunction

      e) Not recommended for women with increased daily alcohol ingestion

d. Serotonin modulators (SMs)

  1) Nefazodone (Serzone®)—Starting dose: 50 mg daily; usual daily dose: 150–300 mg per day.

  2) Trazodone (Desyrel®)—Starting dose: 50 mg daily; usual daily dose: 75–300 mg/qd in divided doses twice a day.

  3) Major side effects of SMs

      a) Orthostatic hypotension

      b) Anticholinergic symptoms

    c) Sedation

    d) Priapism (trazodone in males)

e. Norepinephrine—Serotonin modulators (NSMs)

    1) Mirtazapine (Remeron®)—Starting dose: 15 mg daily; usual daily dose: 15–45 mg daily.

    2) Major side effects of NSMs

        a) Anticholinergic symptoms

        b) Weight gain

        c) Sedation

        d) Increase in cholesterol levels

        e) Agranulocytosis (discontinue medication)

Tricyclics and MAOs have not been included because of their side effects' profile.

2. Antianxiety Medication

a. Benzodiazepines: Benzodiazepines should be used for short term only (i.e., specific situation known to cause anxiety/panic or sleeplessness, plane flights, recent loss) This category of drugs is habit forming and can quickly lead to dependence.

    1) Alprazolam (Xanax®)—Usual dose: 0.5 mg 3 times a day

    2) Clonazepam (Klonopin®)—Usual dose: 0.5 mg twice a day

    3) Diazepam (Valium®)—Usual dose: 10 mg twice a day

    4) Lorazepam (Ativan®)—Usual dose: 1 mg 3 times a day

    5) Oxazepam (Serax®)—Usual dose: 15 mg 3 times a day

    6) Most common side effects of Benzodiazepines

        a) Frequent: drowsiness, ataxia

        b) Occasional: confusion, amnesia, disinhibition, depression, dizziness

        c) Withdrawal symptoms: delirium/convulsions (with abrupt discontinuation), rebound insomnia or excitement

        d) Discontinue by tapering dose, no more than 25 percent per week decrease in dose

b. Other treatment

    1) Psychotherapy

        a) Cognitive therapy

        b) Interpersonal therapy

        c) Behavioral therapy

    2) Exposure therapy

    3) Biofeedback therapy

c. Other medications

    1) Buspirone hydrochloride (BuSpar®)—Starting dose: 5/10 mg daily; usual daily dose: 10/15/30 mg twice a day.

      2) Most common side effects:
        a) Frequent: headaches, dizziness, nausea
        b) Occasional: nausea, paresthesias, diarrhea
        c) Rare: psychosis, mania
  d. Complementary therapy
      1) St. John's Wort (hypericum perforatum)—Usual daily dosage: 300 mg 3 times a day or 450 mg twice a day for use in depression. Interaction with all medications listed above. Serotonin syndrome of nausea, diarrhea, headaches may occur if used simultaneously.
      2) Essential fatty acids are increasingly used for mood stabilization.
      3) Meditation/relaxation therapy.
      4) Regular exercise program.
      5) Regulation of sleep/wake patterns.
      6) Dietary changes, including decrease or elimination of caffeine.
      7) Light therapy with Seasonal Affective Disorder.

IX. Complications

  A. Untreated
    1. Increased risk for suicide or harm to others
    2. Increased risk for other impulsive and acting-out behavior
    3. Loss of friends, job
    4. Decrease in family harmony
    5. Exacerbation of any of the symptoms previously mentioned
  B. Treated
    1. Behaviors and somatic problems listed above
  C. Consultation
    1. All conditions indicated previously
    2. Failure to improve
    3. Collaboration for an appropriate medication
    4. Medication use in pregnant and lactating women

X. Follow-Up

  A. Monitor response, mood relief from symptoms
  B. Follow-up appointment in 3–6 weeks to monitor response to treatment, adverse reactions.

See Bibliography. Web sites: http://www.nimh.nih.gov; http://www.adaa.org; http://www.cognitivetherapy.com

PART II

Appendixes

Materials in this section: clinical forms, screening tools, patient education information

APPENDIX A

For Your Information: Patient Education Handouts

BACTERIAL VAGINOSIS (BV)

I. Definition

Overgrowth of a variety of anaerobic bacteria, genital mycoplasmas, and gardnerella

II. Transmission

The condition can be sexually transmitted, but it may also be identified in the nonsexually active female

III. Signs and Symptoms
- A. In the female
  1. Fishy, musty odor with a thin, chalk-white to gray watery vaginal discharge
  2. Discharge may cause vaginal and vulvar itching and burning
  3. Burning and swelling of genitals after intercourse
  4. No symptoms in some women
- B. In the male: No male version of BV has been identified

IV. Diagnosis

    A. Female evaluation may include
        1. Vaginal examination to check for bacterial vaginosis
        2. Further laboratory work to rule out Candida, trichomonas, gonococcus, or Chlamydia
        3. Blood test for syphilis
    B. Male evaluation: Rule out other infections such as trichomonas, gonococus, or Chlamydia

V. Treatment

    A. Treatment may be by mouth or with a vaginal cream or gel.
    B. Treatment of partners is not recommended because studies have not shown that their treatment decreases the number of recurrences unless partner is a woman also.
    C. It is very important to report any medical conditions you may have or medications you take regularly (especially for a seizure disorder) before taking any treatment.

VI. Patient Education

    A. Sexual partners should be alerted to the diagnosis and referred for evaluation and possible treatment if the patient has other infections concurrently.
    B. Sexual partners should be protected by condoms until patient's treatment is over. Check with your clinician because some creams weaken the latex of condoms or vaginal diaphragms.
    C. Alcoholic beverages should not be consumed during or for 48 hours after oral treatment.
    D. Minor side effects of oral treatment may include nausea, dizziness, and a metallic taste.
    E. No douching with or after treatment; douching is never recommended.

VII. Follow-up

Return to clinician for a reevaluation if symptoms persist or new symptoms occur.

Special notes:_____

Clinician: _____

For more information call: CDC STD Hotline: 1–800–227–8922: Phone numbers of free (or almost free) STD clinics are listed in the Community Service Numbers in the government pages of your local phone book. http://www.cdc.gov; www.cdc.gov/STD/BV/STDFact-Bacterial-Vaginosis.htm

From Hawkins, Roberto-Nichols, & Stanley-Haney, Guidelines for Nurse Practitioners in Gynecologic Settings, 9th edition, 2007, © Springer Publishing Company.

CANDIDIASIS (MONILIA) YEAST INFECTION

I. Definition

Candidiasis, or monilia, is a yeast-like overgrowth of a fungus called candida albicans (may also be caused by candida tropicalis or candida torulopsis glabrata and rarely by other candida species). Candida can be found in small amounts in the normal vagina but under some conditions it gets out of balance with the other vaginal flora and produces symptoms.

II. Transmission

    A. Usually nonsexual.

    B. Some common causes of candida overgrowth are: use of hormonal contraceptives such as birth control pills, the patch, ring, implant; antibiotics; diabetes; pregnancy; stress; deodorant tampons and other such menstrual products.

III. Signs and Symptoms

    A. In the female
        1. Vaginal discharge: thick, white, and curd-like
        2. Vaginal area itch and irritation with occasional swelling and redness
        3. Burning on urination
        4. Possibly, pain with intercourse
    B. In the male
        1. Itch and/or irritation of penis
        2. Cheesy material under foreskin, underside of penis
        3. Jock itch; athlete's foot

IV. Diagnosis

    A. Female evaluation may include vaginal examination to check for candida and rule out trichomoniasis, bacterial vaginosis, Chlamydia, and gonorrhea.
    B. Male evaluation may include:
        1. Examination of penis to check for irritation and/or cheesy materials

2. Culture for ruling out gonorrhea and Chlamydia
3. Urinalysis

V. Treatment

Prescription medicine: _____;
over the counter medication recommendation _____

_____

VI. Patient Education

A. No intercourse until symptoms subside.
B. Continue prescribed treatment even if menses occurs, but use pads rather than tampons.
C. Ways to prevent recurrent candida (yeast) infections:
   1. Bathe daily (with lots of water and minimal soap)
   2. To minimize the moist environment Candida favors, use:
      a. Cotton-crotched or cotton underwear/pantyhose (or cut out crotch of pantyhose)
      b. Loose-fitting slacks
      c. No underwear while sleeping
   3. Wipe the front first and then the back after toileting.
   4. Avoid feminine hygiene sprays, deodorants, deodorant tampons/minipads, colored or perfumed toilet paper, tear-off fabric softeners in the dryer, etc., any of which may cause allergies and irritation.
   5. Some women have found that vitamin C 500 mg 2–4 x each day helps or taking oral acidophilous tablets 40 million to 1 billion units a day (1 tablet).
D. Over-the-counter medication. Many women choose to try an over-the-counter preparation before seeking an examination. If symptoms do not subside after 1 course of treatment (1 tube or 1 set of suppositories), having an examination for diagnosis is recommended.

VII. Follow-up

Return to clinician for reevaluation if symptoms persist or new symptoms occur after treatment is completed.
Special Notes: _____
Clinician: _____
For more information call: CDC STD Hotline: 1–800–227–8922; Phone numbers of free (or almost free) STD clinics are listed in the Community Service Numbers in the government pages of your local

phonebook. CDC http://www.cdc.gov; http://www.cdc.gov/ncidod/dbmd/diseaseinfo/candidiasis_gen_g.htm

From Hawkins, Roberto-Nichols, & Stanley-Haney, *Guidelines for Nurse Practitioners in Gynecologic Settings,* 9th edition, 2007, © Springer Publishing Company.

CHLAMYDIA TRACHOMATIS

I. Definition

Chlamydia trachomatis is a sexually transmitted disease of the reproductive tract. It is currently believed to be the most common cause of sexually transmitted disease in males and females, more common than gonorrhea.

II. Transmission

Sexual contact with 1 to 3 week incubation period before symptoms present

III. Signs and Symptoms

    A. In the female
        1. Often no symptoms
        2. Possibly, increased vaginal discharge
        3. Cervicitis or an abnormal Papanicolaou smear
        4. Possibly, frequent uncomfortable urination
        5. Advanced symptoms include those of pelvic infection
    B. In the male
        1. Possibly, thick and cloudy discharge from the penis
        2. Possibly, painful urination and/or frequent urination

IV. Diagnosis

    A. Evaluation may include tests to rule out candidiasis, trichomoniasis, bacterial vaginosis, gonorrhea, syphilis, and urinary tract infection
    B. Vaginal and urethral smears are examined for the Chlamydia trachomatis organism

V. Treatment

Prescription medicine: _____

Take all the prescribed medicine, even though the symptoms may decrease early in treatment. Incomplete treatment gives the causative organism a chance to lie dormant and re-infect later.

VI. Patient Education

    A. Any sexual contacts should be advised to seek evaluation and treatment.

    B. Do not have intercourse until you and any sex partner(s) have completed treatment.

    C. In an untreated male or female the disease may progress to further reproductive infection with possible tissue scarring and infertility risks.

    D. Wash all sex toys, diaphragm, cervical cap with soap and water or soak in rubbing alcohol or betadine scrub. Be sure to rinse thoroughly.

VII. Follow-up

Return to clinician if symptoms persist or new symptoms occur.
Special notes: _____
Clinician: _____
For more information call: CDC STD Hotline: 1–800–227–8922:
Phone numbers of free (or almost free) STD clinics are listed in the Community Service Numbers in the government pages of your local phone book. http://www.cdc.gov; http://www.cdc.gov/std/Chlamydia/STDFact-Chlamydia.htm

From Hawkins, Roberto-Nichols & Stanley-Haney, *Guidelines for Nurse Practitioners in Gynecologic Settings,* 9th edition, 2007, © Springer Publishing Company.

CONSTIPATION

Constipation is a common problem and can be related to a number of factors. First, though, it is important to clarify what is meant by the term. Irregularity is another related term—it implies that there is some standard of regularity. Although many of us have been taught that daily bowel elimination (having at least one bowel movement "BM" daily) is normal, in fact for many persons normal is every 2 or 3 days.

Constipation occurs when one's regular pattern (whatever is normal for that person) changes so that the time between bowel movements lengthens, pain and/or straining are associated with them, and/or the bowel movements are very hard. Sometimes bleeding occurs because the fecal material (the stool) is hard and the person has to strain so much that there is damage to the rectum (lowest part of the bowel) or to the opening of the intestinal track (called the anal opening). There are other causes of bleeding, too, so if you ever have bleeding with a bowel movement, you should not ignore it.

Some causes of constipation are:

Stress. Stress can cause spastic constipation meaning tightening or spasm of the muscles in the large intestine; stress can also mean not taking time to eat properly, drink enough fluids, and/or go to the bathroom when your body signals you.

Diet. More about this later, but lack of roughage or fiber in the diet can cause constipation, as can lack of sufficient fluids, notably water.

Lack of Exercise. Having no active exercise on a regular basis can cause constipation.

Medications. Medications such as diuretics (water pills), iron pills, and calcium pills can cause constipation in some people, so pay attention to your body and to changes in your bowel movements when taking any medication.

Symptoms. Some diseases have constipation as a symptom, so be sure to tell your clinician if you continue to be constipated after trying the suggestions here.

What You Can Do About Constipation

1. Eat right. Select foods from those in the table below including lots of roughage or fiber in each day's diet. You can also add coarse bran to a bowl of cereal or to other foods.
2. Time. Take time when your body signals you; don't put off bowel evacuations.
3. Fluids. Fluid intake is very important to your general good health and especially for good bowel and bladder and kidney health. Six to eight glasses of water a day are recommended to prepare fecal material at the proper consistency for bowel elimination. In addition to water, add fruit juices, coffee, tea, and soda; the latter three can be irritating to your bladder or stomach or both (if caffeinated), so try to keep amounts limited and don't substitute these for water.
4. Exercise. Regular exercise (4 to 7 times a week) is important to general good health and also helps us to keep our regular (usual for us) bowel evacuation schedule. Walking, running, bicycling, swimming, working-out, active work routine (walking a lot, lifting and moving things), dancing, skating, sports such as tennis, soccer, touch football, basketball, volleyball, handball, racquetball, all help keep our body and its functions in shape.
5. Flavored or Unflavored Metamucil or store brand psyllium hydrophilic mucilloid fiber is useful if diet, exercise, and fluids

TABLE A.1   From Hawkins, Roberto-Nichols & Stanley-Haney,
Guidelines for Nurse Practitioners in Gynecologic Settings, **9th edition, 2007, © Springer Publishing Company.**

Food Group	Foods to Emphasize	Servings per day
Breads. cereals, grains	whole wheat bread, whole grains, bran cereals, rice, wheat germ, whole wheat pasta, popcorn, oats, rice cakes, granola, wheat bran	3–4 servings 1 cup or more
Fruits, fruit juices	dates, raisins, figs, apples, berries, melons, whole oranges, pears	3 or more fresh fruits
Vegetables	broccoli, cauliflower, peas, green & wax beans, brussel sprouts, lettuce, spinach, cabbage, celery, asparagus, artichokes, carrots, squash, turnips	3 or more , some raw vegetables
Miscellaneous	legumes (dried peas, kidney beans, navy beans)	varies with diet
Seeds, nuts	a variety of seeds and nuts (not tropical)	some each day

don't work for you. Mix a tablespoon in 8 or more ounces of water. Metamucil also comes in wafers (cookies) in several flavors. You can also try over-the-counter stool softeners such as dialose, kasof, and colace. Follow directions carefully about use; it is best to discuss this with your clinician. Stool softeners and sources of fiber are not harmful or habit forming, but you should try diet, fluids, and exercise first.

6. Laxatives. Laxatives, enemas, and drugs to cause you to evacuate your bowels can be harmful in the long run and should be used only after consulting a health care provider to rule out bowel disease as the cause of the constipation and after trying the measures discussed here.

CONTRACEPTIVE PATCH

I. Definition/Mechanism of Action

The contraceptive *patch* is a 3–layer transdermal polyethylene/polyester device about the size of a matchbook with an adhesive on one side. It is impregnated by a synthetic progestin, and a synthetic estrogen, and releases 150 micrograms of the progestin and 20 micrograms of the estrogen every 24 hours. The patch is changed weekly for 3 weeks, then is left off for 1 week. The patch causes suppression of ovulation, changes the lining of the uterus so it is not receptive to an egg, changes the cervical mucus so sperm cannot get through, changes the transportation of the egg down the fallopian tube, and possibly makes sperm less able to penetrate the egg.

II. Effectiveness

   A. 99% effectiveness
   B. Women weighing 90 (kg) or 198 pounds are at an increased risk for pregnancy. An alternative method is recommended.

III. Side Effects and Disadvantages

   A. Minor side effects
      1. Local irritation from patch
      2. Dislocation of patch
      3. Breast discomfort, tenderness
      4. Nausea
      5. Spotting
      6. Decreased menstrual flow (withdrawal bleeding), no bleeding
      7. Depression, mood changes
      8. Headaches
      9. Abdominal pain
   B. Risk factors
      1. Blood clots in legs, lungs, stroke
      2. Hypertension (high blood pressure)
      3. Gallbladder disease
      4. Heart attack (smokers 35 and older)
      5. Smoking increases risk associated with patch use. Women should not smoke and use the patch.

IV. Contraindications

   A. Women with a history of any of the following conditions may not be able to use the patch:
      1. Thromboembolic disorders—blood clots in legs, lungs
      2. Coronary artery disease
      3. Heart disease involving the heart valves with complications
      4. Severe hypertension (high blood pressure)
      5. Diabetes with vascular (blood vessel) involvement
      6. Headaches, migraines with neurological symptoms

7. Major surgery on legs or with prolonged immobility
8. Cancer of the breast or reproductive system
9. Undiagnosed genital bleeding
10. Impaired liver function, liver problems
11. Known or suspected pregnancy
12. Taking certain prescription drugs
13. Smoking
14. Weight equal to or greater than 198 pounds (90 kg); weight decreases effectiveness of patch
15. Skin disorders that may predispose to application-site reactions
16. Breastfeeding—not yet approved

V. Alternative Methods of Birth Control

A. Abstinence
B. Sterilization
C. Natural Family Planning
D. Condoms with contraceptive gel, foam, cream, jelly, suppositories, vaginal film
E. Intrauterine device
F. Diaphragm with contraceptive jelly, cream
G. FemCap, Lea's Shield
H. Contraceptive implant
I. Female condom
J. Depo-Provera injection
K. Progestin-only oral contraceptives
L. Contraceptive sponge

VI. Explanation of Method

A. Ways in which the patch is used
  1. Apply patch on first day of menses or on the first Sunday after bleeding begins; postpartum nonnursing 4 weeks or with resumption of menses. Apply to clean, dry, healthy skin on buttocks, abdomen, upper outer arm, or upper torso. Patch should not be applied to breasts.
  2. Do not use lotions, cosmetics, creams, powders, or other topical products in area of patch or area where patch will be applied.
  3. Press down firmly on patch for at least 10 seconds and then check that the edges adhere.
  4. Check patch daily.
  5. If patch detaches, immediately apply a new patch. Supplemental tapes or adhesives should not be used.

6. Apply a new patch the same day of the week 7 days after first patch. Repeat this in week 3.
7. No patch is applied in week 4.
8. Begin a new cycle on the same day of the week for week one and repeat cycle of 3 weeks on and 1 week off.
9. Withdrawal bleed (period) will occur during 4th week.
10. If you forget to apply a new patch and less than 48 hours have passed, you can apply a new patch as soon as you remember and then apply that next patch on the usual renewal day.
11. If more than 48 hours have elapsed, you should stop the current cycle and immediately begin a new 4-week cycle by applying a new patch. The day for patch renewal will now change. Use back-up contraception for 1 week.
12. If missed change day occurs at the end of the 4-week cycle, remove the patch and apply a new patch on the usual change day to begin a new cycle.

VII. Danger Signals Associated With Patch Use

A. Visual problems: Loss or blurring of vision, double vision, spots before eyes, flashing lights
B. Numbness or paralysis in any parts of body or face, even temporary
C. Unexplained chest pain
D. Painful inflamed areas along veins or severe calf pain
E. Severe recurrent headaches or new headaches or worsening of migraines

Note. Concerns have been raised due to higher exposure to estrogen as compared to most birth control pills. The FDA warning has been changed to indicate this. At this time the patch has not been recalled nor has there been an FDA warning to discontinue patch use. If you have concerns regarding this, consult your clinician.

Contact us at _____ if you develop any of the above problems.

From Hawkins, Roberto-Nichols, & Stanley-Haney, *Guidelines for Nurse Practitioners in Gynecologic Settings,* 9th edition, 2007, © Springer Publishing Company.

CONTRACEPTIVE VAGINAL RING (NUVARING)

I. Definition of Mechanism of Action

The contraceptive vaginal ring is flexible, transparent, colorless, and about 2 inches in diameter. It is impregnated with a synthetic progestin and a synthetic estrogen and releases 120 micrograms of progestin and 15 micrograms of estrogen every 24 hours over a period of 3 weeks. The ring is removed at the end of the third week and a new ring is inserted at the beginning of a new cycle, 1 week later. The ring causes suppression of ovulation, changes the lining of the uterus so it is not receptive to an egg, changes the cervical mucus so sperm cannot get through, changes the transportation of the egg down the fallopian tube, and possibly makes sperm less able to penetrate the egg.

II. Effectiveness

   A. 98–99% effectiveness

III. Side Effects and Disadvantages

   A. Minor side effects
      1. Vaginal irritation from the ring
      2. Dislocation of the ring
      3. Sensation of something in the vagina
      4. If ring is out more than 3 hours, need to use back-up contraception for 7 days

IV. Contraindications

   A. Women with a history of any of the following conditions may not be able to use the ring:
      1. Blood clots in your legs (thrombosis), lungs (pulmonary embolism), or eyes now or in the past
      2. Chest pain (angina pectoris)
      3. Heart attack or stroke
      4. Severe high blood pressure
      5. Pregnancy or suspected pregnancy
      6. Diabetes with complications of the kidney, eyes, nerves, or blood vessels
      7. Headaches with neurological symptoms
      8. Need for a long period of bedrest following major surgery
      9. Known or suspected cancer of the breast or cancer of the lining of the uterus, cervix, or vagina (now or in the past)
      10. Unexplained vaginal bleeding
      11. Yellowing of the whites of the eyes or of the skin (jaundice) during pregnancy or during past use of oral contraceptives (birth control pills)
      12. Liver tumors or active liver disease
      13. Disease of the heart valves with complications
      14. Allergic reaction to any of the components of the rings

15. Smoking and over age 35 (15 cigarettes a day or more)
16. Weight greater than or equal to 198 pounds (90 kg); excess weight decreases effectiveness of the ring
17. A prolapsed (dropped) uterus, dropped bladder (cystocele), or rectal prolapse (rectocele)
18. Under 35 and a heavy smoker (≥ 15 cigarettes/day)
19. Breast-feeding—not yet approved for use

V. Alternative Methods of Birth Control

A. Abstinence
B. Sterilization
C. Natural Family Planning
D. Condoms with contraceptive gel, foam, cream, jelly, suppositories, vaginal film
E. Intrauterine device
F. Diaphragm with contraceptive jelly, cream
G. FemCap, Lea's Shield
H. Female condom
I. Depo-Provera contraceptive injection
J. Contraceptive Patch
K. Oral contraceptives
L. Contraceptive implant
M. Contraceptive sponge

VI. Explanation of Method

A. Ways in which the ring is used
   1. Insert ring into vagina between day 1 and day 5 of menstrual cycle and note start day
   2. Keep ring in place for 3 weeks in a row
   3. Remove ring for one week for withdrawal bleeding
   4. If ring is removed from the vagina and is out for more than 3 hours, use back-up contraception for the next 7 days, except for the week with no ring

VII. Danger Signals Associated With Ring Use

   1. Visual problems
      a. Loss or blurring of vision, double vision
      b. Spots before eyes, flashing lights
   2. Numbness or paralysis in any parts of body or face, even temporary
   3. Unexplained chest pain
   4. Painful inflamed areas along veins or severe calf pain

5. Severe recurrent headaches or new headaches or worsening of migraines

Contact us at _____ if you develop any of the above problems. Web Site for ring information: http://www.organoninc.com; http://www. nuvaring.com.

From Hawkins, Roberto-Nichols, & Stanley-Haney, *Guidelines for Nurse Practitioners in Gynecologic Settings,* 9th edition, 2007, © Springer Publishing Comp

CONTRACEPTIVE SHIELD: LEA'S SHIELD

I. Definition/Mechanism of Action

Lea's Shield is a silicone device similar to a diaphragm that is used to hold spermicide and to provide a partial barrier to sperm when placed over the cervix. It is an elliptical bowl in shape and the posterior end has a reservoir for spermicide. There is a valve in the middle to allow cervical secretions to drain and also to relieve pressure against the cervix. There is a molded loop to aid in removal. Insertion is similar to using a diaphragm.

II. Effectiveness and Benefits

    A. 86% effectiveness—has not been in use long, so information is scarce
    B. May be inserted before intercourse and left in place for up to 48 hours
    C. Latex free
    D. Reusable for more than a year

III. Side Effects and Disadvantages

    A. Minor side effects
        1. Vaginal irritation from the device
        2. Vaginal irritation from the spermicide used with the device
        3. Sensation of something in the vagina
        4. Difficulty in removing
        5. Requires prescription

IV. Contraindications

    A. Allergy to spermicide
    B. Allergy to silicone
    C. Partner allergy to silicone or spermicide
    D. Device is expelled repeatedly during use

E. Cannot be used during menses
F. Known or suspected uterine or cervical cancer
G. History of toxic shock syndrome
H. Current infection of vagina or cervix, PID
I. Cannot be used during postpartum or after an abortion for 6 weeks

V. Alternative Methods of Birth Control

A. Abstinence
B. Sterilization
C. Natural Family Planning
D. Condoms with contraceptive gel, foam, cream, jelly, suppositories, vaginal film
E. Intrauterine device
F. Diaphragm with contraceptive jelly, cream, FemCap, sponge
G. Female condom
H. Depo-Provera injection
I. Contraceptive Patch, Ring, implant
J. Oral contraceptives

VI. Types

A. Available in 1 size

VII. Fitting

A. Pelvic examination to rule out any problems that might occur with use and to evaluate size and position of cervix
B. Follow-up for any concerns, problems; annual examination
Web site: http://www.leasshield.com.
From Hawkins, Roberto-Nichols, & Stanley-Haney, *Guidelines for Nurse Practitioners in Gynecologic Settings*, 9th edition, 2007, © Springer Publishing Company.

SPERMICIDES AND CONDOMS

Spermicides

I. Definition/Mechanism of Action

Spermicides are a barrier method of birth control. All contain an inert base or vehicle and an active ingredient, most commonly a surfactant such as nonoxynol-9 that disrupts the integrity of the sperm membrane (acts as a spermicide).

II. Effectiveness and Benefits

    A. Method: 96% effectiveness rate
    B. User: 60% effectiveness rate
    C. Inexpensive and readily available

III. Side Effects and Disadvantages

    A. Local irritation from spermicide
    B. Can necessitate interruption of lovemaking
    C. Emotional difficulty with touching ones own body

IV. Types

    A. Creams, jellies, gels
    B. Foams
    C. Foaming tablets
    D. Suppositories
    E. Vaginal film

V. How to Use

    A. Instructions should be read prior to using any spermicide. Method of insertion, time of effectiveness, time needed prior to intercourse, etc., will vary with each type
    B. Use new insertion of spermicide with each intercourse
    C. After each use, wash the applicator with soap and water
    D. When using a spermicide, partner should always use a condom unless you use female condom

VI. Follow-up

    A. Yearly physical examination with Papanicolaou smear is recommended

Condoms

I. Definition/Mechanism of Action

Condoms are thin sheaths, most commonly made of latex (female condoms are made of polyurethane; male polyurethane condoms are now on the market) that prevent the transmission of sperm from the penis to the vagina.

II. Effectiveness and Benefits

    A. Method: 97 to 98% effectiveness rate, providing the method is used correctly

B. User: 70 to 94% effectiveness rate

C. Inexpensive and readily available

D. Offer protection against sexually transmitted disease. Only latex condoms provide protection against the AIDS (HIV) virus. The female condom is made of thick polyurethane so it does offer protection.

E. Encourage male participation in birth control

III. Side Effects and Disadvantages

A. Allergic reaction to latex (rare). (Female condom is polyurethane as are some male condoms.)

B. Use necessitates interruption of lovemaking for application

C. May decrease tactile sensation

D. Psychological impotency with male condom

E. If latex allergy is a problem, double condom use is an option. If the woman is allergic, the male can wear a latex condom with a skin or polyurethane condom covering it. If the man is allergic, he can wear a polyurethane or skin condom with a latex condom over it. Skin condoms should not be worn alone since they do not offer protection from HIV.

IV. Types

Condoms vary in color, texture (smooth, studded, or ribbed), shape, and price; they come lubricated and plain; some have spermicide; some are extra strength, some sheerer and thinner, some have a unique shape; some are scented or flavored.

V. How to Use Male Condom

A. Always pull the male condom on an erect penis and before there is any sexual contact. Use for every act of intercourse.

B. Do not pull the male condom tightly over the end of the penis; leave about an inch extra for ejaculation fluid and to avoid breakage; some condoms have a reservoir tip.

C. Withdraw before the penis becomes limp and hold the open end of the condom tightly while withdrawing.

D. Partner should always use a contraceptive spermicide along with condom.

E. Condoms should be used only once.

VI. How to Use Female Condom

The female condom comes pre-lubricated.

A. Pinch ring at closed end of pouch and insert like a diaphragm covering the cervix; adding 1 to 2 drops of additional lubricant makes insertion easier and decreases or eliminates squeaking noise and dislocation during intercourse.

B. Adjust other ring over labia.

C. Can be inserted several minutes to 8 hours prior to intercourse.

D. Remove before standing up by squeezing and twisting the outer ring and pulling out gently.

If the condom breaks or slips off, check Web site http://not-2 late. com for emergency contraception information. Plan B is now available over the counter for women 18 years of age and older.

From Hawkins, Roberto-Nichols, & Stanley-Haney, *Guidelines for Nurse Practitioners in Gynecologic Settings,* 9th edition, 2007, © Springer Publishing Company.

CYSTITIS (BLADDER INFECTION)

Cystitis, a bladder infection, is usually caused by bacteria. Women are more prone to cystitis because the urethra (connection between the bladder and the outside through which we urinate or pee) is short and the vagina and rectum are close to the opening of the urethra, called the urethral meatus. However, men can also develop cystitis.

Symptoms

1. Frequent urination of small amounts of urine; often you will experience urgency feeling of needing to urinate and then just urinating a little
2. Burning, pain, or difficulty in urinating
3. Blood in the urine
4. Pain in the lower part of the abdomen (pelvic pain) around the pubic bone
5. Chills, fever

Treatment

Treatment of cystitis is with an antibiotic. It is important that you tell your clinician if you are allergic to any antibiotics or to sulfonamides so that you are given a suitable medication.

You may be asked to give what is called a clean catch urine specimen prior to the diagnosis (as opposed to just urinating in a paper cup for the specimen). For the clean catch specimen, you will be given special wipes to use on your perineal area and instructions on collecting the urine specimen in a sterile container. This specimen will be sent to the laboratory to evaluate the bacteria in the urine and to see what sulfonamides or antibiotics will be effective against the bacteria.

It is important to take the entire prescription given to you even if symptoms disappear quickly. Follow the directions for times to take the medication and try not to skip a dose as this may allow the bacteria to increase in number. You may also be given a prescription for a bladder pain medication or information about over-the-counter medication (Aso-Standard, Uristat) to take away the bladder pain. These bladder pain medications are to be used with, and not instead of, the antibiotic or sulfonamide as they only relieve bladder pain and have no effect on the bacteria causing your cystitis.

Things You Can Do About Cystitis (Bladder Infection)

There are several things you can do to avoid cystitis and to help your body heal when you have cystitis, more commonly known as a bladder infection.

1. After going to the bathroom, wipe from front to back, or wipe the front first and then the back, so as not to carry bacteria from your rectal area to the vaginal area where your urethral opening (opening into the bladder) is located. A woman's urethra is quite short, so bacteria can travel into the bladder quite easily.
2. If your lovemaking includes vaginal or oral contact after anal contact, you might consider washing off your genitals and those of your partner before proceeding with vaginal and/or oral sex.
3. During a tub bath, it is better not to use bath oils and bubble bath, because these help bacteria travel up your urethra.
4. Try to empty your bladder before sex, and after sex empty your bladder as soon as you can to wash bacteria from your urethra, particularly if you seem to get cystitis easily (several times a year).
5. Tight clothing, especially clothes made of synthetic fabrics such as polyester, helps bacteria grow more easily by creating a warm, dark, moist environment. Cotton underpants and loose clothing help your body breathe and discourage bacterial growth.
6. Always urinate when you have the urge; don't put it off until you are desperate. Bacteria grow better in urine that is sitting in your bladder for a long period of time.
7. Drink 6–8 glasses of water and juice a day; cranberry juice helps to decrease cystitis. Cranberry is also available as Azo-Cranberry® cranberry juice capsules with 450 milligrams of cranberry juice concentrate; the dose is 1–4 capsules per day with meals.
8. Caffeine is a bladder irritant, meaning it can cause bladder pain or spasms (cramps), so the less caffeine you take in, the less bladder irritation you will experience. Caffeine is in coffee, tea,

chocolate, and many carbonated beverages even if they are not colas. Check labels.

9. Smoking (nicotine) is also very irritating to the bladder.
10. A well-balanced diet including 6 or more servings of fresh fruits and vegetables a day and 3–4 servings of whole grain breads, cereals, and pasta, will increase your resistance to infection.

Cystitis is the least serious of the urinary tract infections. Untreated, it can lead to infection of the rest of the urinary tract including the ureters (connecting bladder and kidneys) and the kidneys. Prompt and correct treatment of cystitis will help you avoid having a more serious urinary tract infection. If your symptoms worsen or do not get better with the treatment prescribed by your clinician, call or return to the health care setting for further help.

Web sites: http://www.mayoclinic.com/health/cystitis/DS00285; http://www.niddk.nih.gov/health/urolog/pubs/cystitis/cystitis.htm.

From Hawkins, Roberto-Nichols, & Stanley-Haney, *Guidelines for Nurse Practitioners in Gynecologic Settings,* 9th edition, 2007, © Springer Publishing Company, LLC.

FEMCAP

I. Definition of Mechanism of Action

The contraceptive FemCap is a prescription-only contraceptive device that is used to hold spermicide and to provide a partial barrier to sperm when placed over the cervix. Available in 3 sizes: 22 mm, 26 mm, 30 mm. Your clinician will examine you and advise on size.

II. Effectiveness

    A. 96–98% effectiveness

III. Side Effects and Disadvantages

    A. Minor side effects
        1. Vaginal irritation from the device
        2. Vaginal irritation from the spermicide used with the device
        3. Sensation of something in the vagina
        4. Requires a pelvic examination and prescription for the device

IV. Contraindications

    A. Allergy to spermicide

B. Allergy to material device is made of
C. Partner allergy to device or spermicide
D. Device is expelled repeatedly during use
E. Cannot be used during menses
F. Known or suspected uterine or cervical cancer
G. History of toxic shock syndrome
H. Current infection of vagina or cervix
I. Abnormality of cervix, uterus, or vagina
J. Cannot be used during postpartum or after an abortion for 6 weeks

V. Alternative Methods of Birth Control

A. Abstinence
B. Sterilization
C. Natural Family Planning
D. Condoms with contraceptive gel, foam, cream, jelly, suppositories, vaginal film
E. Intrauterine device
F. Diaphragm with contraceptive jelly, cream, Lea's Shield, sponge
G. Female condom
H. Depo-Provera injection
I. Contraceptive Patch, Ring, implant
J. Oral contraceptives

VI. Explanation of Method

A. Ways in which the device is used (FemCap comes with instructional video)
   1. Insert spermicide into the device according to directions by manufacturer and place in the vagina over the cervix before any sexual arousal.
   2. Keep device in place for at least 6 hours after last act of intercourse.
   3. Add additional spermicide to outside of device for each repeated act of intercourse within next 48 hours. Do not remove device to add spermicide.
   4. Remove FemCap by squatting and bearing down. Slip finger between the dome and the removal strap and pull gently.
   5. Wash device thoroughly with antibacterial hand soap, rinse thoroughly in clear water, and allow to air dry.

Contact us at _____ if you have any questions or develop any problems. You will need to return for a Pap smear after first three months of use.

From Hawkins, Roberto-Nichols, & Stanley-Haney, *Guidelines for Nurse Practitioners in Gynecologic Settings,* 9th edition, 2007, © Springer Publishing Company.

GENITAL HERPES SIMPLEX

I. Definition

The herpes *simplex* virus is one of the most common infectious agents of humans. It is transmitted only by direct contact with the virus from an active infected oral or genital lesion. The herpes simplex virus (HSV) is of two types:

HSV Type 1: Usually affects body sites above the waist (mouth, lips, eyes, fingers)
HSV Type 2: Usually involves body sites below the waist, primarily the genitals.

Genital herpes may be caused by either HSV 1 or 2. If oral sex is practiced, remember that cold sores are herpes lesions and can be spread to the genital area. The cause, symptoms, complications, diagnosis, treatment, and patient education are the same for males and females.

II. Symptoms
 A. Painful, itchy sores similar to cold sores or fever blisters, surrounded by reddened skin, that appear around the mouth, nipples or genital areas 4 to 7 days up to 4 weeks after contact
 B. Fever or flu-like symptoms
 C. Burning sensation during urination
 D. Swollen groin lymph nodes
 E. Symptoms may last 2 to 3 weeks

III. Diagnosis
 A. Examination based on your clinical symptoms and history
 B. Laboratory analysis of discharge from the lesions to identify virus
 C. Blood test for HSV-1, HSV-2 antibodies in your blood

IV. Treatment
 A. Tepid bath with or without the addition of iodine solution
 B. Unrestrictive clothing

C. Prevent secondary infection
D. Medication for pain
E. There are topical and oral medications that do not cure the infection but can shorten the duration and severity of symptoms and decrease recurrence; these medications may, in some cases, be taken on a long-term basis to suppress virus

V. Complications

A. Secondary infection of herpes lesions
B. Severe systemic and life-threatening infections in infants born vaginally during an episode of herpes in the mother

VI. Recurrences

Herpes sores may never recur after the first episode or there may be occasional flare-ups, not as painful as the initial infection, lasting up to 7 days. Recurring infections may be related to stress (physical or emotional), illness, fever, overexposure to sun, or menstruation. Recurrences are due to a reactivation of the virus already present in the nerve endings of your body.

VII. Patient Education

A. After urinating, wash the genital area with cool water.
B. If urinating is difficult, sit in a tub of warm water to urinate.
C. Cool, wet tea bags applied to the lesions may offer some relief.
D. Avoid intercourse when active lesions are present. If intercourse does occur, condoms should be used.
E. Women with chronic herpes should have a Pap smear yearly.

Medication: _____
Special notes: _____
Clinician: _____

For more information:

1. CDC STD Hotline: 1–800–227–8922: Phone numbers of free (or almost free) STD clinics are listed in the Community Service Numbers in the government pages of your local phone book.
2. Seek out local rap and support groups
3. Try resources on the Internet: http://www.cdc.gov; alt.support. herpes (usenet news group); http://www.herpes.com; http://www.ashastd.org/herpes/hrc.html

From Hawkins, Roberto-Nichols, & Stanley-Haney, *Guidelines for Nurse Practitioners in Gynecologic Settings,* 9th edition, 2007, © Springer Publishing Company.

GENITAL WARTS (CONDYLOMATA ACUMINATA)

I. Definition

Genital warts, or condylomata acuminata, may occur on either the male or female genital areas. The virus family causing the warts is believed to be sexually transmitted, although warts have been found on individuals whose partner has no history or sign of warts. The human papilloma virus family has more than 150 types, some of which cause warts on the genitals, nipples, umbilicus, hands, soles of the feet, cervix, vagina, penis, scrotum, and rectal area. Some HPV types are associated with cancers of the cervix, penis, mouth, anus, lungs, and other parts of the body.

II. Signs and Symptoms

Warts may not appear until two weeks to many months (or even years after exposure).

    A. In moist areas, the warts are small, often itchy bumps or lumps, sometimes with a cauliflower-like top, appearing singly or in clusters.

    B. On dry skin (such as the shaft of the penis), the warts commonly are small, hard, and yellowish-gray, resembling warts that appear on other parts of the body.

    C. On the female, the warts are commonly found on or around the vaginal opening, vaginal lips, in the vagina, around the rectum, and on the cervix.

    D. On the male, the warts can be found on any part of the penis, scrotum, or rectal area.

III. Diagnosis

    A. The diagnosis is usually obvious on the basis of appearance of the warts, but sometimes a microscopic examination is necessary to identify minute lesions.

    B. Laboratory tests may include checking for gonorrhea, Chlamydia, and syphilis, HIV/AIDS, and a Papanicolaou smear if none within a year.

IV. Treatment

    A. If small, the warts may be treated by several weekly applications of medication by you or your clinician.

    B. Patients with large, persistent warts or warts in the vagina or on the cervix may be referred to a physician for treatment. Some treatments include cryotherapy (freezing) and lasering the warts.

V. Patient Education

    A. Always advise sexual partners to see a clinician for examination.

    B. Having warts may increase vaginal discharge; have it checked and treated.

    C. Treatment medication is applied weekly by the clinician in office or clinic. Some of the drugs used must be rinsed off in 4 hours. Your clinician will advise you. Certain treatment medication should never be used in pregnant patients. If pregnancy is suspected, tell your clinician.

    D. You may be given medication for self-treatment and separate instructions on how to do this.

    E. Recurrence is possible without re-infection, as treatment does not always eradicate very small warts. Microscopic examination and treatment by a specialist may be necessary.

    F. A woman with a history of warts, especially if on the cervix, is encouraged to have an annual gynecological examination with a Pap smear as recommended by her clinician (often twice a year).

    G. A vaccine Gardasil is now available for girls who are pre-adolescent, adolescents, and young women. It protects against 4 types of HPV—two associated with genital warts and two associated with cervical cancer.

Special notes: _____

Clinician: _____

For more information and/or care for friends:

CTD STD Hotline: 1–800–227–8922 Phone numbers of free (or almost free) STD (VD) clinics are listed in the Community Service Numbers in the government pages of your local phone book. Web sites: http://www. nci.nih.gov; http://www.ashastd.org; http://www.cdc.gov/std/hpv/; http://www.cdc.gov/std/hpv/STDFact-HPV-vaccine-hcp.htm.

From Hawkins, Roberto-Nichols, & Stanley-Haney, *Guidelines for Nurse Practitioners in Gynecologic Settings*, 9th edition, 2007, © Springer Publishing Company.

Self-Treatment for Genital Warts (Condylomata Acuminata)

Condylox® is a prescription treatment for genital warts that you can use at home. Fill your Condylox® prescription at any drugstore or the pharmacy in a department store. The Condylox® package contains directions for use of the medication.[1] Please read these carefully and use the medication as directed. It is important to follow these directions and those of your clinician to assure the maximum possible effect from the medication.

Condylox® works by destroying the wart tissue. This does not happen all at once, but gradually. The wart will change in color, from skin color to a dry, crusted, dead appearance, and then disappear. You may feel some pain or burning when applying the Condylox® as these changes occur. You may also see some redness, have some soreness or tenderness at the wart sites, and may even see small sores in that area. These symptoms usually disappear within a week after you have completed the treatment. If any of these changes are severe or concern you, stop the treatment and contact your clinician.

Treating Your Warts

Treat your warts twice a day with Podofilox (Condylox®). (It is okay to do so even if you get your menstrual period during the time you are treating your warts.) Plan a time in the morning and again in the evening to apply the medication. Repeat the twice-a-day treatments for 3 days and then do not treat the warts again for 4 days. You can repeat this pattern of treatment—3 days of medication and then 4 days off—for up to 4 weeks. Stop the treatment, however, as soon as the warts disappear. It is important that you do not treat the warts in any week for more than 3 days as such treatment will not help them to disappear faster and may cause you to have side effects from the medication.

If you have completed 4 weeks of treatment and still have warts, return to your clinician for further evaluation, and do not use Condylox® until you have this check-up.

Remove any clothing over the affected area and wash your hands before treating your warts. Open the bottle of Condylox® and place it on a flat surface so it will not spill while you are treating your warts. It may be helpful to use a hand mirror to locate the warts so that you can treat them. Good light is also important so that you do not get medication on skin that is free of warts.

Holding onto the bottle to steady it, dip the tip of one cotton tip applicator (Q-tip) into the medication. The tip should be wet with the medication, but not dripping. Remove any excess medication by pressing the applicator tip against the inside of the bottle. Apply the Condylox® only to those areas you and your clinician have identified as warts.

Try not to get any Condylox® on any area of your skin that is not a wart. If the wart is on a skin fold, gently spread the skin with one hand to flatten out the wart and touch the medication applicator to the area with the other hand. Allow the Condylox® to dry before letting skin folds relax into normal position and before putting clothing over the affected area.

After application, throw away the Q-tip. Close the bottle tightly to prevent evaporation of the medication and wash your hands carefully when you are finished with the treatment.

If you are using Condylox® gel, follow the same treatment schedule as for the liquid. Wash your hands before treating your warts. Squeeze out a small amount of gel (about half the size of a pea) onto your fingertip. Dab a small amount of the gel onto the warts or the areas your clinician has instructed you to treat. Try not to get any of the gel on normal skin areas. For warts in skin folds, spread the folds apart and apply the gel to the wart, letting the area dry before you return the skin folds to their normal position. Wash your hands carefully after completing the treatment.

The area you have treated may sting when you apply the gel. It may also become red, sore, itchy, or tender after treatment.

Precautions in Self-Treatment

Podofilox (Condylox®) is intended only for treatment of venereal warts and only on the outside of the body. It is not safe to use podofilox on any other skin condition. If you have severe pain, bleeding, swelling, or itching, stop the treatment and contact your clinician. Do not get this medication in your eyes. If you do so accidentally, flush your eyes immediately with running water and call your clinician. The effects of podofilox on pregnancy are unknown, so it is not safe to use this medication during pregnancy.

Follow-up Care

It is important to return for a check-up as suggested by your clinician or if you have completed 4 weeks of treatment and still have warts. If the warts reappear after you have completed treatment, contact your clinician prior to restarting treatment. Your partner should also be checked and treated for any warts; otherwise, you can be reinfected.

Web site: www.rxlist.com/cgi/generic/podofil_ids.htm.

Self-treatment With Imiquimod Cream 5% (Aldara®)[2]

Aldara® is a prescription treatment for genital warts that you can use at home. Fill your Aldara® prescription at any drugstore or pharmacy in a department store. The Aldara® package contains directions for use of the medication. Please read these carefully and use the medication only as directed.

Aldara® probably works by boosting your body's immune response to the wart virus (there are over 150 types of wart virus, called human papilloma virus or HPV). Aldara® should be used only on warts outside the vagina, on the labia, and the area around your anus.

Treating Your Warts

Careful handwashing before and after application of the cream is recommended so that you do not experience a secondary bacterial infection in the wart area and get the cream on other parts of your body. Apply Aldara® three times a week just prior to your normal sleeping hours. Apply a thin layer of the cream to all external genital warts and rub it in until it is no longer visible. Leave Aldara® on the skin for 6–10 hours. Don't cover the treated area. Following this treatment period, remove the cream by washing the treated area with mild soap and water. Continue treatment until the warts disappear. Do not continue treatment past 16 weeks without consulting your clinician.

Precautions in Treatment

Aldara® cream may weaken condoms and vaginal diaphragms, so do not use these while you are treating your warts. Sexual (genital) contact should be avoided while the Aldara® cream is on the skin. Common reactions to Aldara® include redness, burning, swelling, itching, rash, soreness, stinging, and tenderness. If any of these occur, wash the cream off with mild soap and water. Do not re-treat until these symptoms are gone. For any questions, call your clinician. A very small percentage of persons have flu-like symptoms, fever, fatigue, headache, diarrhea, and/or achy joints. If you experience any of these, call your clinician.

Web site: www.3m.com/us/healthcare/pharma/aldara/index.jhtm.

From Hawkins, Roberto-Nichols, & Stanley-Haney, *Guidelines for Nurse Practitioners in Gynecologic Settings,* 9th edition, 2007, © Springer Publishing Company.

GONORRHEA

I. Definition

Gonorrhea is an acute infection that is spread by sexual contact and involves the genitourinary tract, throat, and rectum of both sexes. It is caused by the organism Neisseria gonorrhoea.

II. Important Information

    A. The highest incidence of gonorrhea occurs in males between the ages of 20 and 24 and in females from 18 and 24. Gonorrhea is usually contracted from an infected person who has ignored symptoms or has no symptoms. This source can reinfect the patient, or possibly infect others unknowingly.

    B. Incubation: 1 to 13 days. Symptoms can occur 3 to 30 days after sexual contact; average is 2 to 5 days after exposure.

III. Usual Signs and Symptoms

    A. Females
        1. Up to 80% have no symptoms
        2. Abnormal, thick green vaginal discharge
        3. Frequency, pain on urination
        4. Urethral discharge
        5. Rectal pain and discharge
        6. Unilateral labial pain and swelling
        7. Abnormal menstrual bleeding; increased dysmenorrhea (menstrual cramps)
        8. Lower abdominal discomfort
        9. Sore throat
    B. Males
        1. 4–10% have no symptoms
        2. Frequency, pain on urination
        3. Burning sensation in the urethra
        4. Whitish discharge from the penis (early); may appear only as a drop during erection
        5. Yellow or greenish discharge from the penis (late)
        6. Sore throat

IV. Diagnosis (for Both Sexes)

    A. History of sexual contact with a person known to be infected with gonorrhea

    B. Smears and cultures taken from infected areas (cervix, penis, rectum, and throat)

V. Treatment for Males and Females

Antibiotics will be prescribed and are effective if taken according to directions. Be sure to tell your clinician if you are allergic to any antibiotic.

VI. Complications

    A. Females: If gonorrhea goes untreated, it may lead to pelvic inflammatory disease (PID). PID involves severe abdominal cramps, pelvic pain, and high fever that will lead to scarring and possible blockage of the fallopian tubes, the risk of tubal pregnancy, and infertility.

    B. Males: If gonorrhea goes untreated, scar tissue may form on the sperm passageway causing pain and sterility.

    C. Females and males: The infection may spread throughout the body causing arthritis, sometimes with skin lesions.

VII. Patient Education (for Both Sexes)

    A. All medication must be taken as directed.

    B. No intercourse until treatment of self and partner(s) is completed.

    C. Return to the clinician for reevaluation if symptoms persist or new symptoms occur after treatment is complete.

    D. Important: The responsible lover informs all partners immediately upon finding out about exposure to sexually transmitted disease so that all persons involved can be evaluated adequately and treated immediately.

Special notes: _____

Clinician: _____

For more information and for care of friends: CDC STD Hotline, 1-800-227-8922. For phone numbers of free (or almost free) STD clinics see the Community Service Numbers in the government pages of your local phone book. Web sites: http://www.cdc.gov; http://www.cdc.gov/std/Gonorrhea/STDFact-gonorrhea.htm.

    From Hawkins, Roberto-Nichols, & Stanley-Haney, *Guidelines for Nurse Practitioners in Gynecologic Settings,* 9th edition, 2007, © Springer Publishing Company.

HORMONE THERAPY (HT)

I. Definition

Hormone therapy is the use of synthetic hormones (estrogen, progesterone, and/or testosterone) by postmenopausal women. Now known as HT, the use of hormones after menopause was once known as estrogen therapy (ET) because women were given synthetic estrogen only.

II. Reasons for Taking HT

A woman's body produces declining amounts of estrogens, progesterones, and androgens during the perimenopausal period, culminating
in the cessation of menstrual cycles (ovulation and bleeding). After 12
months without any bleeding (periods), you can consider that you are
postmenopausal. A woman is said to have gone through surgical menopause if she has had her tubes, ovaries, and uterus removed.

Some natural estrogen production does continue after natural menopause; heavier women produce more estrogen because fat cells convert
body chemicals called precursors to estrone, the most common form of
natural estrogen in menopause.

Decline in natural estrogen production contributes to such menopausal symptoms as loss of elasticity of the vagina, a less lush vaginal lining causing a feeling of itching or burning or dryness, and pain around the
urethra (the opening to the urinary bladder). Hot flashes or hot flushes,
including night sweats, characterize menopause for some women. There
may also be a relationship between menopause and loss of bone density
leading to osteoporosis.

III. What You Should Know When Considering HT

IIT should never be taken by women who have vaginal bleeding after menopause until the cause of the bleeding is discovered. Pregnant
women or perimenopausal women who suspect pregnancy cannot take
HT. If you have ever had a stroke, heart attack, or a blood clot in your
legs or lungs, liver disease, or any problems with the function of your
liver, you may not be an HT candidate. Women with known or suspected cancer of the breast, ovaries, uterus, or cervix may not be good
candidates for HT.

A number of conditions require special evaluation to determine if
taking HT will be safe. These include undiagnosed vaginal bleeding,
known or suspected pregnancy, a history of blood clots in your lungs
or legs, known or suspected cancer of the breast or reproductive tract
or malignant melanoma, history of bleeding disorder treated with blood
transfusion, active gallbladder disease, family history of breast cancer,
migraine headaches, elevated triglycerides, a ratio of good to bad cholesterol that is concerning, and endometriosis.

Considering HT is a decision that is yours to make if you and your
clinician decide you have no contraindications to its use. To make the best
decision, you and your clinician will discuss whether you are at greater
risk of loss of bone density leading to osteoporosis because of your family
or personal history, whether you have risk factors for developing osteoporosis, and your personal and family medical history including heart

disease. Your desire for taking HT as well as your access to health care for monitoring HT will be considered. Some clinicians recommend that a sample of the lining of your uterus be analyzed before beginning HT, with a repeat of this test, called an endometrial biopsy, every year. An annual mammogram for women 40 and older, as well as a Pap smear, based on your medical and surgical history, are important to your well-being.

IV. Evaluating Your Physical Risks and Benefits in Taking HT

In addition to a careful personal and family history, your clinician will recommend that you have a complete physical exam including a pelvic (internal) exam and Pap smear, and testing for infections such as vaginitis, sexually transmitted diseases, and bladder infection (cystitis) if you have any signs or symptoms. Testing might also include: a mammogram if you have not had one in the past year, examination of hormone levels, an endometrial biopsy, a lipid profile to determine your cholesterol level and the ratio of low density lipids (LDL—the bad ones) to high density lipids (HDL—the good ones), a hematocrit and/or hemoglobin to see if you are anemic, a bone density scan, and an electrocardiogram (EKG) if you have never had one and/or have a family history of heart disease. Other testing will depend upon findings from the physical exam and your personal and family health history.

For some women, the benefits of taking HT outweigh the risks. For others, the risks and benefits balance, and for still others, the risks outweigh the benefits.

V. Taking HT

If your uterus has been removed (hysterectomy) you will take estrogen only without progestin. You and your clinician will decide which estrogen is best for you, both the amount and the way you take it (in pill form, the patch, or as a vaginal cream, suppository, or vaginal ring). If you still have your uterus, you may take both estrogen and a progestin patch, pill, or intrauterine device. Some women bleed when taking progestin, so you and your clinician will need to decide what is best for you.

As androgen levels drop with menopause, some women also take a small amount of male hormone (androgen), which may help women whose menopausal symptoms are not resolved with estrogen or estrogen and progestin alone, have a decreased sense of well-being, a lower libido (sex drive), and/or generalized loss of energy (lethargy).

VI. Consider Alternatives and Adjuncts to HT

All women need a diet with at least 6–8 servings of fruit and vegetables a day, several servings of complex carbohydrates such as breads and pasta; sources of protein including dairy products, eggs, meat, fish, and poultry; and legumes such as beans, peas, and calcium. Women also need to decrease fat to 30 percent or less of total calories daily through using nonfat dairy products (rich in protein and calcium), limiting red meat, and eating lean meat, poultry, and fish. Whole grain pastas, cereals and breads, bran, vegetables, and fruit add roughage to the diet. Most women need calcium supplements. Postmenopausal women need a total of 1500 milligrams each day of calcium as well as 400–800 international units of vitamin D. Six to eight 8-ounce glasses of water daily will help keep all tissues healthy and promote both bowel and bladder health. Consider adding phytoestrogens to diet and essential fatty acids in recommended amounts.

Regular weight-bearing exercise and strength training are critical to maintenance of bone density; 30 to 45 minutes four to six times a week is recommended. Some women build this exercise into their daily routines by walking on errands and at work and using stairs instead of elevators. Botanicals, Chinese remedies, vitamins, nonhormonal vaginal lubricants such as KY jelly, KY liquid, Lubrin®, Vagisil®, Replens®, and Astroglide®, naturalistic interventions, and homeopathic preparations can be helpful supplements to or alternatives to HT. Because herbs and homeopathic remedies can interact with each other and with prescription and over-the-counter medications, it is best to consult a practitioner who specializes in their use. Your local library, health food store, bookstore, and health care providers are all sources of information about caring for yourself after menopause.

Menopause: Another change of life, http://www.ppfa.org.ppfa/menopub/html; National Institute on Aging, http://www.pueblo.gsa.gov/cic-text/health/other/menopause.txt; Power Surge, http://www.dearest.com/refer.htm; http://www.allwise.com

From Hawkins, Roberto-Nichols, & Stanley-Haney, *Guidelines for Nurse Practitioners in Gynecologic Settings,* 9th edition, 2007, © Springer Publishing Company.

LICE (PEDICULOSIS)

I. Definition

Pediculosis means having the skin infested with lice, particularly on hairy areas such as the scalp, underarms, and the pubic area. Three types of lice prey on humans: head lice *(p. capitis),* body lice *(p. corposis),* and pubic lice or crab lice *(p. pubis).*

II. Transmission

Lice are transmitted by lice-infected shared clothing, bedding, brushes, towels, pillows, and upholstered furniture, or by close personal contact with an infected person. Head lice move from head to head. Adult pubic lice probably survive no more than 24 hours off their host.

III. Signs and Symptoms

    A. Intense itching
    B. Observing the lice or, more easily, their nits (eggs), which are greenish-white ovals attached to hair shafts in eyebrows, eyelashes, scalp hair, pubic hair, and other body hair.
    C. Known exposure to household member or intimate partner with lice
    D. Crusts or scabs on body from scratching
    E. Enlargement of lymph nodes (swollen glands) in the neck, an allergic response to lice
    F. Body lice found on clothing, especially in the seams, as lice are rarely found on the body
    G. Black dots (representing excreta) on skin and underclothing

IV. Diagnosis

See Signs and Symptoms above. Lice can best be detected by using a magnifying glass or microscope

V. Treatment

    A. General measures
        1. Wash clothing, towels, etc., with hot water, or dry clean contaminated items or run them through a dryer on heat cycle to destroy nits and lice; wash combs and hairbrushes in hot, soapy water. Items can also be sealed in a plastic bag for 2 weeks; lice will suffocate. Or items can be put outside in cold weather for 10 days.
        2. Spray couches, chairs, car seats, and items that can't be washed or dry cleaned with over-the-counter products (A-200 Pyrinate®, Triplex®, RID, or store brand products); alternative is to vacuum carefully to pick up lice and nits.
    B. Specific measures
        1. Head lice
            a. Thoroughly wet hair with Permithin 1% cream rinse applied to affected areas and washed off after 10 minutes or Triplex Kit (Pronto (piperonyl), RID shampoo or R&C shampoo or End Lice; work up lather, adding water as necessary; shampoo thoroughly leaving shampoo on head for 5 minutes; rinse, or use Pronto shampoo/conditioner or

Clear® lice killing shampoo and lice egg remover per directions on product or Klout® per directions on product.

   b. Rinse thoroughly, towel dry.

   c. Remove remaining nits with fine-tooth metal comb or tweezers (use of vinegar solution and hair conditioner or olive oil make combing easier).

2. Body lice

   a. Bathe with soap and water if no lice are found.

   b. Wash with hot water and dry in dryer all clothing, bedclothes, towels, etc.

   c. Dry clean items that cannot be washed; for items that cannot be washed or dry cleaned, seal in a plastic bag for 1 week: lice will suffocate (in cold climates put bags outside for 10 days; temperature change kills lice).

   d. If evidence of lice is found or you are not relieved by a. and b. above, use Malathion 0.5% lotion applied for 8–12 hours, and thoroughly rinsed off.

3. Pubic lice

   a. NIX rinse applied to affected area and washed off after 10 minutes; OR

   b. RID, Clear, A-200, Pronto, generics applied to affected area and washed off after 10 minutes; OR

   c. Malathion 0.5% lotion applied for 8–12 hours, and thoroughly rinsed off.

   d. If pregnant or breastfeeding: use same products as above.

   e. Inform any sexual partners within past month that they need to be treated too.

   h. Wash in hot water and thoroughly dry on heat cycle or dry clean all clothing, bed linen, towels, etc., or remove from body contact for at least 72 hours.

VI. Patient Education

   A. Carefully check family and household members and close contacts for evidence of lice contamination and if found, treat as above.

   B. Call your clinician if signs of infection from scratching occur (redness, swelling of skin, discharge that looks like pus, bleeding, fever).

   C. Stop using the treatment and call your clinician if you or your family members experience sensitivity to the treatment (pain, swelling, rash).

D. Consult with your clinician if you have lice on the eyelashes as the treatments cannot be used near eyes. Ophthalmic (eye) ointment must be applied to the eyelashes twice a day for 10 days.

VII. Follow-up

Contact your clinician if itching, redness or other problems listed above persist or recur.

Special notes: _____

Clinician: _____

Web site: http://www.health.state.ny.us/diseases/communicable/pediculosis/fact_sheet.htm.

From Hawkins, Roberto-Nichols, & Stanley-Haney, *Guidelines for Nurse Practitioners in Gynecologic Settings,* 9th edition, 2007, © Springer Publishing Company.

NATURAL FAMILY PLANNING TO PREVENT OR ACHIEVE PREGNANCY*

Modern natural family planning methods use normally occurring signs and symptoms of ovulation for both the prevention and achievement of pregnancy. No drugs or devices are used. The couple that uses one of the natural methods to prevent pregnancy makes the choice not to have intercourse during the method defined fertile phase. Natural methods of family planning are 75%-99% effective in preventing pregnancy, depending on the method used and on how well the information is taught and applied. The monitoring of fertility signs also provides invaluable information for couples seeking pregnancy or struggling with infertility. Successful use of natural methods depends on competent instruction and follow up, correct and consistent charting and patient compliance with rules.

Commonly Used Methods of Natural Family Planning

1. Cervical mucus method based on detectable changes in cervical mucus throughout the cycle.
2. Basal body temperature method based on changes in the temperature of the woman's body at rest.
3. Symptothermal method is based on the changes in the body temperature, cervical mucus, and other bodily signs. To become knowledgeable about natural family planning methods requires

instruction and can be a pleasant, healthy way to learn to avoid or achieve pregnancy and be aware of your individual fertility pattern.

Terminology Used In a Natural Family Planning Class

abstinence: not having vaginal sexual intercourse
fertile days: the days in the menstrual cycle when pregnancy (conception) is possible
genitals or genitalia: organs of the reproductive system in both male and female
genital-to-genital contact: penis *touching* or coming into close contact with the vaginal area
hormone: a substance that causes special changes in the body; may be naturally occurring or synthetically produced
infertile days: the days in the menstrual cycle when pregnancy (conception) cannot occur
menstruation: bleeding that occurs when the lining of the uterus breaks down and is released; this happens about 12 to 16 days after ovulation
menstrual cycle: the time from the first day of menstrual bleeding to the day **before** the next menstrual bleeding begins; may vary normally from 21 to 40 days in length
ovulation: release of the egg (ovum) from the ovary about 12 to 16 days **before** the onset of the next menstrual period (the day bleeding begins)
ovum: female sex cell, egg
sperm: male sex cell (spermatozoa) found in the semen of a man

Review of the Menstrual Cycle

The menstrual cycle is controlled by hormones. The cycle begins on the *first* day of menstrual bleeding and ends the day *before* menstrual bleeding begins again.

Following menstruation, eggs (ova) are usually maturing in the follicles of the ovaries. As they grow, estrogen (a hormone known as the female sex hormone) is produced in increasing amounts, and certain changes take place:

1. The lining of the uterus builds up the blood supply needed for pregnancy to occur.
2. Cervical mucus is produced and changes in character to become more hospitable to sperm so sperm can live and travel in the uterus.

3. The cervix becomes higher in the pelvis and softer as the cervical os opens to allow sperm to enter the uterus.
4. Basal body temperature (BBT) is low.

As the time of ovulation nears, some women may experience one or more of the following changes:

1. Clearer complexion and less oily hair
2. Increase in energy level
3. Spotting of blood
4. Pain or aching in the pelvic area
5. Breast tenderness and/or fullness

Once ovulation has occurred, there is an increase in the production of progesterone (another hormone important to the menstrual cycle and to pregnancy), and the following changes occur during the 12 to 16 days before menstruation begins:

1. Basal body temperature (BBT) rises
2. Mucus becomes inhospitable to sperm so they cannot live and travel into the uterus
3. Cervix becomes lower, firmer, and the opening closes to prevent sperm from going into the uterus
4. Increased progesterone maintains the lining of the uterus in place for 12 to 16 days. As menstruation approaches, women may also experience one or more of the following changes:
   1. Cramps
   2. Headaches
   3. Oily hair and complexion, acne, or increase in acne
   4. Mood changes
   5. Decrease in energy level
   6. Desire to eat foods with sugar and/or salt
   7. Breast tenderness
   8. Pelvic aching or pain
   9. Low back pain; joint pain or aches

Cervical Mucus Method

Cervical mucus is produced by tiny cells in the cervix. As the ovum is maturing, the mucus will change in a special way that helps keep sperm alive and makes it easier for sperm to travel into the uterus. The mucus loses this quality within a day after the ovum leaves the ovary. The quality or condition of the cervical mucus is an excellent indicator of the days in the menstrual cycle when the woman can become pregnant.

A. How to check the cervical mucus
   1. Begin checking for cervical mucus when the menstrual bleed-
       ing ends or becomes light enough to let you be able to deter-
       mine its presence.
   2. As you go through the day, note mentally whether the area
       around the vaginal opening feels dry, moist, or wet.
   3. Check sensation and for the presence of mucus each time
       you use the bathroom since the character of the mucus can
       change during the day. Cervical mucus should be checked
       before and after urination.
   4. Fold a piece of toilet tissue and wipe over the vaginal open-
       ing. If the tissue slides across the vaginal opening the sensa-
       tion is wet. If the tissue drags, pulls, or chafes across the
       vaginal opening the sensation is dry. If the tissue sticks a little
       to the vaginal opening or if the sensation is neither wet nor
       dry it is a moist sensation.
   5. After wiping, observe the tissue for the presence of cervical
       mucus. Note the color, texture, and stretchiness of the mu-
       cus. The best way to observe its characteristics is to place it
       between two fingers and slowly open the two fingers. The
       woman who does not want to touch the mucus can assess
       its traits by holding the tissue in both hands, then pulling it
       apart (see Figure A.1).
B. How to Chart Information about the Mucus
   1. A new cycle starts the first day of the menstrual bleeding,
       regardless of the time of the day the flow begins. Write the
       date that bleeding begins in the space on the natural family
       planning chart.
   2. Record each day of bleeding with a star.
   3. When the period ends, if the vaginal sensation is dry, chart a
       dry day using the letter D.
   4. Continue to use the letter D each day until a moist or wet
       sensation is experienced. Chart a moist sensation using the
       letter M and a wet sensation by using the letter W.
   5. Note the color and texture of any mucus found or observed
       on toilet tissue.
   6. Write an X through the W on the last day of wet vagi-
       nal sensation and/or slippery or stretchy mucus. The last
       day of slippery or stretchy mucus and/or wet sensation is
       called the Peak Day. This day will not be noted until the
       following day when the mucus will no longer be slippery
       or stretchy and the vaginal sensation will have changed to
       moist or dry.

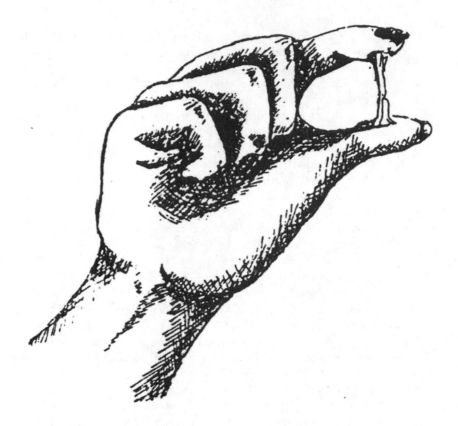

Mucus Check

FIGURE A.1   Mucus check.
Artist: Glen Hawkins

Summary of Mucus Descriptions (By the late Eleanor S. Tabeek, RN, CNM, PhD, updated by Mary Finnigan, BA, MA.)

	D	M	W	W
menses	dry	moist	wet	Peak Day
	sensation	sensation	sensation	

Colors: yellow, white, cloudy, clear
Texture: pasty, creamy

Sticky: stretches but stretches less than ½ inch

Slippery/stretchy: Stretches more than ½ inch

Always chart the most fertile sensation and the most fertile characteristics of the mucus

    C. How to Chart Other Symptoms

        1. Record intercourse by a check mark.

        2. Record any other changes in your body, (e.g., pain with ovulation, breast tenderness, etc.) in the column under "Notes."

Basal Body Temperature (BBT) Method

Basal body temperature is the temperature of the body at rest. As the ova are maturing, the temperature is low. At some time shortly before, during, or after the ovum leaves the ovary, the temperature will usually rise about ³⁄₁₀ths to one full degree higher than it had been. This change in temperature tells you when the ovum has left the ovary, that is, that ovulation has taken place.

    A. How to Take Basal Body Temperature

        1. Begin taking temperature the first day of menstrual bleeding.

        2. Take temperature about the same time every day, usually in the morning when you first awake.

        3. Take temperature before eating, drinking, smoking, and any physical activity.

        4. The thermometer can be placed in the mouth. Always take temperature the same way every day. Record temperature on the Natural Family Planning Chart (see Figure A.2).

    B. Change in Daily Events

Occasionally, a woman may become ill, drink alcoholic beverages, or change the usual time she takes her temperature. Since such events or any change in lifestyle may affect the temperature, when and if they happen, take and record the temperature anyway. In the "Notes" column on the Natural Family Planning Chart, record the possible reason for any change in the usual temperature.

Circle your temperature each day on the Natural Family Planning Chart and connect the circles with a line (see Figure A.3).

    C. To adjust temperatures not taken at usual or base time

        1. Pick a base time.

        2. For every **half hour** earlier than the base time **add** ¹⁄₁₀ of a degree to thermometer reading before it is recorded on the temperature graph.

        3. For every **half hour** later than the base time, **subtract** ¹⁄₁₀ of a degree from the thermometer reading before it is recorded on the temperature graph.

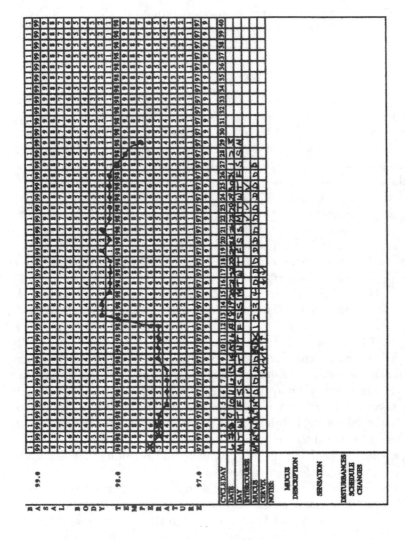

FIGURE A.2　Natural family planning chart.

To record your temperature . . . .
Circle your temperature each day on the
Natural Family Planning Chart
and connect the circles with a line.

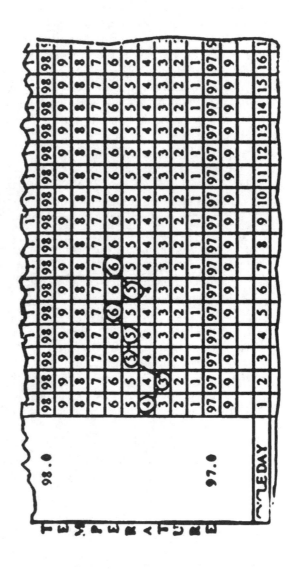

FIGURE A.3   Natural family planning chart (fragment).

The Cervix

After menses, the cervix is low in the vaginal canal, the opening is closed, and it feels firm or pointed, like the tip of a nose. As the ovum is developing and being released, the cervix will rise, soften, and the opening will become wide. These changes help sperm travel into the uterus. Within a few days after the ovum leaves the ovary (ovulation) the cervix will lower in the vaginal canal; it will feel firm or pointed and the opening will close up. These changes help prevent sperm from traveling into the uterus. It is not necessary to check the cervix in order to use a natural method. However, observing and charting the cervical changes can give interested women additional information about their fertile and infertile days. The information can be particularly useful for the breastfeeding or premenopausal woman.

    A. How to Check Status of the Cervix
        1. Begin checking the cervix after the menstrual bleeding ends.
        2. Check the cervix while in a comfortable position such as squatting or standing with one foot on a stool or chair. Use the same position each time you check the cervix.
        3. Check in the evening.
        4. Wash your hands before placing a finger in the vagina.
        5. When feeling the cervix, check for: position in vagina: high (may be difficult to feel) or low (usually easy to feel) softness or firmness opening: open or closed
        6. Chart the most fertile cervical sign of the day.
    B. How to Chart Information About the Cervix
        1. Use circles to represent the sizes of the cervical opening. Place the circles in different positions in the boxes on the Natural Family Planning Chart to represent the rising and lowering of the cervix. Another way the position of the cervix can be noted is through using arrows:
rising cervix ↑
lowering cervix ↓
        2. You can also use the letter "F" to represent a firm cervix and the letter S to represent a soft cervix (see Figure A.4):

Symptothermal Method

Combining use of all the information described to this point.

Natural Family Planning Rules

By following the natural family planning rules, women will know on which days they are fertile and infertile during each menstrual cycle. It is

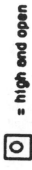 = low and closed   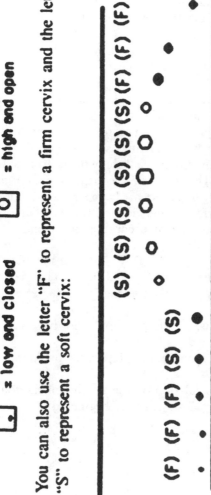 = high and open

2. You can also use the letter "F" to represent a firm cervix and the letter "S" to represent a soft cervix:

(S) (S) (S) (S) (S) (F) (F) (F)

(F) (F) (F) (S) (S)

(Closed circles represent a closed cervical opening–as the. cervix opens. the circles are larger.)

3. Another way the position of the cervix can be noted is through using arrows
   - a high cervix ➤
   - a lowering cervix ➤
   - a cervix tilted to the side = ➤ (right side) or ➤ (left side)

FIGURE A.4 Firm and soft cervix chart.

important for women to check with their instructor or health care provider before following any of the rules.

Ovulation Method (Observing and charting cervical mucus)

A. To Avoid Pregnancy:
   Avoid intercourse during menses.
B. Every Other Dry Day Rule (to determine which days before ovulation are infertile).

Intercourse can take place on the evening of every other dry day. Fertility begins when mucus is observed or the sensation changes to moist or wet.

Intercourse is restricted to the evening so that the woman can observe her cervical mucus during the day undisturbed by intercourse.

It is common for some of the man's semen to be in the woman's vagina on the day after intercourse. If cervical mucus starts to be produced on that day, the presence of semen may prevent the woman from seeing or feeling the presence of mucus. This is why intercourse should not take place on consecutive evenings and why abstinence from intercourse should be followed the day after intercourse has taken place. If the day after the abstinence day is a dry day, intercourse may occur on that evening.

Dry Day	Abstinence	Dry Day	Abstinence
Intercourse in the evening	No intercourse the next day	Intercourse in the evening	No intercourse the next day

When the fertile phase begins, the couple should not have vaginal intercourse until the fertile phase ends.

C. Peak Day Rule (To determine which days after ovulation are infertile).

The fertile phase ends after ovulation on the evening of the fourth day after Peak Day. This infertility lasts until the beginning of the next menses.

Remember: The Peak Day is the last day of wet sensation and/or slippery or stretchy mucus.

   a. Mark the Peak Day on the chart with an "X"
   b. Number the days after Peak Day 1, 2, 3, 4. The sensation on these days must be moist or dry. There may be no mucus present or it may be pasty, sticky, or creamy. It may be cloudy, white, or yellow in color.

D. To achieve pregnancy:

Follow the every other dry day rule until the mucus sign indicates fertility. This allows the woman to accurately chart her mucus sign and to identify the start of the fertile phase.

Intercourse should occur on days identified as fertile by the cervical mucus. Particular attention should be paid to the days of wet sensation *and* clear or slippery/stretchy mucus. It is important for the couple to begin intercourse at the first signs of fertility because the fertile phase is limited in length.

Basal Body Temperature Method (observing and charting basal body temperature)

A. To Avoid Pregnancy
   1. Shortest Cycle Rule (To determine which days before ovulation are infertile days)
      This rule cannot be used until there is a record of at least six, normal menstrual cycles.

Shortest Past Cycle	Assume Infertile	Fertility Begins Abstinence Begins
26 days or longer	first six days of cycle	day 7
23 to 25 days	first 5 days of cycle	day 6
22 days or fewer	0 days	day 1

   2. Earliest Temperature Rise Rule (To determine which days before ovulation are infertile days)
      This rule cannot be used until there is a record of at least six, normal menstrual cycles.
      Subtract 7 days from the earliest recorded day of temperature rise. The result is the first day of Fertility/Abstinence.
      Example: Earliest recorded day of temperature rise Day 15: 15−7 = 8
      The first 7 days of the menstrual cycle are infertile beginning with the first day of menstrual bleeding. Intercourse can take place at any time during these days. Fertility/Abstinence begins on day 8. If a shorter cycle is recorded, the formula needs to be recalculated.
   3. Thermal Shift Rule (To determine which days after ovulation are infertile)
      Fertility ends after ovulation on the evening of the fourth consecutive temperature above the temperature cover line.
      1. Identify the temperature rise. Watch for the temperature rise—three temperatures in a row that are higher than the six preceding temperatures. Find the highest of the six temperatures immediately preceding the rise.

2. Draw the temperature coverline. Draw a line across the chart $^{1}/_{10}$ degree above the highest of the six temperatures immediately preceding the rise. Number the first four temperatures above the temperature coverline.

B. To Achieve Pregnancy

The basal body temperature pattern does not give any indication as to the start of the fertile phase. Previous charts can be reviewed to predict when a temperature rise might occur. Intercourse should occur on the days before an anticipated temperature rise.

Sympto-Thermal Method (observing and charting basal body temperature, cervical mucus, and other bodily signs)

C. To Postpone Pregnancy (To determine which days before ovulation are infertile days)

Use any of the following rules:

Shortest Cycle Rule

Earliest Temperature Rise Rule

Every Other Dry Day Rule

Abstinence should begin if mucus appears at any time during the days determined infertile by the above rules.

Sympto-Thermal Rule (To determine which days after ovulation are infertile)

Fertility ends after ovulation on the evening of the third day after Peak Day or on the evening of the third day of temperature above the coverline, whatever occurs last.

1. Identify Peak Day. Peak day is the last day of wet sensation and/or slippery stretchy mucus. Mark Peak Day with an "X" and number the three days after Peak Day 1,2,3.

2. Identify the temperature rise. Watch for the temperature rise—three temperatures in a row that are higher than the six preceding temperatures. Find the highest of the six temperatures immediately preceding the rise

3. Draw the temperature coverline. Draw a line across the chart 1/10 degree above the highest of the six temperatures immediately preceding the rise. Number the first three temperatures above the temperature coverline.

To Achieve Pregnancy or See corresponding section under Ovulation Method.Web site for Standard Days Method : http://www.cyclebeads.com.

OSTEOPOROSIS

I. Definition

Osteoporosis is characterized by decreased bone mass (loss of bone density), deterioration of bone microarchitecture, and an increase in bone fragility and risk for bone fractures (broken bones).

II. Etiology

Humans have two types of bone—cortical and trabecular. Cortical bone is very compact; it forms the outer shell of bones and makes up 80 percent of the skeletons of adults. Trabecular bone, also called spongy or cancellous bone, makes up the remaining 20 percent and forms the interior of bones. For bones to develop properly and maintain bone mass, we need adequate calcium and phosphorus and other minerals in our diets. We also need other vitamins and adequate Vitamin D for our bodies to absorb calcium from our diets and enable the body to maintain our bones.

We reach our peak bone mass at about age 35. Estrogen seems to play a role in enabling women's bones to retain calcium and the other minerals necessary to build bone and preserve bone mass. From age 35 or so, some sources say that we lose about 2 percent of bone density each year. After menopause, the loss of bone mass may accelerate during the first 5 or 6 years. Thereafter, rate of loss returns to previous level. If bone mass loss becomes too great, the woman becomes very susceptible to fractures.

III. Risk Factors

The risk of developing osteoporosis is greater for women than for men (women begin with less bone mass), and increases with age. Women who have never had children, had early menopause (before age 50), are of Northern European or Asian descent, have a thin body frame, blond or red hair, fair skin and freckles, curvature of the spine (scoliosis), are unable to digest milk or dairy products, smoke, have a high alcohol intake, low calcium diet, high salt diet, not enough vitamin D, drink more than 2 or 3 cups of caffeinated beverages a day, do not exercise or exercise excessively, live in a northern climate, have little fluoride in their drinking water, and have a family history of osteoporosis are at greater risk than women with none of these risks.

IV. Prevention

We cannot change our heritage, family history, gender, our body build, hair, or skin colors, the time at which we go through natural menopause, or our inability to drink milk or eat milk products. But we can exercise an appropriate amount, stop or never start smoking, limit alcohol intake, choose a diet with the amount of calcium we need (1200–1500 milligrams daily at ages 11–24 or when pregnant or breast feeding, 1000 milligrams between ages 25 and 49, and 1500 milligrams at age 50+), take vitamin D supplements (400–800 international units after menopause), decrease or eliminate caffeine, and decrease daily salt intake.

Calcium-rich foods include: broccoli; bok choy; collard, mustard, and turnip greens; kale; and oranges. Dairy products, sardines, and salmon with bones, shrimp paste, dried anchovies, soy products (tofu, soy milk, etc.), and almonds are all high in calcium. Vitamin D (400–800 international units is the recommended daily dose) can be obtained from 5 to 10 minutes in the sun each day, drinking the equivalent of a quart of vitamin D fortified milk, or taking a vitamin D supplement. Foods rich in vitamin D include fatty fish, butter, vitamin D-fortified margarine, egg yolks, and liver.

We can help prevent osteoporosis by changing what we can change in our lifestyles and by considering hormone therapy after menopause. Hormone therapy, known as HT, is not for every woman and is a decision each should make very carefully with her health care provider.

If you do not choose to use HT, in addition to all the lifestyle changes discussed above, you may also consider the use of vitamins—especially 400 units of vitamin E each day, and exploring botanicals or other homeopathic products with knowledgeable persons.

V. Treatment for Osteoporosis

If you have osteoporosis, you can prevent further loss of bone mass and, in some cases, actually restore bone mass with a regimen of exercise prescribed by a clinician specializing in osteoporosis therapy.

Calcium supplements, adequate vitamin D, hormonal and nonhormonal drug therapy, changes in lifestyle including smoking cessation, decreasing or eliminating caffeine, and lowering alcohol intake can also improve the health of your bones.

Making your home as safe as possible will help you avoid fractures. Nurses and physical therapists who specialize in working with persons with osteoporosis can help you reduce or eliminate those hazards.

From Hawkins, Roberto-Nichols, & Stanley-Haney, *Guidelines for Nurse Practitioners in Gynecologic Settings*, 9th edition, 2007, © Springer Publishing Company.

POLYCYSTIC OVARY SYNDROME (PCOS)

I. Definition

PCOS is a complex condition of the endocrine system (including the ovaries). It is one of the most common reproductive tract problems in women under 30 years of age. Some women, when examined with laparoscopy (a lighted scope for viewing the inside of the abdomen and pelvic area), have ovaries with a thickened capsule and multiple cysts of the follicles (which develop and release eggs). The causes of PCOS are unknown, but theories include genetic factors.

II. Signs and Symptoms (only 20–30% of women have these)

    A. Menstrual cycles without ovulation
    B. Infertility—inability to conceive
    C. No menses (periods) or very scanty menses
    D. Prolonged menses, sometimes unpredictable or irregular menses
    E. Increase in body and facial hair
    F. Increase in or appearance of acne
    G. Loss of hair especially at the crown
    H. Whitish breast discharge
    I. Change in body shape—increased waist to hip ratio
    J. Increase in skin pigment at nape of neck, in axillae (under arms), groin area

III. Diagnosis

    A. The diagnosis is made on the basis of signs and symptoms, laboratory tests, ultrasound of the ovaries, and imaging the adrenal glands.
    B. Laboratory testing can include measures of androgens (male hormones), function and hormone level tests for thyroid, adrenal, and pituitary glands.

IV. Treatment

    A. Weight loss and exercise program
    B. Low dose oral contraceptives to restore menstrual cycles
    C. Possibly prescription drugs to reduce excessive hair growth and acne
    D. Medications for type 2 (noninsulin dependent) diabetes seem to help symptoms
    E. Electrolysis and/or depilatories for excessive hair
    F. Medications to induce ovulation when pregnancy is desired

V. Patient Education

    A. Education about PCOS and lifestyle alterations

    B. Education about pharmacologic (prescription drug) interventions

    C. Education about fertility

Special Notes:_____

Clinician:_____

For more information: http://www.pcosupport.org

From Hawkins, Roberto-Nichols, & Stanley-Haney, *Guidelines for Nurse Practitioners in Gynecologic Settings,* 9th edition, 2007, © Springer Publishing Company.

POSTABORTION CARE

1. Someone should accompany you to the facility and wait there to take you home if you have an elective surgical abortion.

2. After the abortion, seek emergency treatment if: you are bleeding (soaking through two thick full-sized sanitary pads per hour for two consecutive hours); you have pelvic pain uncontrolled with medication regimens recommended; you have a fever greater than 100.4 degrees F or higher that lasts for more than 4 hours; severe abdominal pain; weakness, nausea, vomiting or diarrhea more than 24 hours after taking Misoprostol® (if you had a medical abortion).

3. Normal physical activities may be resumed as soon as you feel ready.

4. You may be given some medication (methergine or ergotrate and/or an antibiotic) to take after your abortion. The first two medications will help your uterus return to its normal size and decrease bleeding. Antibiotics will help prevent infection. Follow the directions on how to take the pills. You may experience some uterine cramping (similar to menstrual cramps) with or without the methergine or ergotrate. It is okay to take acetaminophen (Tylenol, Datril, Tempra, Valadol, Valorin, Acephen) for cramps, or ibuprofen (Motrin, Advil).

5. Because of the risk of infection, it is important not to have intercourse or to insert anything into the vagina for 2 to 3 weeks. Other forms of sexual activity or orgasm will not be harmful to your body. Do not douche at all and do not use tampons for 2 to 3 weeks after the procedure, or until you stop bleeding. You

may also be given 3 to 5 days of antibiotics to help prevent infection. Be sure to complete this medication.

6. Bleeding will probably cease after 3 to 4 days, but may last up to 3 weeks. There may be no bleeding at all. If bleeding exceeds two sanitary pads an hour or if you have a fever, call your clinician or the facility where the procedure was performed.

7. Menstruation (period) should resume in 4 to 6 weeks but may take as long as 8 weeks and as short as 2 weeks.

8. You will be given an appointment with a clinician 2 to 3 weeks after your abortion. The clinician will check to see that your body is back to normal and will provide you with your desired form of contraception or schedule an appointment for a diaphragm or cap fitting 6 weeks after the abortion. An IUD can be inserted immediately after or within 3 weeks of a first trimester miscarriage or abortion. Depo-Provera® may be given the day of the abortion or within 5 days of the procedure. This appointment will also give you an opportunity to discuss your feelings. A friend or partner is welcome to see the clinician with you if you wish.

9. If you have chosen to use a hormonal contraceptive method, begin on the Sunday following the abortion procedure. If not, be sure to use another form of contraception such as spermicide and condoms when you resume sexual relations. Remember, you will probably ovulate before you resume menses; you can become pregnant any time after your abortion. If you received Depo-Provera® after your abortion, it is still important to return for your after-abortion check-up 2 to 3 weeks after the procedure. You can then schedule your next Depo-Provera shot.

10. If you have a problem or concern, call the clinician or office at:

Web sites: http://www.fwhc.org/abortion/medical-ab.htm; http://www.nlm.nih.gov/medlineplus/ency/article/001512.htm.

From Hawkins, Roberto-Nichols, & Stanley-Haney, *Guidelines for Nurse Practitioners in Gynecologic Settings,* 9th edition, 2007, © Springer Publishing Company.

PRECONCEPTION SELF-CARE

The purpose of preconception self-care is to help you be at your healthiest as you plan a pregnancy. Advanced planning can help reduce your risk of having a low birth weight or premature baby. Working with your clinician, you can identify any medical condition or medications you are taking that need to be considered when contemplating a pregnancy. You may also wish to have a genetic consultation if you or your partner have a family history of inherited disorders such as cystic fibrosis, Tay-Sachs disease, hemophilia, or birth defects in the family. Infections such as sexually transmitted diseases and tuberculosis may affect the health of a pregnancy, or even your ability to conceive.

Good health is important for a successful pregnancy and healthy baby. A complete health history and physical examination including a Pap smear, pelvic exam, and screening for sexually transmitted diseases, as well as other communicable diseases such as hepatitis B and C and HIV prior to conception will ensure that your body is in an optimal state for a pregnancy. Having your immunizations up to date will protect you and your baby. Evaluation of your nutritional state, diet and exercise patterns, and your toxin exposure at work and at home will help you prepare your body for conception.

Smoking and using alcohol and/or street drugs can have serious consequences for the health of a pregnancy and baby. At least 1 month before attempting to conceive, women who smoke, drink alcohol, or use street drugs should stop. If you use prescription or over-the-counter drugs, limit them to those your clinician approves of. Also check with your clinician about use of herbals, homeopathics, and vitamins.

Protect yourself from exposure to toxins as much as possible. These include pesticides, household cleaning products, gases, lead, solvents, and radiation. Modify, undertake, or continue your program of exercise. Bring your immunizations up-to-date (although some are contraindicated in pregnancy, so it is best to do this 3 months before trying to conceive).

Eat a balanced diet, paying particular attention to fresh fruits and vegetables (5–9 or more servings a day); whole grain breads, cereals, and pasta; protein (especially fish,[3] poultry, legumes, eggs, and nonfat dairy products), and drink 6–8 glasses of water a day. Avoid eating raw fish or raw meat. Decrease or eliminate caffeine from your diet (including coffee, tea, and carbonated soft drinks). Begin taking 400 micrograms of folic acid a day; a prenatal vitamin that includes at least 400 micrograms of folic acid is fine. Increase your calcium intake to the equivalent of 1 quart of milk a day (1200 to 1500 milligrams of calcium). In general, avoid food with lots of preservatives and artificial sweeteners.

Avoid hot tubs and saunas as these bring your body temperature above 102 degrees F, which can limit or eliminate sperm production. Avoiding such excessive heat will also protect the baby once conception has occurred.

If you are on hormonal contraceptives, stop using them at least 1 month before you plan to conceive to allow your body to resume cycling. Several months are advised, as it often takes that long to resume ovulatory (fertile) cycles. You can use spermicides and condoms until you wish to try to conceive.

In order to maximize the health of their sperm, men planning to father children should stop smoking and using street drugs, drink only in moderation (1/day) and avoid toxin exposure at least 3 months before attempting conception. They should also have their infectious disease status checked through a sexually transmitted disease screen and hepatitis B and C and HIV testing. One-half of the baby's genetic material comes from the father, so he needs to be in good health.

Discuss with your partner your feelings about parenting, your expectations of him or her, and what parenting means to you. How do you expect your life to change? How will having a child change your relationship, the way your household functions, your work schedule, your expectations, and those of your partner? Who will be the primary parent? Will one or both of you have maternity/parenting leave? How will your finances be affected by having a child? How do you plan to integrate a new baby into the household with other children, extended family, and other members of the household?

Planning for a pregnancy will help you be at your best when you conceive. It will also help you consider the changes pregnancy and a baby will have on your life and the lives of those close to you.

For resources on genetic counseling, nutrition, prenatal care, and prenatal classes, as well as information on conception and pregnancy, ask your clinician and check your community library, your local bookstore, and on line such as: March of Dimes Birth Defects Foundation: http://www.modimes.org; Ask NOAH about: Pregnancy: http:/Avww.noah.cuny.edu/pregnancy/Pregnancy.html

From Hawkins, Roberto-Nichols, & Stanley-Haney, *Guidelines for Nurse Practitioners in Gynecologic Settings,* 9th edition, 2007, © Springer Publishing Company.

PREMENSTRUAL SYNDROME (PMS)

I. Definition

The premenstrual syndrome consists of a group of behavioral and cognitive dysfunctions and physical symptoms associated with the menstrual cycle.

II. Signs and Symptoms

    A. Usually appear 1 week prior to menses but may also appear up to 2 weeks or just several days before menses, and include:

1. Mood fluctuations—anxiety, crying, persistent anger
2. Depression, feeling hopeless
3. Fatigue, lethargy; joint or muscle pain
4. Weight gain
5. Headache
6. Irritability
7. Breast tenderness
8. Increased appetite, craving for sweets and/or salt
9. Insomnia/sleep disturbance
10. Inability to concentrate, reduced interest in usual activities
11. Constipation
12. Palpitations
13. Hot flashes
14. Abdominal bloating
15. Acne
16. Changes in sex drive

B. If you are bothered by these changes, make an appointment with your clinician for a consultation. A complete history will be taken and a diet and exercise regimen suggested. You may be asked to document your temperature and symptoms daily in a journal. You will also be scheduled for a complete physical.

III. Treatment

Treatment consists of alleviating the signs and symptoms described above with a diet and exercise plan and/or medication.

A. Diet recommendations
1. Limit your salt intake to 3 gm or less per day, i.e., avoid using the saltshaker
2. Limit your intake of alcohol
3. Avoid caffeine, i.e., coffee, tea, chocolate, soft drinks
4. Increase your intake of complex carbohydrates, i.e., fresh fruit, vegetables, whole grains, pasta, rice, potatoes
5. Consume moderate protein and fat. Limit your red meat consumption to 2 x weekly.

B. Exercise recommendations
1. Exercise 3 times per week for 30–40 minutes. Examples: brisk walking, jogging, aerobic dancing, swimming.

C. Medications
1. Vitamins, calcium supplements, and other medications as prescribed or recommended by your clinician.

D. Consider complementary therapies such as meditation, botanicals, aroma or muscle therapy, energy healing, and acupuncture. Talk with your clinician about these.

You may be evaluated monthly x 3 months to determine the effects of diet, exercise, vitamins, and your symptoms. If there is no improvement at that time, a more extensive work-up may be done with possible referral.

From Hawkins, Roberto-Nichols, & Stanley-Haney, *Guidelines for Nurse Practitioners in Gynecologic Settings*, 9th edition, 2007, © Springer Publishing Company.

SCABIES

I. Definition

Scabies is a highly contagious skin rash whose chief symptom is itching. Scabies is caused by the scabies mite (Sarcoptes scabiei), which burrows into the skin and deposits its eggs along the tunnel it has made. The eggs hatch in 3 to 5 days and gather around hair follicles. Newly hatched females burrow into the skin, mature in 10 to 19 days, then mate and start a new cycle.

II. Transmission

    A. Scabies among adults may be sexually transmitted.

    B. Persons living in close proximity with others, in dormitories, and in crowded living spaces are more likely to incur scabies if one person amongst them becomes infested with the mite. Persons sharing clothing or towels are at increased risk.

III. Signs and Symptoms

    A. May appear 4 to 6 weeks after contact with scabies from another person, because it takes several weeks for sensitization to develop. In persons previously infected, symptoms may appear 1 to 4 days after repeat exposure to the scabies mite.

    B. Itching, becoming worse at night or at times when the body temperature is raised such as after exercise. Itching begins first, before other signs and symptoms.

    C. Lesions are usually on the webs between fingers, the inner aspects of the wrists and elbows, areas surrounding the nipples, umbilicus (belly button), belt line, lower abdomen, genitalia, and cleft between the buttocks; can be all over the body. These lesions look like little burrows about ½ to ¾ inch in length ending in a raised red area (papule) or a raised area filled with fluid (vesicle). These lesions can become scaly and become crusted over. When scratched, the areas become raw looking and become infected.

III. Diagnosis

    A. Diagnosis is made through examination of lesions and of those areas of the body most frequently involved.

    B. Linear burrows can be seen in the affected area.

    C. Scaling, crustation lesions, furuncles (boils), and/or scratches may be visible with secondary infection.

    D. When scrapings from the lesions are examined under low power with a microscope, the mites can sometimes be seen.

IV. Treatment

    A. Treatments to kill mites
        1. 5% permethrin cream (Elimite), applied to all areas of the body from neck down and washed off after 8 to 14 hours OR
        2. Ivermectin 200 µg/Kg orally, repeated in 2 weeks (not for children under 2 or less than 33 pounds or for pregnant or breastfeeding women)
        3. Do not use Lindane (Kwell) without consulting a clinician as it can be toxic.

    B. Treatments to relieve symptoms. Antihistamines may be taken to relieve itching. (These do not kill the mites but may make you feel better.)

    C. General measures to decrease risk of re-infestation
        1. Clothing, towels, and bed linens should be laundered (hot cycle) and dried on heat cycle or dry cleaned on day of treatment with medication.
        2. If clothing items cannot be washed or dry cleaned, separate them from the cleaned clothes and do not wear for at least 72 hours. Mites cannot exist for more than 2 to 3 days away from the body. You can decontaminate mattresses, sofas, and rugs with over-the-counter sprays or powders.
        3. Sexual partner and close personal or household contacts within the past month should be informed and referred to a clinician for examination and treatment.

V. Patient Education

    A. Follow the treatment regimen carefully.

    B. Itching may persist for several weeks. If you do not respond to therapy and itching persists after 1 week, contact your clinician to decide if further therapy is necessary.

    C. Call clinician if the infested areas bleed, do not seem to be healing, are swollen or warm to the touch, or have drainage that looks like pus. You may have a secondary infection and need additional treatment.

D. Discontinue treatment and call your clinician if you develop a rash after using medication.

VI. Follow-up

A. Call your clinician if
    1. Lesions do not begin to resolve with treatment or you are getting new lesions.
    2. The treatment has brought out another skin condition, one you had previously, such as eczema or psoriasis.
    3. Lesions appear to be spreading and increasing in size.
    4. Lesions appear crusted.
B. Return to your clinician if symptoms persist or new symptoms occur.
C. Return to your clinician for evaluation of the success of the treatment, the need for re-treatment.

Web site: http://www.cdc.gov/NCIDOD/DPD/parasites/scabies/factsht_scabies.htm.

From Hawkins, Roberto-Nichols, & Stanley-Haney, *Guidelines for Nurse Practitioners in Gynecologic Settings,* 9th edition, 2007, © Springer Publishing Company.

STOP SMOKING

Smoking is the leading cause of preventable illness and early death in the United States. If you stop you can expect an increase in your life expectancy and improvement in your health.

Smokers are at greater risk for:

Strokes
Cancer of the larynx
Oral cancers—tongue, lip, gum
Lung disease
Chronic obstructive pulmonary disease
Heart disease and heart attack
Cervical cancer
Possibly breast cancer

Smokers also develop other smoking-related problems:

Pregnancy complications and losses
Sinus infections
Cataracts
Impotence and infertility

Abnormal Papanicolaou smears (dysplasia)
Osteoporosis and bone density problems
Premature skin wrinkling
Gum disease and dental cavities
Stained teeth and bad breath
Poor circulation
Poor tolerance for exercise
High blood pressure

Family members are at greater risk for:

Lung cancer and heart disease
Children of smokers have higher incidences of sudden death syndrome, asthma and other lung problems, ear infections, colds, learning delays
The rewards of quitting are experienced quickly and long-term

Within several weeks of quitting smoking:

Blood pressure drops
Circulation improves
Lung function improves
Coughing, sinus infections, fatigue, and shortness of breath improve
Number of colds decreases
Energy level improves

After 1 year of quitting smoking:

Excess risk of heart disease improves to half that of a smoker

After 5 years of quitting smoking:

Lung cancer death rate decreases by almost half
Risk of cancer of the mouth, throat, and esophagus is half that of a smoker

After 5–15 years of quitting smoking:

Stroke risk is reduced to that of a nonsmoker

After 10 years of quitting smoking:

Lung cancer death rate is similar to that of a nonsmoker

After 15 years of quitting smoking:

The risk of coronary heart disease is that of a nonsmoker

Do you think you have a dependence on nicotine? Ask yourself the following questions:

- Do you smoke a cigarette first thing in the morning?
- Do you wake up to smoke a cigarette during the night?
- Do you smoke 5 or more cigarettes a day?
- Do you find it hard to not smoke in places where it is forbidden? Do you leave such places to smoke?
- Do you smoke more cigarettes in hours after you wake up than during the rest of the day?
- Do you smoke when you are ill?

If you answer yes to any of these questions you can consider yourself as having a nicotine problem.

Want to quit? The following suggestions may help:

Make the decision to stop smoking

Think about why you want to stop smoking. Make a list of those reasons and the rewards associated with quitting. Keep this list with you and review it when you feel the urge to smoke.

Talk to your friends and family; ask for their support and encouragement.

Keep a journal. You can start it when you are making the decision to quit. Record each cigarette smoked, the time, the place, and the intensity of the craving and the reward of the cigarette. Think about the social cues associated with smoking and about how you will deal with these after you stop smoking. Record your thoughts and feelings. Doing this can help you identify your smoking "triggers" and assist you in adapting strategies and skills to get past those triggers. Continue recording your feelings in the journal after you have quit smoking.

Avoid drinking alcohol. Alcohol will weaken your resolve.

Clean your clothes, car, drapes, and furniture to rid them of the smell of smoke.

Throw out all cigarettes, ashtrays, and smoking paraphernalia.

Avoid being around other smokers.

If possible, establish living space as "no smoking."

Increase exercise level (walking, weight lifting, yoga, Tai Chi). This assists in weight management, stress reduction, and general sense of well-being.

Change your daily routine to avoid smoking triggers.

Keep oral substitutes handy. Use low calorie vegetables and fruits; sugarless gum; toothpicks.

Engage in activities that make smoking difficult, such as exercising, gardening, washing the car.

Spend time in places where smoking is prohibited.

Join a support group. Such groups are offered by Nicotine Anonymous, American Cancer Society, the American Lung Association, and your local hospital or health care center.

Make an appointment with your clinician to talk about your desire to stop smoking. Your clinician can help you choose the most appropriate method to assist in breaking your habit. Choices available include:

- Nicotine replacements: gum, transdermal patches, nasal sprays, inhaler
- Zyban® or Wellbutrin® SR—a non-nicotine oral medication for smoking cessation treatment
- Chantix® (Varenicline)—an oral medication

Good luck in your journey to a smoke-free life. Remember, if you have a relapse and start smoking again, you can quit again. Many people need to try several times before they are successful. If this happens to you, don't be too hard on yourself. Review the above suggestions and begin again!

From Hawkins, Roberto-Nichols, & Stanley-Haney, *Guidelines for Nurse Practitioners in Gynecologic Settings*, 9th edition, 2007, © Springer Publishing Company.

STRESS OR URGE INCONTINENCE (LOSS OF URINE)

Stress and urge incontinence are caused by relaxation of the muscles and ligaments of the pelvic floor, that is, the muscles and ligaments that support the bladder, uterus, urethra (tube leading from the bladder to the outside), lower bowel, and vagina. Due to this relaxation, which is commonly the result of stretching due to childbirth and normal loss of muscle elasticity with aging, any stress such as laughing, coughing, or sneezing can cause involuntary loss of urine or the need to urinate urgently.

Urine can be irritating to the skin, so it is important to wash it off as soon as possible. The ammonia odor from urine leakage may be distressing also. Cotton underwear, the use of nondeodorized, unscented panty liners, and use of wipes especially designed for the perineal area, such as baby wipes, will all help to prevent irritation, rashes, and cracking of skin. Skin cracking, irritation, and rashes will often increase the possibility of bacterial infection, especially in the warm, moist, genital area. Dusting with cornstarch will protect the skin from irritation. Only mild unscented soaps should be used, and used sparingly, as soap can be drying to skin. Perfumes (which are alcohol based) can increase the drying effect also and may cause an allergic reaction or chemical irritation to sensitive skin. Avoid bubble baths, vaginal hygiene products, and perfumed powders and talcums for the same reasons. Also avoid caffeine and smoking—both are bladder irritants (see Figure A.5).

Diary of Incontinence

Code numbers for WHEN	*Code letters for AMOUNT*
1. coughing/sneezing	a. a drop or two
2. laughing/crying	b. a teaspoonful
3. blowing nose	c. a tablespoonful
4. climbing stairs	d. more than a tablespoonful
5. bending over	e. unable to estimate
6. sitting or resting	
7. washing hands or dishes	
8. other times	

Kegel (Pelvic Floor Muscle Strengthening) Exercises

Practice contracting, holding, and relaxing each time you urinate until you can stop the flow completely and start and stop at will. Then proceed to this exercise program.

Day One: Repeated contracting, holding, and relaxing of pubococcygeus muscle (muscle band of perineal area) 4 times this day, 10 contractions and 10 relaxations each time.

Day Two: Increase to 20 contractions and 20 relaxations, 4 times this day.

Day Three: Increase to 30 contractions and 30 relaxations, 4 times this day.

Day Four: Increase to 40 contractions and 40 relaxations, 4 times this day.

Day Five: Increase to 70 contractions and 70 relaxations, 4 times this day.

Continue with Day Five regimen, so you are now doing the exercise 4 times each day, contracting and relaxing 70 times at each of the 4 exercise periods (see Figure A.6).

You may want to ask your clinician about vaginal cones or sphere to help you practice. Graduated weighted cones are available to assist in Kegel exercises; a cone is inserted in the vagina and Kegels are performed using the cones' feedback; when weight of one cone can be maintained 15

**Log of Times of Urine Loss,
Circumstances of Loss, and Amount**

	S	M	T	W	T	F	S
Week 1							
Week 2							
Week 3							
Week 4							

FIGURE A.5   Log of times of urine loss, circumstances of loss, and amount.

Log for Pelvic Floor Exercise

(Place a checkmark in box for each exercise period each day)

	S	M	T	W	T	F	S
Week 1							
Week 2							
Week 3							
Week 4							

FIGURE A.6   Log for pelvic floor exercises.

minutes when walking or standing, move to next weight. The sphere is inserted in the vagina to strengthen pelvic muscle tone. You can do Kegel exercises with the sphere in place as well.

From Hawkins, Roberto-Nichols, & Stanley-Haney, *Guidelines for Nurse Practitioners in Gynecologic Settings,* 9th edition, 2007, © Springer Publishing Company.

SURGICAL POSTABORTION CARE

1. Someone should accompany you to the facility where you are to have the abortion and wait there to take you home.

2. You may resume normal physical activities according to the post-operative care instructions you will be given and as soon as you feel ready.

3. You may be given some medication (methergine or ergotrate and/or an antibiotic) to take after your abortion. The first two medications will help your uterus return to its normal size and decrease bleeding. Antibiotics will help prevent infection. Follow the directions on how to take the pills. You may experience some uterine cramping (similar to menstrual cramps) with or without the methergine or ergotrate, as each of these medications causes the uterus to contract to help it to return to pre-pregnancy size. It is okay to take acetaminophen (Tylenol®, Datril®, Tempra®, Valadol®, Valorin®, Acephen®) for cramps, or ibuprofen (Motrin®, Advil®).

4. Because of the risk of infection, it is important not to have intercourse or to insert anything including fingers into your vagina for 2–3 weeks. Other forms of sexual activity or orgasm will not be harmful to your body. Do not douche at all and do not use tampons for 2–3 weeks after the procedure, or until you stop bleeding. You may also be given 3 to 5 days of antibiotics to help prevent infection. Be sure to complete this medication.

5. Bleeding will probably cease after 3–4 days, but may last up to 3 weeks. There may be no bleeding at all. If bleeding exceeds two sanitary pads an hour, if you have a fever, or are passing clots the size of a quarter or larger, call your clinician or the facility where the procedure was performed. If you continue to have bright red bleeding longer than 3 days, call your clinician. Bleeding should change from bright red to darker red and then to pink and then whitish mucousy discharge by the end of 3 weeks, and it should decrease in amount.

6. Menstruation (period) should resume in 4–6 weeks but may take as long as 8 weeks and as short as 2 weeks. You will probably ovulate (produce an egg) before you have a period, so protect yourself from pregnancy or abstain from vaginal penile intercourse until you are using a contraceptive method.

7. You will be given an appointment with a clinician 2–3 weeks after your abortion. The clinician will check to see that your body is back to normal and will provide you with your desired form of contraception or schedule an appointment for a diaphragm or FemCap® fitting 6 weeks after the abortion. An IUD can be inserted immediately after or within 3 weeks of a first trimester miscarriage or abortion. Depo-Provera® may be given the day of the abortion or within 5 days of the procedure. This appointment will also give you an opportunity to discuss your feelings. A friend or partner is welcome to see the clinician with you if you wish.

8. If you have chosen to use a hormonal contraceptive method, begin on the Sunday following the abortion procedure. If not, be sure to use another form of contraception such as spermicide and condoms when you resume sexual relations. Remember, you can become pregnant any time after your abortion if you are not using contraception. If you received Depo-Provera® after your abortion, it is still important to return for your after-abortion check-up 2 to 3 weeks after the procedure. You can then schedule your next Depo-Provera® shot.

9. If you have a problem or concern, call the clinician clinic or office at: _____

Web site: http://www.emmagoldman.com/services/abortion/care.htm.

From Hawkins, Roberto-Nichols, & Stanley-Haney, *Guidelines for Nurse Practitioners in Gynecologic Settings,* 9th edition, 2007, © Springer Publishing Company.

SYPHILIS

I. Definition

Syphilis is a sexually transmitted disease that can affect any organ in the body such as the bones, brain, or heart. It is spread by sexual contact and can also be passed on from mother to unborn baby. It is caused by the organism Treponema pallidum (T. pallidum).

II. Important Information

    A. Any sexually active person can get infected with syphilis. An untreated person can spread syphilis for 1 year after being infected.

    B. Symptoms can occur 10 to 90 days after sexual contact; average is 21 days.

III. Usual Signs and Symptoms. What You May Experience

    A. *Primary Syphilis.* The first sign of syphilis is a painless chancre (sore) at the site of entry of the syphilis organism. The chancre may occur on the vulva, labia, opening to vagina, clitoris, cervix, nipple, lip, roof of mouth, opening to the urethra on the head of the penis, the shaft of the penis, the anal area, or the scrotum. You may notice painful and/or swollen glands in your groin area, on your neck, or under your arms. The chancre will last 1 to 5 weeks and will go away even if not treated. If you are not diagnosed and treated you will progress to secondary syphilis.

    B. *Secondary Syphilis.* In 2 to 8 weeks or as long as 6 months after the chancre appears (average is 6 weeks), you will notice a rash on any part of your body. It can even appear on the palms of your hands or the soles of your feet. You may also have some hair loss so that your head has a moth eaten look and you may lose part of your eyebrows. You may notice swollen glands in any part of your body, have a low-grade fever, a sore throat, headache, feel tired, have loss of appetite, and your joints may feel sore. This will last about 6 weeks and go away without treatment. If you are not diagnosed and treated you will progress to latent syphilis.

    C. *Latent Syphilis.* You will have no symptoms, although 25 percent of persons may have a chancre again. During primary and secondary syphilis and early latency you are infectious to sexual partners. After 12 months have passed from the date of the initial infection, you are no longer infectious but the organism is in your blood. If you are not diagnosed and treated, you may remain in the latent stage for the rest of your life.

    D. *Tertiary Syphilis.* One-third of persons infected with syphilis and not treated will go into the tertiary stage. In this stage your bones, skin, heart, or nervous system including your brain, can be affected. Persons with tertiary syphilis can become unable to work or care for themselves and have a shortened life.

IV. Diagnosis

    A. History of sexual contact with a known infected person.

    B. Blood tests and examination of material from a chancre under a special microscope to see the syphilis organism.

V. Treatment

The treatment of choice is penicillin given by injection. For those allergic to penicillin, other antibiotics can be used. The amount and treatment will depend on the stage of the syphilis.

VI. Complications

    A. Progression of the disease to tertiary stage.
    B. Transmission of syphilis from a woman to her unborn baby causing congenital syphilis in the baby. Congenital means present at birth. Congenital syphilis can cause permanent damage to the baby.

VII. Patient Education

    A. Follow-up for second dose of medications as instructed by health care provider.
    B. Use barrier contraception (condom) each time you have sexual intercourse.
    C. Look at your partner before having sex. If you see a sore (chancre), rash, swelling, or discharge, consider a check up for both of you before having sex.
    D. If you think you may have contracted syphilis or any other sexually transmitted disease (STD), avoid having sex and visit a local STD clinic.
    E. If you are diagnosed with syphilis, report any sexual partners to your clinician so they can be notified and treated, or notify them to seek treatment.
    F. Return for testing after treatment for primary or secondary syphilis at 6 and 12 months; for latent syphilis, at 6, 12, and 24 months.
    G. There is no immunity to syphilis, so you can be reinfected by an infected partner. Return for treatment if you believe you have been infected again.

Special Notes:_____

Clinician: _____

For more information for yourself or friends: CDC (Centers for Disease Control) STD Hotline 1-800-227-8922; on line: http://www.cdc.gov. For phone numbers of free (or almost free) STD clinics see the Community Service Numbers in the government pages of your local phone book. http://www.cdc.gov/node.do/id/0900f3ec80007600

From Hawkins, Roberto-Nichols, & Stanley-Haney, *Guidelines for Nurse Practitioners in Gynecologic Settings,* 9th edition, 2007, © Springer Publishing Company.

TRICHOMONIASIS (TRICH)

I. Definition

Trichomoniasis is a parasitic infection occurring in the female vagina or urethra, or male urethra and prostate. The infection is believed to be sexually transmitted although it has been identified in non-sexually active women.

II. Signs and Symptoms

    A. May appear 5 to 30 days after contact

    B. In the female, symptoms include
       1. Odorous, greenish-yellow, frothy vaginal discharge (often fishy)
       2. Painful intercourse or urination
       3. Discomfort on tampon insertion
       4. Itchiness, redness, and irritation of the vulva and upper thigh
       5. Papanicolaou smear may be abnormal
       6. Some patients may not have any symptoms

    C. In the male, symptoms include:
       1. Mild itch or discomfort in penis
       2. Moisture at tip of penis disappearing spontaneously
       3. Slight early morning discharge from penis before first urination

    D. Untreated symptoms in the female or male can progress to infection of neighboring urinary and reproductive organs

III. Diagnosis

    A. Female evaluation may include
       1. Vaginal examination to check for trichomoniasis and to rule out yeast infections and bacterial infections such as gonorrhea or bacterial vaginosis
       2. Blood test to rule out syphilis

    B. Male evaluation may include
       1. Examination for gonorrhea or urinary tract infection
       2. Blood test for syphilis

IV. Treatment

The male should seek treatment after exposure to a partner with the infection. He may have no symptoms but could harbor the parasite in his urethra or prostate.

It is very important to report any medical conditions you have (especially seizure disorder) or medication you take regularly before taking any treatment.

V. Patient Education

A. Take no alcohol during the 48 hours after treatment (medication)
B. For minor side effects of medication (nausea, dizziness, or metallic taste), take medication with some food or milk
C. Advise sexual contact(s) to seek simultaneous treatment
D. Use condoms until all partners are treated

VI. Follow-up

Return to clinician if symptoms persist or new symptoms occur.
Special notes: _____
Clinician: _____
For more information, call: CDC STD Hotline: 1-800-227-8922: Phone numbers of free (or almost free) STD clinics are listed in the Community Service Numbers in the government pages of your local phone book. http://www.cdc.gov; www.cdc.gov/NCIDOD/dpd/parasites/trichomonas/default.htm

From Hawkins, Roberto-Nichols, & Stanley-Haney, *Guidelines for Nurse Practitioners in Gynecologic Settings,* 9th edition, 2007, © Springer Publishing Company.

VAGINAL CONTRACEPTIVE SPONGE

I. Definition/Mechanism of Action

The vaginal contraceptive sponge looks like a small doughnut with the hollow in the center. The hollow area fits over the cervix. The sponge measures about 1 ¾ of an inch in diameter. Across the bottom is a string loop to provide for easy removal. The sponge is polyurethane and contains the spermicide Nonoxynol 9. It provides a barrier between sperm and the cervix, traps sperm within the sponge, and releases spermicide to inactivate sperm over 24 hours.

II. Effectiveness and Benefits

A. 89–90.8% effectiveness
B. May be inserted before intercourse and left in place for up to 24 hours

    C. Latex free

    D. Over-the-counter—no prescription needed

    E. No need to add extra spermicide within 24 hours

III. Side Effects and Disadvantages

    A. Vaginal irritation from the sponge

    B. Vaginal irritation from the spermicide in the sponge

    C. Sensation of something in the vagina

    D. Difficulty in inserting or removing sponge

    E. Some concern about sponge using increasing the risk of toxic shock syndrome if not used as directed. Use with care or do not use during menses.

    F. Frequent use of Nonoxynol 9 can cause genital irritation and increase the risk of HIV and other STDs

IV. Explanation of Method

    A. How to insert

       1. Read instructions carefully before using

       2. Wash your hands before opening the package

       3. Open package carefully to avoid tearing sponge

       4. Wet sponge with water

       5. Insert in vagina as you would a tampon

       6. The sponge can be inserted any time up to 24 hours before sexual intercourse. There is no need to add spermicide once the sponge has been moistened with water and inserted.

       7. Sponge can be left in place for up to 24 hours from the time you inserted it and offers protection for each act of intercourse

    B. How to remove

       1. Read printed instructions carefully

       2. Wash your hands with soap and water

       3. Remember to remove sponge slowly to avoid tearing it

       4. Do not flush the sponge down the toilet

       5. Special removal instructions

          a. If the sponge appears to be stuck, relax your vaginal muscles and bear down, and you should be able to remove it without difficulty

          b. The sponge may turn upside down in the vagina making the string more difficult to find. To find the string, run your finger around the edge on back side of the sponge until you feel the string. If you cannot find the loop, grasp the sponge between your thumb and forefinger and remove it slowly.

    C. Remember the sponge cannot get lost in the vagina

V. Additional Information

    A. It is okay to use the sponge while swimming or bathing

    B. The sponge should be used only once and then discarded.

VI. Danger signs of toxic shock syndrome

    A. Fever (temperature 101 degrees and above)

    B. Diarrhea

    C. Vomiting

    D. Muscle aches

    E. Rash (sunburn-like)

Yearly physical examination including Papanicolaou smear is recommended.

Web site: http://www.todaysponge.com.

VAGINAL DISCHARGE

All women have a normal discharge called leukorrhea; the amount and consistency vary with each individual. This discharge is generally of a mucus-like consistency and tends to increase during the menstrual cycle up to 2 weeks before menstruation. A normal vaginal discharge may vary slightly in color, although it is usually clear or white, has no unpleasant odor, and is not itchy or irritating to the skin. Occasionally a woman may notice a fishy or musty smelling discharge if she has recently had vaginal intercourse. This may be due to dead sperm being cleansed from the vagina. If this occurs persistently, don't confuse it with a bacterial infection or overgrowth called vaginosis. Have it checked by a clinician. Some methods of birth control may affect the amount of normal vaginal discharge.

Hints for Prevention of Vaginal Infection

    1. Even under the best conditions, vaginal infections sometimes occur. Don't panic if you discover that you have such an infection. Treat it with common sense: cleanliness, pelvic rest (no intercourse), and prescribed medications, and wear sensible clothing (cotton panties, cotton crotch panties, no panty hose under slacks, no underwear to bed).

    2. Cleanliness and personal hygiene are very important. Keep clean by bathing (shower or tub, but be sure you disinfect the tub before and after use) with soap and water. Vaginal deodorants can be irritating and are worthless in treating or preventing an infection. Avoid all use of feminine hygiene sprays and deodorants

as well as deodorant or scented tampons, pads, panty liners, and toilet paper because these products tend to alter the natural environment of the vagina and make it more susceptible to irritation and/or infection.

3. *Douching is never recommended.* It can be harmful if done when an infection is already present. For example, the pressure of the douche solution may cause the infection to spread into the womb (uterus) and become even worse. Also, the douche solution removes the natural cleansing secretions of the vagina that normally help to maintain an environment that prevents infections. Indiscriminate douching with various commercial products may aggravate existing conditions, set up a chemical vaginitis (inflammation, irritation of the vagina), or contribute to a pelvic infection.

4. To prevent both vaginal and bladder infections from occurring, wear cotton underwear or underwear with a cotton crotch and no underwear while sleeping; change tampons or sanitary napkins after each urination or bowel movement; wipe yourself in the front first and then the back after going to the bathroom; urinate after intercourse and/or genital stimulation; and drink lots of fluids: at least 6 glasses of water a day; cranberry juice or cranberry tablets may be helpful in avoiding infection.

Rules to Follow if You Have A Vaginal Infection (Vaginitis) or a Vaginosis

1. Take the entire course of medication exactly as prescribed. If you do not, the infection may go underground temporarily and then return and be more troublesome than before.

2. If you are treating an infection with vaginal cream or suppositories, remain lying down in bed for at least 15 minutes after insertion to allow the medication to spread deeply around the cervix, where it is needed. Standing up may cause the medicine to seep outward toward the vaginal opening.

3. Do not use tampons for protection because they will absorb the medication and reduce its effectiveness. Instead, use unscented external pads or small minipads to prevent staining underwear.

4. If you have a vaginal infection and use a diaphragm, soak diaphragm for 30 minutes with Betadine® scrub (not solution) or 70% rubbing alcohol, after using prescribed medication for 2 days and again when medication is completed. Use alcohol for your FemCap or Lea's Shield.

5. Sexual relations should be avoided for at least 1 week, and preferably throughout the entire course of treatment. Intercourse

can be very irritating to the inflamed vagina and cervix during an infection and can slow down the healing process. Also, the germs that cause your infection might spread to your partner; if the partner is male, he should use a condom during the entire treatment period.

6. Insufficient lubrication prior to intercourse may contribute significantly to vaginal infections (and bladder infections). Water-soluble jelly can be used for lubrication. There are also vaginal lubricants and moisturizers especially for peri- and postmenopausal women.

From Hawkins, Roberto-Nichols, & Stanley-Haney, *Guidelines for Nurse Practitioners in Gynecologic Settings,* 9th edition, 2007, © Springer Publishing Company.

NOTES

1. Adapted from manufacturer's literature Oclassen Pharmaceuticals, 1990: Watson Laboratories, 1998.
2. Adapted from the Aldara manufacture's literature, 3M pharmaceuticals.
3. Follow current recommendations for pregnancy due to mercury content.

Informed Consent Forms

(Includes Patient Information)

Hormonal Contraception
Diaphragm
IUD
Emergency Contraception

HORMONAL CONTRACEPTIVES

(May also be used as informational handout)

I. Mechanism of Action

    A. A systemic method of preventing conception that acts by
        1. Suppressing ovulation
        2. Producing changes in the endometrium that make it unreceptive to implantation
        3. Producing a thickened cervical mucus; interference with sperm reaching the egg

II. Benefits of the Method

    A. Highly effective: 99.66% for combination hormonal contraceptives (0.1 pregnancy/year); 97% for progestin-only hormonal contraceptives

    B. Sexual spontaneity
    C. Regulated menstrual flow
    D. Lighter flow and less cramping
    E. Decreased incidence of uterine and ovarian cancers
    F. Relief of symptoms associated with peri-menopause

III. Risk of Method: Applies to combination oral contraceptives, patch, and ring

    A. Minor side effects (these are rare and usually subside after several months of method use; may be alleviated by changing type of hormonal contraception or discontinuing). Listed are a few more common, although rare, side effects:
        1. Nausea (if using oral contraceptive try taking pill with a meal or with milk; with severe nausea/vomiting, use back-up method of birth control such as condoms)
        2. Spotting
        3. Decreased menstrual flow and sometimes missed periods
        4. May have more problems with yeast infections or vaginal discharges
        5. Depression or mood changes
        6. Acne or increase in acne
        7. Headaches (not severe)
    B. Major side effects (rare in women under 40 who are non-smokers)
        1. Blood clots in legs, lungs; stroke
        2. Hypertension (high blood pressure)
        3. Gallbladder disease
        4. Heart attack (smokers age 35 and older)
        5. Smoking doubles risk factors associated with hormone use. These side effects are characterized by the following danger signals (if they occur, seek medical care *IMMEDIATELY*): pain, redness, or swelling of the legs or a localized tender red spot warm to the touch may indicate a blood clot in a vein; persistent and severe headaches; chest pain and/or difficulty breathing; blurred vision, flashing vision; blindness; abdominal pain

IV. Contraindications

Women with a history of any of the following conditions may not be able to use hormonal contraceptives containing estrogen
    A. Thromboembolic disorders (blood clot) in leg, lungs
    B. Impaired liver function at present time; liver problems
    C. Cancer of breast or reproductive system (uterus, ovaries, cervix)

D. Hypertension (high blood pressure); uncontrolled, or smoking and high blood pressure
E. Hyperlipidemia (high cholesterol)
F. Stroke
G. Coronary artery disease
H. Major surgery on legs or with prolonged immobility
I. 35 years or older and currently a smoker
J. Pregnancy—known or suspected
K. Undiagnosed genital bleeding
L. Taking certain prescription drugs
M. Diabetes with vascular (blood vessel) disease
N. Headaches, migraines with neurological symptoms

V. Alternate Methods of Birth Control

A. Abstinence
B. Sterilization; natural family planning
C. Condom used with contraceptive cream, jelly, or foam, contraceptive suppositories or tablets, vaginal film, contraceptive gel, sponge
D. Intrauterine device (IUD)
E. Diaphragm with contraceptive cream or jelly, FemCap, Lea's Shield
F. Female condom
G. Contraceptive patch, ring (if estrogen is not a problem)
H. Progestin only methods: progestin only pill, Mirena® IUD, Implant [Implanon®], Depo-Provera®

VI. Inquiries are encouraged

Please ask us questions; a change in decision does not create a problem.

VII. Explanation of method

A. Way in which hormonal contraceptives are prescribed
   1. A complete physical examination is done, including blood pressure, weight, urinalysis, gynecologic examination with Papanicolaou smear (unless one was done within the past year)
   2. Review side effects and dangers of use; review packet if using oral contraceptives
   3. If requested to do so by your clinician, review and sign an informed consent for hormonal contraceptives
   4. You may transfer your records from another clinic or clinician's office

B. Way in which oral contraceptives are taken
   1. Start taking your first package of pills as directed by your clinician
   2. Oral contraceptive pills are *usually* started initially at the same time as your period; you begin the Sunday of the week your period starts even if you are still bleeding
   3. Swallow one pill at the *same time* daily
   4. A second form of contraception is recommended for the first 7 days after starting the pill (unless specified differently)
   5. Some medications can decrease effectiveness or cause other pill-related problems (e.g., spotting). Always mention to your clinician and pharmacist that you are on oral contraceptives and the type prior to starting any other medication. Also tell us if you are on any medications prior to starting oral contraceptives. Use a back-up method of birth control if you have any doubts about the possibility of a drug interaction.
   6. If you are taking prescribed antibiotics for an illness, you should continue your pill but use a back-up method.
   7. Breakthrough bleeding (spotting) is common during the first few months a woman is on an oral contraceptive; do not be alarmed if the following occurs:
      a. If you experience spotting after several months of pill use, make sure you are taking the pill correctly, as directed below. But make sure you discuss this at the time of your first pill check.
      b. If the pill is taken improperly, breakthrough bleeding may occur. You must make every effort to take your pill at the same time *every day*.
         1) If you take your pill more than 6 hours late, take the pill when you remember it; you are also advised to use a second method of birth control for the next 7 days.
         2) If you miss one pill: take the pill when you remember and then take the scheduled pill at the regular time. A second method of birth control is recommended for 7 days.
         3) If you miss 2 pills in the first 2 weeks of a pill pack: take two pills at the regular time and then take two pills at the regular time the next day, and use a second method of birth control for 7 days.
         4) If you miss 2 pills in the third week, or if you miss 3 or more pills at any time, and you start packets on Sunday, take a pill each day until Sunday, then discard the remainder of that pack and start a new pack immediately,

omitting the hormone-free week (if there is one). If you don't start a new pack on Sundays, throw away the rest of the pill pack and start a new pack that day. A back-up method of birth control should be used for the first 7 days of this new pill pack.

   5) If you miss 1 or more pills and used no back-up method and have no period, call to discuss possible pregnancy test.

   6) If you aren't sure what to do about missed pills, use a back-up method any time you have sex and keep taking a birth control pill (hormone pill) each day until you can talk with your clinician.

C. Occasionally, withdrawal bleeding (your period) does not occur during the week of nonhormone pills (placebos).

   1. If this happens to you and all pills have been taken properly, continue with next pill cycle. If you miss two periods, start your third pill cycle but call your clinician for advice.

   2. If this happens to you and you have taken your pill late or forgotten to take it, and did not use a second birth control method, start your next pill packet but call your clinician for advice.

D. If you experience severe vomiting and/or diarrhea, use a back-up method of birth control since the pill may not have been absorbed properly.

I have read the above material; it has been fully explained. I have been given the opportunity to ask questions, and I understand the information. I have chosen to use an oral contraceptive.

   Signed _____ Date _____
   Witness _____ Date _____

Danger Signals Associated with Hormonal Contraceptive Use

Abdominal pain (severe)
Chest pain (severe) or shortness of breath
Headaches (severe)
Eye problems such as blurred vision or loss of vision
Severe leg pain (calf or thigh)

   Contact us at ( ) _____ if you develop any of the above problems.

   NOTE: Birth control pills can be used as emergency contraception. Ask your health care provider; check directions in pill packet; call 1-888-NOT-2-LATE; http://not-2-late.com. Plan B® Emergency

Contraception is available over the counter at a pharmacy (no prescription) if you are 18 or older.

From Hawkins, Roberto-Nichols, & Stanley-Haney, *Guidelines for Nurse Practitioners in Gynecologic Settings*, 9th edition, 2007, © Springer Publishing Company.

INJECTABLE CONTRACEPTION (DEPO-PROVERA®)[1]

(May also be used as an informational handout)

I. Definition

Depo-Provera® is a hormonal substance that prevents ovulation from occurring. It is injected intramuscularly or subcutaneously every 12 weeks into the muscle of the upper arm or buttocks.

II. How It Works

The hormones in the injection suppress ovulation (egg production) for 12 weeks.

III. How Effective Is It?

Failure rate is less than one pregnancy per 100 women per year when women return for injections every 12 weeks (Depo) and when injection is done in the first 5 days of menses (bleeding).

IV. Why Choose This Method?

  A. Consider use of other methods and whether their side effects make you prefer this method
  B. Desire for long-term contraceptive—12-week coverage
  C. Desire for reversible method (ability to stop injections)
  D. Desire for method disconnected from intercourse; nothing to take or put in

V. Why You Might Not Be a Candidate

  A. Known or suspected pregnancy
  B. Unexplained abnormal vaginal bleeding
  C. Known breast cancer
  D. Known sensitivity to Depo-Provera® or any of its ingredients (have you ever had an allergic reaction to local anesthetic at the dentist?)

VI. Things to Consider Before Choosing Depo-Provera®

    A. Depression
    B. Abnormal mammogram
    C. Kidney disease
    D. Hypertension (high blood pressure)
    E. Planned pregnancy in near future
    F. Gallbladder disease
    G. Mild cirrhosis (liver disease)
    H. Do you regularly use any prescription drugs or herbals—we need to check possible interactions with Depo-Provera®

VII. Side Effects You Might Experience

    A. Weight gain or loss; change in appetite
    B. Menstrual irregularity—possibly no periods by second or third shot
    C. Headaches
    D. Abdominal bloating
    E. Breast tenderness
    F. Tiredness, weakness
    G. Dizziness
    H. Depression, nervousness
    I. Nausea
    J. No hair growth or loss or thinning of hair; increased hair growth on face or body
    K. Skin rash or increased acne
    L. Increased or decreased sex drive

VIII. Explanation of Method and Assessment

Depo-Provera® is injected intramuscularly or subqutaneously in one dose every 12 weeks for as long as contraceptive effect is desired. It is injected in the first 5 days of the menstrual cycle (after onset of menses), within 5 days postpartum.

IX. Use of This Method and Warning Signs

    A. Drug interactions are possible when using Depo-Provera® with other prescription drugs. Always check with your physician or nurse practitioner and pharmacist for such possible interactions before taking any other prescription drug; Depo-Provera® is a medication and you need to list it in your health history.
    B. Warning signs to report to your clinician (physician or nurse practitioner):

1. Sharp chest pain, coughing of blood, sudden shortness of breath
2. Sudden severe headache, vomiting, dizziness, or fainting
3. Visual disturbance (double vision, blurred vision, spots before your eyes or speech disturbance (slurred, unable to speak)
4. Weakness or numbness in arm or leg
5. Severe pain or swelling in calf or leg
6. Unusually heavy vaginal bleeding (unlike usual periods)
7. Severe pain or tenderness in lower abdomen, pelvis
8. Persistent pain, pus, or bleeding at injection site

X. Follow-up Care of Yourself

A. Visit your clinician every 12 weeks for injection of Depo-Provera
B. The first visit should take place during first 5 days of your menses (period)
C. Review any side effects or danger signs with your clinician
D. Review your menstrual cycles with your clinician
E. Have a Pap smear every year along with a complete physical examination including pelvic and breast examinations
F. Depo-Provera® provides no protection against sexually transmitted diseases (including AIDS) or vaginal infections, so consider using condoms to protect yourself.
G. Depo-Provera® contains no estrogen. Estrogen is needed for strong bones. While using this birth control method, you need to be sure you get enough calcium and vitamin D in your diet. Your clinician will advise you on how to do this.

I have read the above and have been given a copy of this consent form and the manufacturer's information, and I agree to have Depo-Provera®

Patient's signature _____ Date _____

Witness's signature _____ Date _____

From Hawkins, Roberto-Nichols, & Stanley-Haney, *Guidelines for Nurse Practitioners in Gynecologic Settings,* 9th edition, 2007, © Springer Publishing Company.

DIAPHRAGM

(May also be used as an informational handout)

I. Mechanism of Action

A contraceptive diaphragm is a shallow rubber cup with a flexible rim that is placed in the vagina so as to cover the cervix. It functions as both a mechanical barrier and a receptacle for spermicidal cream or jelly or vaginal film that must be used to ensure effectiveness.

II. Benefits of the Method

    A. Effectiveness rate ranges from 80–95%: theoretically, 95%. 80–85% use effectiveness (due to user failure)

    B. No chemicals are taken internally

III. Risks of the Method

    A. Allergic response to the rubber and/or spermicidal agent

    B. Foul-smelling discharge from leaving diaphragm in place too long (diaphragm should not be left in place longer than 24 hours)

    C. Toxic shock syndrome has been reported in association with diaphragm use during the menstrual period. To avoid this, do not leave your diaphragm in place for more than 24 hours and follow use precautions at the end of these instructions.

IV. Contraindications

    A. Inability to achieve satisfactory fitting

    B. You are unable to learn correct insertion technique

    C. Allergy to rubber or spermicidal agent

    D. Inconvenience of method (e.g., lack of sexual spontaneity, timing, messiness, etc.)

    E. Repeated bladder infections (cystitis)

    F. Chronic constipation (causes discomfort for some users)

V. Alternative Birth Control Methods

    A. Abstinence

    B. Sterilization

    C. Oral contraceptives (birth control pills, mini pills)

    D. Intrauterine device

    E. Condom used with contraceptive cream, foam, gel, suppositories, vaginal film or sponge

    F. FemCap, Lea's Shield

    G. Natural family planning

    H. Female condom

    I. Depo-Provera® contraceptive injection

    J. Contraceptive patch, ring, Implant [Implanon®]

VI. Explanation of the Method

    A. How a diaphragm is prescribed

        1. A complete physical examination including Papanicolaou smear is necessary unless one has been done within the past year. A pelvic examination (bimanual) will be done at the time the diaphragm is fitted.

2. If required by your clinician, review and sign an informed consent similar to this one prior to your initial prescription.

B. How a diaphragm is used
1. How it works
   a. Inserted prior to intercourse to fit snugly in vagina
   b. Holds spermicidal cream or jelly or vaginal film against cervix and kills sperm
   c. Diaphragm is to be left in place for 8 hours after last intercourse
   d. No douching for 8 hours after intercourse
   e. Prior to repeated intercourse, additional jelly or cream should be applied with applicator to outside of diaphragm or another vaginal film should be inserted
   f. Effective immediately upon insertion and up to 4 hours without adding more cream or jelly or film, or for one intercourse (some sources suggest 6 hours for c., d., and f.)

2. Technique for use
   a. Empty your bladder, wash your hands carefully whenever you insert or remove your diaphragm.
   b. Apply approximately 1 tablespoon spermicidal cream or jelly into the dome of the diaphragm and spread around the dome; cream or jelly need not be spread on the rim or outside of diaphragm.
   c. Fold in half and insert into vagina like a tampon.
   d. With index finger check rim at pubic arch and make sure cervix is covered.
   e. To remove (at proper time), hook finger around rim and pull diaphragm out.

3. Care of diaphragm
   a. Wash with warm water and mild soap after removal.
   b. Dry thoroughly.
   c. Store in dry place (allowing it to dry thoroughly before putting it in a case keeps rubber in better condition longer and prevents odor; powder lightly with cornstarch).
   d. Soak in rubbing alcohol (70%) for 30 minutes after use following treatment for vaginal infection.

VII. Diaphragm Check

A. We encourage you to return to the office 1 week after fitting for diaphragm check.
B. If you lose or gain 10–15 pounds (or if diaphragm fit seems to change).

C. If you have a miscarriage, abortion, or a baby.
D. If you have any kind of pelvic surgery.
E. If you experience problems urinating or trouble moving your bowels with diaphragm in place.

VIII. Inquiries are Encouraged

Please feel free to ask us questions at any time!

You may change your mind about a birth control method at any time.

I have read the above material; it has been explained fully. I have been given the opportunity to ask questions and I understand the information. I have chosen to use the diaphragm.

Patient's signature _____ Date _____
Witness's signature _____ Date _____

Toxic Shock Syndrome

Toxic shock syndrome has been reported in association with diaphragm use during menses. It is recommended that if you use your diaphragm during menses, you observe hand washing recommendations carefully, use tampons only during heaviest days (not super-absorbent type—see tampon package labeling), and monitor yourself carefully for any signs of toxic shock syndrome.

Danger Signals Associated with Possible Toxic Shock Syndrome

Fever (temperature 100 degrees F and above)
Diarrhea
Vomiting
Muscle ache
Rash (sunburn-like)

Contact us at ( )_____ if you develop any of the above problems (and don't use your diaphragm—remove at once)

If your diaphragm slips out of place or comes out, you can call 1-888-NOT-2-LATE for information on emergency contraception. Web sites: http://not-2-late.com; http://www.go2planB.com.

Emergency contraception Plan B® is available over the counter (no prescription) at pharmacies if you are 18 or older.

From Hawkins, Roberto-Nichols & Stanley-Haney, *Guidelines for Nurse Practitioners in Gynecological Settings*, 9th edition, 2007, © Springer Publishing Company.

INTRAUTERINE DEVICE (IUD)

(May also be used as informational handout)

I. Definition/Mechanism of Action

An intrauterine device consists of a sterile body placed in the uterus to prevent fertilization. This is accomplished through several mechanisms of action, depending on the type of device:

    A. A local sterile inflammatory response to the foreign body (the IUD) causes a change in the cellular makeup of the uterine lining

    B. A possible increase in the local production of prostaglandins may increase endometrial activity

    C. Alteration in uterine and tubal transport of egg

    D. Change in cervical mucus causing barrier to sperm penetration

    E. Mirena® may stop release of an egg but this is not the primary way it works

II. Benefits of the Method

    A. Encourages sexual spontaneity

    B. Effectiveness rate, theoretically, 97–99%

    C. Semi-permanent (depending on the type of device); replacement time varies but all devices are effective for at least 5 years; one device lasts 10 years

III. Risks of Method

    A. Major risks
        1. Involuntary expulsion (approximately 6%)
        2. Pelvic inflammatory disease
        3. Ectopic pregnancy (outside of the uterus)
        4. Uterine perforation
        5. Pregnancy

    B. Minor risks
        1. Increased menstrual flow
        2. Increased dysmenorrhea (cramps)
        3. String may cause some discomfort to partner

IV. Reasons for Not Using an Intrauterine Device (IUD)

    A. Active pelvic infection (acute or subacute) including known or suspected gonorrhea or Chlamydia

    B. Known or suspected pregnancy

    C. Recent or recurrent pelvic infection

   D. Purulent cervicitis, untreated acute cervicitis, or vaginosis

   E. Undiagnosed genital bleeding

   F. Uterine cavity not suitable for IUD insertion

   G. History of ectopic pregnancy (pregnancy outside uterus)

   H. Diabetes mellitus can use ParaGard® IUD

   I. Allergy to copper (known or suspected) or diagnosed Wilson's Disease; can use Mirena® IUD

   J. Abnormal Pap; cervical or uterine cancer, precancer

   K. Impaired response to infection (diabetes, steroid treatment, immunocompromised patients such as those with HIV/AIDS)

   L. Presence of previously inserted IUD

   M. Genital actinomycosis; chronic infection of genital area

V. Reasons IUD May Not Be Best Choice or Require Careful Monitoring With Clinician

   A. Multiple sexual partners or partner has multiple partners

   B. In very rural areas, emergency treatment difficult to obtain

   C. Cervical opening resistant to inserting IUD

   D. Impaired blood clotting response

   E. Uterine cavity too small, too large

   F. Endometriosis

   G. Fibroids in uterus

   H. Polyps in uterine lining (endometrium)

   I. Severe dysmenorrhea (Mirena® IUD may help)

   J. Heavy or prolonged menstrual bleeding without anemia; consider oral iron or nutritional changes to prevent anemia

   K. Unable to check for IUD string

   L. Concerns for future fertility

   M. Postpartum or infected abortion within the past 3 months

   N. History of pelvic uterine infection

   O. Valvular heart disease infection

VI. Alternatives

   A. Abstinence

   B. Sterilization

   C. Birth control pills

   D. FemCap, Lea's Shield, contraceptive sponge

   E. Natural family planning

   F. Depo-Provera®

   G. Female condom

   H. Contraceptive ring, patch, implant

   I. Diaphragm and spermicidal cream or jelly, film, sponge

  J. Condom used with contraceptive cream, foam, suppositories, gel, or vaginal film

VII. Explanation of the Method

  A. How the intrauterine device may work (no one is quite sure), but there are several theories:
    1. Motility of the egg in fallopian tube is altered
    2. A sterile inflammatory response to the IUD causes a change in the cells of the uterine lining
    3. A change in the cervical mucus causing a barrier to sperm
  B. What you should know about caring for your IUD
    1. Know the type of device you have in place
    2. Know when your device should be replaced
    3. Learn how to check the string that extends from the center of the cervix into the vaginal canal
    4. Check the string frequently the first few months and then after each period
    5. Do not let your partner pull on the string
    6. Never try to remove IUD yourself
    7. Return for your 6-week check-up after insertion of the device
    8. Get a check-up every year including a Pap smear
    9. Depending on your normal menstrual cycle, if you miss a period, consult your clinician for possible pregnancy
  C. What to expect
    1. Possible increase in menstrual flow, menstrual cramping
Remember: if this condition becomes intolerable, you have the option of having your IUD removed by a clinician
  D. Side effects to be reported *immediately*
    1. Late period or absence of period
    2. Abdominal or pelvic pain (severe)
    3. Elevated temperature, chills (not due to illness)
    4. Unpleasant vaginal discharge (smelly, foul, bloody, or greenish color)
    5. Unusual vaginal bleeding (heavy period, clotting)
  E. Insertion
    1. IUDs usually inserted within 7 days of menses
    2. Should have negative gonococcus and Chlamydia cultures prior to insertion (within 30 days); consider culture for Strep. Group B
    3. Must have recent (within the year) normal Pap smear
    4. May have some discomfort and dizziness with insertion
    5. May have spotting for several months after insertion

6. Although the IUD is effective immediately, it is recommended that intercourse not take place for 24 hours

VII. Inquiries are encouraged! Ask us questions at any time.

I have read the above material; it has been explained fully. I have been given the opportunity to ask questions and I understand the information. I have chosen to use the IUD _____ type
Signed _____ Witness _____
Date _____

Danger Signals Associated with the Use of the IUD

Late period or absence of period
Abdominal pain (severe)
Elevated temperature, chills (not due to illness, e.g., flu)
Unpleasant vaginal discharge (smelly, foul, bloody, or greenish color)
Unusual vaginal bleeding (heavy period, clotting)

Contact us or a clinician immediately if above danger signs develop!
From Hawkins, Roberto-Nichols, & Stanley-Haney, *Guidelines for Nurse Practitioners in Gynecologic Settings,* 9th edition, 2007, © Springer Publishing Company

INFORMATION HANDOUT FOR EMERGENCY CONTRACEPTION (EC)

I. Definition

Emergency contraception (EC), often known as the morning after pill, is the use of birth control pills to prevent pregnancy after a contraceptive method has failed or because there was no contraception. Currently in the United States there is one product available just for EC, Plan B®.

II. How It Works

If used within the first 120 hours after unprotected sexual intercourse, EC probably works because of one or more of the following reasons:
A. Progestational hormones in Plan B pills interfere with the sperm's ability to travel up through the uterus and into the fallopian tube to fertilize the egg; also they affect the growth of the ovary's follicles
B. Combination hormones are thought to interfere with or disrupt ovulation (release of an egg by the ovary)

III. How Effective Is It?

If used within the first 72 hours after sex without birth control protection, EC is greater than 90 percent effective. EC literature says that EC may be used up to 120 hours after unprotected sex; however, the earlier the pills are taken, the more effective they will be.

IV. Benefits

    A. Pregnancy prevention
    B. Inexpensive
    C. Relatively noninvasive

V. Disadvantages

    A. May not be appropriate for women with certain medical conditions
    B. Pregnancy may occur due to:
       1. Fertilized egg already implanted in the uterus
       2. Too much time between unprotected sex and taking EC
       3. Failure of the emergency contraception
       4. Must be used within 72 or at most 120 hours of unprotected sex

VI. Risks and Side Effects

    A. Nausea and/or vomiting
    B. Breast tenderness
    C. Irregular bleeding
    D. Headache

VII. You May Not Be Able to Take Combination Birth Control Pills as EC if You Have:

    A. An active liver disease
    B. Unexplained bleeding from the vagina
    C. An already established pregnancy
    D. History of blood clots, inflammation in the veins, or cancer of the breast, uterus, or ovaries

VIII. Alternative EC

    A. Progestin-only oral contraceptives used as EC
    B. Insertion of an IUD

IX. How EC is Prescribed

    A. Pelvic examination as appropriate (to be determined by you and your clinician)

B. If rape or sexual assault occurred, specimens can be collected if desired by you and your clinician

C. Pregnancy test

D. Testing for sexually transmitted diseases (STDs) if desired, or if recommended by clinician

E. Blood pressure

X. Ways in which EC is taken

A. Take one Plan B pill within 72–120 hours of unprotected intercourse and follow directions D to F. Take second pill 12 hours later. Or you can take both pills at the same time. (EC is indicated in the packet for up to 120 hours; however, the earlier you take it, the greater the efficacy.)

B. Take ____ birth control pills within 72–120 hours of unprotected intercourse. Do not take the pills on an empty stomach: eat a snack such as juice or milk and crackers and take the pills 20 minutes later. Take _____ birth control pills 12 hours after the first dose.

C. If you vomit within an hour after taking the birth control pills, follow the instructions your clinician gives you.

D. Talk with your clinician about methods of contraception you might be interested in for ongoing protection. Emergency contraception is just that—for emergencies—and is not recommended for routine use. Some birth control methods can be started immediately or the day after using EC. Methods vary in how soon they become effective.

E. Report any of the warning signs listed below to your clinician at once.

F. After using EC, return to your clinician as directed for a check-up, particularly if you have not had a normal menstrual period.

*Plan B is now available over-the-counter if you are 18 or older. Check with your pharmacy.

I have read the above material. I have been given the opportunity to ask questions and I fully understand the information. I have chosen to use emergency contraception.

Signed _____ Date _____
Witness _____ Date _____

Danger Signals Associated with EC

Abdominal pain (severe)
Chest pain (severe), arm pain, or shortness of breath
Headaches (severe)

Eye problems such as blurred or double vision, loss of vision
Severe leg pain (calf or thigh)

    Contact us at ( )_____ if you develop any of the above danger
signals
    Emergency Contraception hotline: 800-584-9911, 888-NOT-2-LATE;
Web sites http://not-2-late.com; http://www.go2planB.com.
    From Hawkins, Roberto-Nichols, & Stanley-Haney, *Guidelines for
Nurse Practitioners in Gynecologic Settings,* 9th edition, 2007, © Springer
Publishing Company.

NOTE

1. U.S. Boxed Warning from the FDA: Prolonged use of medroxyprogesterone contraceptive injection may result in a loss of bone mineral density (BMD). Loss is related to the duration of use, and may not be completely reversible on discontinuation of the drug. The impact on peak bone mass in adolescents should be considered in treatment decisions. U.S. Boxed Warning: Long-term use (i.e., >2 years) should be limited to situations where other birth control methods are inadequate. Consider other methods of birth control in women with (or at risk for) osteoporosis. Web sites: http://www.merck.com/mmpe/lexicomp/medroxyprogesterone.html; http://www.fda.gov/bbs/topics/ANSWERS/2004/ANS01325.html

APPENDIX C

Abuse Assessment Screen

1. Have you EVER been emotionally or physically abused by your partner or someone important to you? YES NO
2. **WITHIN THE LAST YEAR,** have you been hit, slapped, kicked, or otherwise physically hurt by somcone? YES NO

If YES, by whom? _____

Total number of times

3. **SINCE YOU'VE BEEN PREGNANT,** have you been hit, slapped, kicked, or otherwise physically hurt by someone? YES NO

If YES, by whom? _____

Total number of times

Mark the areas of injury on a body map (Figure C.1).

Score each incident according to the following scale

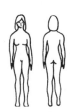

　　　1 = Threats of abuse including use of a weapon

　　　2 = Slapping, pushing; no injuries, and/or lasting pain

FIGURE C.1　Body map.

　　　3 = Punching, kicking, bruises, cuts, and/or continuing pain

　　　4 = Beating up, severe contusions, burns, brokcn bones

　　　5 = Head injury, internal injury, permanent injury

　　　6 = Use of weapon; wound from weapon

If any of the descriptions for the higher number apply, use the higher number.

4. **WITHIN THE LAST YEAR** has anyone forced you to have sexual activities? YES NO

If YES, by whom?_____Total number of times_____

5. **ARE YOU AFRAID** of your partner or anyone in your life? YES NO

Developed by the Nursing Research Consortium on Violence and Abuse. Readers are encouraged to reproduce and use this assessment tool. Adapted by Pregnancy Support Project, Boston College, William F. Connell School of Nursing

Danger Assessment

Jacquelyn C. Campbell, PhD, RN, FAAN

TABLE 1. Danger Assessment

Several risk factors have been associated with increased risk of homicides (murders) of women and men in violent relationships. We cannot predict what will happen in your case, but we would like you to be aware of the danger of homicide in situations of abuse and for you to see how many of the risk factors apply to your situation.

Using the calendar, please mark the approximate dates during the past year when you were abused by your partner or ex partner. Write on that date how bad the incident was according to the following scale:

1. Slapping, pushing; no injuries, and/or lasting pain

2. Punching, kicking; bruises, cuts, and/or continuing pain

3. "Beating up"; severe contusions, burns, broken bones, miscarriage

4. Threat to use weapon; head injury, internal injury, permanent injury, miscarriage

5. Use of weapon; wounds from weapon

(If **any** of the descriptions for the higher number apply, use the higher number.)

Mark **Yes** or **No** for each of the following.

("He" refers to your husband, partner, ex-husband, ex-partner, or whoever is currently physically hurting you.)

Yes　　　**No**

　　　　　　　1. Has the physical violence increased in severity or frequency over the past year?

　　　　　　　2. Does he own a gun?

3. Have you left him after living together during the past year?

3a.   (If have never lived with him, check here___)

4. Is he unemployed?

5. Has he ever used a weapon against you or threatened you with a lethal weapon?

5a.   (If yes, was the weapon a gun?____)

6. Does he threaten to kill you?

7. Has he avoided being arrested for domestic violence?

8. Do you have a child that is not his?

9. Has he ever forced you to have sex when you did not wish to do so?

10. Does he ever try to choke you?

11. Does he use illegal drugs? By drugs, I mean "uppers" or amphetamines, speed, angel dust, cocaine, "crack", street drugs or mixtures.

12. Is he an alcoholic or problem drinker?

13. Does he control most or all of your daily activities? (For instance: does he tell you who you can be friends with, when you can see your family, how much money you can use, or when you can take the car?)

   (If he tries, but you do not let him, check here: __)

14. Is he violently and constantly jealous of you?

   (For instance, does he say "If I can't have you, no one can"?)

15. Have you ever been beaten by him while you were pregnant?

   (If you have never been pregnant by him, check here: ____)

16. Has he ever threatened or tried to commit suicide?

17. Does he threaten to harm your children?

18. Do you believe he is capable of killing you?

19. Does he follow or spy on you, leave threatening notes or messages on answering machine, destroy your property, or call you when you don't want him to?

20. Have you ever threatened or tried to commit suicide?

Total "Yes" Answers

Thank you. Please talk to your nurse, advocate or counselor about what the Danger Assessment means in terms of your situation.

Self-Assessment of AIDS (HIV) Risk

1. Do you use injectable drugs? Does your sexual partner(s)? Do you or your partner(s) have a partner(s) who uses injectable drugs? How about in the past?
2. If you or your partner(s) use injectable drugs, do you ever share needles or syringes? How about in the past? Have you ever used intranasal drugs (snorted)?
3. Did you or your partner(s) have a blood transfusion between 1975 and 1985 or have sexual exposure to partners who did?
4. Do you have or have you had a hemophiliac partner(s) who received blood or blood products between 1975 and 1985?
5. Do you or your partner(s) use latex condoms/female condoms whenever you have vaginal or anal sex?
6. Do you ever let your partner(s) ejaculate (cum) in your mouth? Do you ever have oral sex with a female partner during menses?
7. Have you ever had unprotected sex with a man who has had sex with another man?
8. Do you ever share sex toys (such as a vibrator)?
9. If you are a clinician, have you ever experienced a needle stick, exposure to a patient's blood, or exposure to amniotic fluid on your unprotected hands or face?
10. Are you and your partner mutually monogamous? How long have you been so?
11. Have you ever traded sex for money, shelter, food, or drugs?
12. Have you ever had unwanted or forced (nonconsensual) sex?

13. How many sexual partners have you had in the past 12 months?
14. How many sexual partners in your whole life?
15. Have you ever exchanged money for sex in the past 12 months?
16. Have you ever had sex with somebody you did not know about at the time (casual sex)?
17. How often do you use drugs?
18. How often do you use alcohol?
19. Have you ever been tested for HIV?
20. Have you ever had a tattoo?
21. Have you ever had a sexually transmitted disease (STD)?
22. Have you ever had sex with someone who is HIV positive?

If your answer to any of the yes/no questions except 5 and 10 is yes, you may be at risk and might consider being tested.

Assessment tool courtesy of Richard S. Ferri, PhD, ANP, ACRN, and updated by Rosanna DeMarco, PhD, APRN BC, ACRN, Associate Professor, Community Health, William F. Connell SON, Boston College

From Hawkins, Roberto-Nichols, & Stanley-Haney, *Guidelines for Nurse Practitioners in Gynecologic Settings,* 9th edition, 2007, © Springer Publishing Company.

Women and Heart Disease: Risk Factor Assessment

Nonmodifiable

1. Age: postmenopausally, the risk for women increases dramatically; mortality is high for ages 35 to 44 and 75 to 84.
2. Race or ethnicity: black women have a higher rate of death than white women; 5-year survival rate is lower and black women younger than 55 have > 2x the death rate of white women; rates of diabetes and hypertension in black women are higher than those in white women.
3. Family history of the disease especially heart attack < 50
4. Gender: attenuating advantage of being a woman especially premenopausally (premenopausally, women's risk is lower than men's)
5. Socioeconomic status: inverse association with morbidity and mortality

Modifiable

1. Lifestyle
   a. Exercise: aerobic exercise can increase HDLs (brisk walking; jogging) > 30 minutes daily or most days; sedentary life increases risk for heart disease almost 2 fold

b. Chronic diseases: diabetes increases risk 3–7 times, obesity—especially waist > 38 inches, high blood pressure major risk factor

c. Nutrition: cholesterol levels, lipid profile (HDL vs. LDL); high fat vs. low fat diet; < 20% of all calories from fat; < 2.4 g/day of sodium and maintain body mass index between 18.5 to 24.9, modifying effects of antioxidants (5 to 9 servings vegetables, fruits/day; 6 servings of grains/day; dietary fiber 25 grams/day)

d. Cigarette smoking
   1. Smoking and OC use (combination hormonal contraception) increases rate of atherosclerosis
   2. Women (under 40 years old) who have MIs are mainly smokers
   3. Older women who smoke have a 50% greater chance to experience sudden death than older nonsmokers
   4. Acts synergistically with hyperlipidemia
   5. Women with hypertension using hormonal contraception or estrogen therapy postmenopausally increase risk 10–15 fold

2. Internal and external environmental factors
   a. Comorbidities: hypertension, diabetes, obesity; poor management of these chronic diseases increases risk while good management decreases risk. Blood pressure maintain at < 120/80.
   b. Psychosocial concerns: stress and social support; high stress and low social support increase morbidity and mortality; lower level employees (such as clerks, cashiers) have two times the likelihood of heart disease than women in white collar jobs.
   c. Access to health care: unequal access appears to be a factor in morbidity and mortality.

Web sites: American Heart Association, http://www.Americanheart.org; Women's Health Initiative, http://www.nhlbi.nih.gov/whi/; http://www.womenheart.org.

From Hawkins, Roberto-Nichols, & Stanley-Haney, *Guidelines for Nurse Practitioners in Gynecologic Settings,* 9th edition, 2007, © Springer Publishing Company.

APPENDIX G

Body Mass Index Table

TABLE 2. BODY MASS INDEX TABLE

BMI	19	20	21	22	23	24	25	26	27	28	29	30	31	32	33	34	35
Height (inches)							Body Weight (pounds)										
58	91	96	100	105	110	115	119	124	129	134	138	143	148	153	158	162	167
59	94	99	104	109	114	119	124	128	133	138	143	148	153	158	163	168	173
60	97	102	107	112	118	123	128	133	138	143	148	153	158	163	168	174	179
61	100	106	111	116	122	127	132	137	143	148	153	158	164	169	174	180	185
62	104	109	115	120	126	131	136	142	147	153	158	164	169	175	180	186	191
63	107	113	118	124	130	135	141	146	152	158	163	169	175	180	186	191	197
64	110	116	122	128	134	140	145	151	157	163	169	174	180	186	192	197	204
65	114	120	126	132	138	144	150	156	162	168	174	180	186	192	198	204	210
66	118	124	130	136	142	148	155	161	167	173	179	186	192	198	204	210	216
67	121	127	134	140	146	153	159	166	172	178	185	191	198	204	211	217	223
68	125	131	138	144	151	158	164	171	177	184	190	197	203	210	216	223	230
69	128	135	142	149	155	162	169	176	182	189	196	203	209	216	223	230	236
70	132	139	146	153	160	167	174	181	188	195	202	209	216	222	229	236	243
71	136	143	150	157	165	172	179	186	193	200	208	215	222	229	236	243	250
72	140	147	154	162	169	177	184	191	199	206	213	221	228	235	242	250	258
73	144	151	159	166	174	182	189	197	204	212	219	227	235	242	250	257	265
74	148	155	163	171	179	186	194	202	210	218	225	233	241	249	256	264	272
75	152	160	168	176	184	192	200	208	216	224	232	240	248	256	264	272	279
76	156	164	172	180	189	197	205	213	221	230	238	246	254	263	271	279	287

TABLE 3. BODY MASS INDEX TABLE

BMI	36	37	38	39	40	41	42	43	44	45	46	47	48	49	50	51	52	53	54
Height (inches)								Body Weight (pounds)											
58	172	177	181	186	.191	196	201	205	210	215	220	224	229	234	239	244	248	253	258
59	178	183	188	193	198	203	208	212	217	222	227	232	237	242	247	252	257	262	267
60	184	189	194	199	204	209	215	220	225	230	235	240	245	250	255	261	266	271	276
61	190	195	201	206	211	217	222	227	232	238	243	248	254	259	264	269	275	280	285
62	196	202	207	213	218	224	229	235	240	246	251	256	262	267	273	278	284	289	295
63	203	208	214	220	225	231	237	242	248	254	259	265	270	278	282	287	293	299	304
64	209	215	221	227	232	238	244	250	256	262	267	273	279	285	291	296	302	308	314
65	216	222	228	234	240	246	252	258	264	270	276	282	288	294	300	306	312	318	324
66	223	229	235	241	247	253	260	266	272	278	284	291	297	303	309	315	322	328	334
67	230	236	242	249	255	261	268	274	280	287	293	299	306	312	319	325	331	338	344
68	236	243	249	256	262	269	276	282	289	295	302	308	315	322	328	335	341	348	354
69	243	250	257	263	270	277	284	291	297	304	311	318	324	331	338	345	351	358	365
70	250	257	264	271	278	285	292	299	306	313	320	327	334	341	348	355	362	369	376
71	257	265	272	279	286	293	301	308	315	322	329	338	343	351	358	365	372	379	386
72	265	272	279	287	294	302	309	316	324	331	338	346	353	361	368	375	383	390	397
73	272	280	288	295	302	310	318	325	333	340	348	355	363	371	378	386	393	401	408
74	280	287	295	303	311	319	326	334	342	350	358	365	373	381	389	396	404	412	420
75	287	295	303	311	319	327	335	343	351	359	367	375	383	391	399	407	415	423	431
76	295	304	312	320	328	336	344	353	361	369	377	385	394	402	410	418	426	435	443

Source: NHLBI Obesity Education Initiative, U.S. Department of Health and Human Services, Public Health Service, National Institutes of Health, National Heart, Lung and Blood Institute. 2000 NIH Pub#00-408.

Bibliographies

ABDOMINAL AND PELVIC PAIN

Bird, S. (2005). Failure to diagnose ectopic pregnancy. *Australian Family Physician, 34,* 175–176.

Carter, J.F.S. (2000a). Chronic pelvic pain: Are you overlooking its nongynecologic causes? *Womens Health in Primary Care, 3*(9), 649–661.

Carter, J.F.S. (2000b). Diagnosing and treating nongynecologic chronic pelvic pain. *Womens Health in Primary Care, 3*(10), 708–725.

Cheong, Y., & Stones, R.W. (2006). Chronic pelvic pain: Aetiology and therapy. *Best Practice & Research Clinical Obstetrics and Gynaecology, 20,* 695–711.

Kriebs, J. M., & Fahey, J. O. (2006). Ectopic pregnancy. *Journal of Midwifery & Womens Health, 51,* 431–439.

Miller, S. K. & Alpert, P.T. (2006). Assessment and differential diagnosis of abdominal pain. *The Nurse Practitioner, 31* (7), 38–47.

Zhang, J., Gilles, J. M., Barnhart, K., Creinin, M. D., Westhoff, C., Frederick, M. M., et al. (2005). A comparison of medical management with misoprostol and surgical management for early pregnancy failure. *The New England Journal of Medicine, 353,* 761–769.

ABORTION

Andrist, L. C., Simmonds, K., Liebermann, E., & Healey, K. (2006). Womens experiences of medical abortion. *The American Journal of Nurse Practitioners, 10* (7–8), 59–65.

Beal, M. W. (2007). Update on medication abortion. *Journal of Midwifery & Womens Health, 52,* 23–30.

Beal, M. W., & Simmonds, K. (2002). Clinical uses of mifepristone: An update for womens health practitioners. *Journal of Midwifery & Womens Health, 47,* 451–460.

Clark, W. H., Gold, M., Grossman, D., & Winikoff, B. (2007). Can mifepristone medical abortion be simplified? A review of the evidence and questions for future research. *Contraception, 75,* 245–250.

Davey, A. (2006). Mifepristone and prostaglandins for termination of pregnancy: Contraindications for use, reasons and rationale. *Contraception, 74,* 16–20.

Esteve, J.L.C., Mari, J. M., Valero, F., Llorente, M., Salvador, I. Varela, L., et al. (2006). Sublingual versus vaginal misoprostol (400 ug) for cervical priming in first-trimester abortion: A randomized trial. *Contraception, 74,* 328–333.

Foster, A. M., Wynn, L., Rouhana, A., Diaz-Olavarrieta, C., Schaffer, K., & Trussell, J. Providing medication abortion information to diverse communities: Use patterns of a multilingual web site. *Contraception, 74,* 264–271.

Goldberg, A. B., Greenberg, M. B., & Darney, P. D. (2001). Misoprostol and pregnancy. *New England Journal of Medicine, 344*(1), 38–47.

Marions, L. (2006). Mifepristone dose in the regimen with misoprostol for medical abortion. *Contraception, 74,* 21–21.

Robinson, D. L., Dollins, A., & McConlogue-O'Shaughnessy, L. (2000). Care of the woman before and after an elective abortion. *The American Journal for Nurse Practitioners, 4*(3), 17–29.

Rue, V. M., Coleman, P. K., Rue, J. J., & Reardon, D. C. (2004). Induced abortion and traumatic stress: A preliminary comparison of American and Russian women. *Medical Science Monitor, 10* (10), SR5–16.

Schaff, E. A., Fielding, S. L., Westhoff, C., Ellertson, C., Eisinger, S. H., Stadalius, L. S., et al. (2000). Vaginal misoprostol administered 1, 2, or 3 days after mifepristone for early medical abortion. *Journal of the American Medical Association, 284*(15), 1948–1953.

Abuse and Violence

Campbell, J. C. (2002). Health consequences of intimate partner violence. *Lancet, 359,* 1331–1336.

Campbell, J. C., Webster, D., Koziol-McLain, J., Block, C. R., Campbell, D. W., Gary, F., et al. (2003). Risk factors for femicide in abusive relationships: Results from a multisite case control study. *American Journal of Public Health, 93,* 1089–1097.

Carpiano, R. M. (2002). Long roads and tall mountains: The impact of motherhood on the recovery and health of domestic abuse survivors. *Health Care for Women International, 23*(5), 442–459.

Cook, S. L. (2002). Self-reports of sexual, physical, and nonphysical abuse perpetration. *Violence Against Women, 8*(5), 541–565.

Davis, K., Taylor, B., & Furniss, D. (2001). Narrative accounts of tracking the rural domestic violence survivors journey: A feminist approach. *Health Care for Women International, 22*(4), 333–347.

Davis, R. E. (2002). Leave-taking experiences in the lives of abused women. *Clinical Nursing Research, 11*(3), 285–305.

D'Avolio, D., Hawkins, J. W., Haggerty, L. A., Kelly, U., Barrett, R., Toscano, S.E.D., et al. (2001). Screening for abuse: Barriers and opportunities. *Health Care for Women International, 22*(4), 349–362.

Dienemann, J., Campbell, J., Landenburger, K., & Curry, M. A. (2002). The domestic violence survivor assessment: A tool for counseling women in intimate partner violence relationships. *Patient Education and Counseling, 46,* 221–228.

Eisikovits, Z., & Winstok, Z. (2002). Reconstructing intimate violence: The structure and content of recollections of violent events. *Qualitative Health Research, 12*(5), 685–699.

Feder, G. S., Hutson, M., Ramsay, J., & Taket, A. R. (2006). Women exposed to intimate partner violence: Expectations and experiences when they encounter health care professionals: A meta-analysis of qualitative studies. *Archives of Internal Medicine, 166,* 22–37.

Garcia-Moreno, C. (2002). Dilemmas and opportunities for an appropriate health-service response to violence against women. *Lancet, 359,* 1509–1514.

Lee, R. K., Thompson, V.L.S., & Mechanic, M. B. (2002). Intimate partner violence and women of color: A call for innovations. *American Journal of Public Health, 92*(4), 530–534.

National Center for Injury Prevention and Control. (2003). *Costs of intimate partner violence against women in the United States.* Atlanta, GA: Centers for Disease Control and Prevention.

BREAST CONDITIONS

Berry, J. A. (2001). Breast pain: All that hurts is not cancer. *The American Journal for Nurse Practitioners, 5*(4), 9–18.

Coleman, E. A. (2001). Clinical breast examination: An illustrated educational review and update. *Clinical Excellence for Nurse Practitioners, 5*(4), 197–204.

Coleman, E. A., Coon, S. K., Fitzgerald, A. J., & Cantrell, M. J. (2001). Breast cancer screening education: Comparing outcome skills of nurse practitioner students and medical residents. *Clinical Excellence for Nurse Practitioners, 5,* 102–107.

Dinkel, H., Gassel, A. M., Muller, T., Lourens, S., Rominger, M., & Tschammler, A. (2001). Galactography and exfoliative cytology in women with abnormal nipple discharge. *Obstetrics and Gynecology, 97*(4), 625–629.

Janowsky, E. C., Kupper, L. L, & Hulka, B. S. (2000). Meta-analyses of the relation between silicone breast implants and the risk of connective-tissue diseases. *New England Journal of Medicine, 342*(11), 781–790.

Johnson, K. C. (2005). Accumulating evidence on passive and active smoking and breast cancer risk. *International Journal of Cancer, 117,* 619–628.

Kinney, A. Y., Emery, G., Dudley, W. N., & Croyle, R. T. (2002). Screening behaviors among African American women at high risk for breast cancer. *Oncology Nursing Forum, 29*(5), 835–844.

Klein, S. (2005). Evaluation of palpable breast masses. *American Family Physician, 71,* 1731–1738.

Smith, R. L., Pruthi, S., & Fitzpatrick, L. A. (2004). Evaluation and management of breast pain. *Mayo Clinic Procedures, 79* (3), 353–372.

Thompson, K. B., & Keehbauch, J. (2006, October). Evaluation and management of common breast complaints. *The Female Patient, 31,* 28–38.

Trock, B. J., Hilakivi-Clarke, L., & Clarke, R. (2006). Meta-analysis of soy intake and breast cancer risk. *Journal of the National Cancer Institute, 98,* 459–471.

Zimmerman, V. L. (2002). BRCA gene mutations and cancer. *American Journal of Nursing, 102*(8), 28–36.

CERVIX, PAPANICOLAOU SMEARS, HPV

Audisio, T., Pigini, T., de Riutort, S., Schindler, L., Ozan, M., Tocalli, C., & Bertolotto, P. (2002). Validity of the Papanicolaou smear in the diagnosis of candida, trichomonas vaginalis, and bacterial vaginosis. *Journal of Lower Genital Tract Disease, 5*(4), 223–225.

Baer, A., Kiviat, N. B., Kulasingam, S., Mao, C., Kuypers, J., & Koutsky, L. A. (2002). Liquid-based Papanicolaou smears without a transformation zone component: Should clinicians worry? *Obstetrics and Gynecology, 99*(6), 1053–1059.

Castellsague, X., Diaz, M., de Sanjose, S., Monoz, N., Herrero, R., Franceschi, S., et al. (2006). Worldwide human papillomavirus etiology of cervical adenocarcinoma and its cofactors: Implications for screening and prevention. *Journal of the National Cancer Institute, 98,* 303–315.

Castle, P. E., Zemlo, T. R., Burk, R. D., Scott, D. R., Sherman, M. E., Lorincz, A. et al. (2001). Cervical HPV DNA detection as a predictor of a recurrent SIL diagnosis among untreated women. *Journal of Lower Genital Tract Disease, 5*(3), 138–143.

Cothran, M. M., & White, J. P. (2002). Adolescent behavior and sexually transmitted diseases: The dilemma of human papillomavirus. *Health Care for Women International, 23*(3), 306–319.

Dickman, E. D., Doll, T. J., Chiu, C. K., & Ferris, D. G. (2001). Identification of cervical neoplasia using a simulation of human vision. *Journal of Lower Genital Tract Disease, 5*(3), 144–152.

Gibson, C. A., Trask, C. E., House, P., Smith, S. F., Foley, M., & Nichols, C. (2001). Endocervical samplings: A comparison of endocervical brush, endocervical curette, and combined brush with curette techniques. *Journal of Lower Genital Tract Disease, 5*(1), 1–6.

Lurie, S., Eliaz, M., Boaz, M., Levy, T., Golan, A., & Sadan,O. (2007). Distribution of cervical intraepithelial neoplasia across the cervix is random. *American Journal of Obstetrics & Gynecology, 196,* 125.e1–125.e3.

Mandelblatt, J. S., Lawrence, W. F., Womack, S. M., Jacobson, D., Yi, B., Hwang, Y., et al. (2002). Benefits and costs of using HPV testing to screen for cervical cancer. *Journal of the American Medical Association, 287,* 2372–2381.

Massad, L. S., Schneider, M., Watts, H., Darragh, T., Abulafia, O., Salzer, E., et al. (2002). Correlating Papanicolaou smear, colposcopic impression, biopsy: Results from the womens interagency HIV study. *Journal of Lower Genital Tract Disease, 5*(4), 212–218.

Moore, S. L., & Seybold, V. K. (2007). HPV vaccine. *Clinician Reviews, 17* (1), 36–41.

Munoz, N., Franceschi, S., Bosetti, C., Moreno, V., Herrero, R., Smith, J. S., et al., for the International Agency for Research on Cancer (IARC) Multicentric Cervical Cancer Study Group. (2002). Role of parity and human papillomavirus in cervical cancer: The IARC multicentric case-controlled study. *Lancet, 359,* 1093–1101.

Nobbenhuis, M.A.E., Helmerhorst, T.J.M., van den Brule, A.J.C., Rozendaal, L., Voorhorst, F. J., Bezemer, P. D., et al. (2001). Cytological regression and clearance of high-risk human papillomavirus in women with an abnormal cervical smear. *Lancet, 358,* 1782–1783.

Schlecht, N. F., Kulga, S., Robitaille, J., Ferreira, S., Santos, M., Miyamura, R. A., et al. (2001). Persistent human papillomavirus infection as a predictor of cervical intraepithelial neoplasia. *Journal of the American Medical Association, 286*(24), 3106–3114.

Solomon, D., Davey, D., Kurman, R., Moriarty, A., O'Connor, D., Prey, M., et al. for the Forum Group Members and the Bethesda 2001 workshop. (2002). The 2001 Bethesda system. *Journal of the American Medical Association, 287*(16), 2114–2119.

Stoler, M. H. (2002). New Bethesda terminology and evidence-based management guidelines for cervical cytology findings. *Journal of the American Medical Association, 287*(16), 2140–2141.

COMPLEMENTARY AND ALTERNATIVE THERAPIES

Egan, C. D. (2002). Addressing use of herbal medicine in the primary care setting. *Journal of the American Academy of Nurse Practitioners, 14*(4), 166–171.

Friedrich, M. J. (2004). To E or not to E, Vitamin Es role in health and disease is the question. *Journal of the American Medical Association, 292,* 671–673.

Kaler, M. M., & Ravella, P. C. (2002). Staying on the ethical high ground with complementary and alternative medicine. *Nurse Practitioner, 27*(7), 38–42.

Kronenberg, F., Cushman, L. F., Wade, C. M., Kalmuss, D., & Chao, M. T. (2006). Race/ethnicity and womens use of complementary and alternative medicine in the United States: Results of a national survey. *American Journal of Public Health, 96,* 1236–1242.

Moss, K., Boon, H., Ballantyne, P., & Kachan, N. (2007). The professionalization of Western herbalists: Response to new product regulations in Canada. *Complementary Therapies in Medicine, 10,* 1–7.

Newton, K. M., Buist, D.S.M., Keenan, N. L., Anderson, L. A., & LaCroix, A. Z. (2002). Use of alternative therapies for menopause symptoms: Results of a population-based survey. *Obstetrics & Gynecology, 100*(1), 18–25.

CONTRACEPTION AND EMERGENCY CONTRACEPTION

Abma, J., Martinez, G., Mosher, W., & Dawson, B. (2004). Teenagers in the United States: Sexual activity, contraceptive use, and childbearing, 2002. National Centers for Health Statistics, Vital Health Stat 23(24). Retrieved January 2, 2007, from http://www.cdc.gov/nchs.nsfg.htm.

Ahrendt, H-J., Nisand, I., Bastianelli, C., Gomez, M. A., Gemzell-Danielsson, K., Urdl, B., et al. (2006). Efficacy, acceptability and tolerability of the combined contraceptive ring, NuvaRing, compared with an oral contraceptive containing 30 ug of ethinyl estradiol and 3 mg of drospirenone. *Contraception, 74,* 451–457.

Albertazzi, P., Bottazzi, M., & Steel, S. A. (2006). Bone mineral density and depot medroxyprogesterone acetate. *Contraception, 73,* 577–583.

American College of Obstetricians and Gynecologists. (2005, December). *Emergency contraception. ACOG Practice Bulletin, Number 69.* Washington, DC: The American College of Obstetrics and Gynecologists.

Anderson, F. D., Gibbons, W., & Portman, D. (2006). Long-term safety of an extended-cycle oral contraceptive (Seasonale): A 2-year multicenter open-label extension trial. *American Journal of Obstetrics and Gynecology, 195,* 92–96.

Anderson, J. E., Santelli, J. S., & Morrow, B. (2006). Trends in adolescent contraceptive use, unprotected and poorly protected sex, 1991–2003. *Journal of Adolescent Health, 38,* 734–739.

Andrist, L. C., Arias, R. D., Nucatola, D., Kaunitz, A. M., Musselman, B. L. Reiter, S. et al. (2004). Women's and providers' attitudes toward menstrual suppression with extended use of oral contraceptives. *Contraception, 70,* 359–363.

Arevalo, M., & Jennings, V. (2002). Efficacy of a new method of family planning: The standard days method. *Contraception, 65,* 333–338.

Axcan Ltee. Department of Research and Development. (1996). *Something new in barrier contraception: The Protective® contraceptive sponge.* Mont-St-Hilaire, Quebec, Canada: Axcan Ltee.

Barreiros, F. A., Guazzelli, C.A.F., de Araujo, F. F., & Barbosa, R. (2007). Bleeding patterns of women using extended regimens of the contraceptive vaginal ring. *Contraception, 75,* 204–208.

Beksinska, M., Joanis, C., Manning, J., Smit, J., Callahaan, M., Deperthes, B. et al. (2007). Standardized definitions of failure modes for female condoms. *Contraception, 75,* 251–255.

Brunton, J., & Beal, M. W. (2006). Current issues in emergency contraception: An overview for providers. *Journal of Midwifery & Women's Health, 51, 457–463.*

Burkman, R. T, Grimes, D. A., Mishell, D. R., & Westhoff, C. L. (2006). Benefits of contraception to women's health: An evidence-based perspective. *Dialogues in Contraception, 10* (3), 1–8.

Clark, L. R., Barnes-Harper, K. T., Ginsburg, K. R., Holmes, W. C., & Schwarz, D. F. (2006). Menstrual irregularity from hormonal contraception: A cause of reproductive health concerns in minority adolescent young women. *Contraception, 74,* 214–219.

Curtis, K. M., & Martins, S. L. (2006). Progestogen-only contraception and bone mineral density: A systematic review. *Contraception, 73,* 470–487.

Dickey, R. P. (2006). *Managing contraceptive pill patients.* 13th ed. Durant, OK: EMIS.

Ellertson, C., Evans, M., Ferden, S., Leadbetter, C., Spears, A., Johnstone, K., & Trussell, J. (2003). Extending the time limit for starting the Yuzpe regimen of emergency contraception to 120 hours. *Obstetrics & Gynecology, 101,* 1168–1171.

Fehring, R. J. (2004). Simple natural family planning methods for breastfeeding women. *Current Medical Research, 15* (1–2), 1–3.

Fehring, R. J. (2005). New low- and high-tech calendar methods of family planning. *Journal of Midwifery and Women's Health, 50,* 31–38.

Fehring, R. J., Raviele, K., & Schneider, M. (2004). A comparison of the fertile phase as determined by the clearplan easy fertility monitor and self-assessment of cervical mucus. *Contraception, 69,* 9–14.

Fehring, R. J., Schneider, M., Raviele, K., & Barron, M. L. (2007). Efficacy of cervical mucus observations plus electronic hormonal fertility monitoring as a method of natural family planning. *Journal of Obstetric, Gynecologic, and Neonatal Nursing, 36,* 152–160.

Gainer, E., Kenfack, B., Mboudou, E., Doh, A. S., & Bouyer, J. (2006). Menstrual bleeding patterns following levonorgestrel emergency contraception. *Contraception, 74,* 118–124.

Georgetown University. (2006). Cycle beads, Retrieved January 12, 2007 from http://www.cyclebeads.com.

Germano, E., & Jennings, V. (2006). New approaches to fertility awareness-based methods: Incorporating the standard days and twoday methods into practice. *Journal of Midwifery & Women's Health, 51,* 417–477.

Gerschultz, K. L., Sucato, G. S., Hennon, T. R., Murray, P. J., & Gold, M. A. (2007). Extended cycling of combined hormonal contraceptive in adolescents: Physician views and prescribing practices. *Journal of Adolescent Health, 40,* 151–157.

Goulard, H., Moreau, C., Gilbert, F., Job-Spira, N., Bajos, N., the Cocon Group. (2006). Contraceptive failures and determinants of emergency contraceptive use. *Contraception, 74,* 208–213.

Grimes, D. A., Raymond, E. G., & Scott Jones, B. (2001). Emergency contraception over-the-counter: The medical and legal imperatives. *Obstetrics and Gynecology, 98,* 151–155.

Grimes, D. A., & Schulz, K. F.(2004). Antibiotic prophylaxis for intrauterine contraceptive device insertion. *The Cochrane Library, Issue 3.* Chichester, UK: John Wiley & Sons, Ltd.

Hatcher, R. A., Trussell, J., Stewart, F., Cates, W., Stewart, G. K., Guest, F., & Kowal, D. (2004). *Contraceptive technology* (19th ed.). New York: Ardent Media.

Helmerhorst, F. M., Belfield, T., Kulier, R., Maitra, N., O'Brien, P., & Grimes, D. (2006). The Cochrane fertility regulation group: Synthesizing the best evidence about family planning. *Contraception, 74,* 280–286.

Holt, V. L., Cushing-Haugen, K. L., & Daling, J. R. (2002). Body weight and risk of oral contraceptive failure. *Obstetrics and Gynecology, 99*(5), 820–827.

Hubacher, D., Lara-Ricalde, R., Taylor, D. J., Guerra-Infante, F., & Guzman-Rodriguez, R. (2001). Use of copper intrauterine devices and the risk of tubal infertility among nulligravid women. *New England Journal of Medicine, 345*(8), 561–567.

Huber, L.R.B., Hogue, C. J., Stein, A. D., Drews, C., Zieman, M. King, J., et al. (2006). Contraceptive use and discontinuation: Findings from the contraceptive history, initiation, and choice study. *American Journal of Obstetrics and Gynecology, 194,* 1290–1295.

Kaunitz, A. M., Miller, P. D., Rice, V. M., Ross, D., & McClung, M. R. (2006). Bone mineral density in women aged 25–35 receiving depot medroxyprogesterone acetate: recovery following discontinuation. *Contraception 74,* 90–99.

Leonard, C. J., Chavira, W., Coonrod, D. V., Hart, K. W. & Bay, R. C. (2006). Study of attitudes regarding natural family planning in an urban Hispanic population. *Contraception, 74,* 313–317.

Marions, L., Hultenby, K., Lindell, I., Sun, X., Stabi, B., & Danielsson, K. G. (2002). Emergency contraception with mifepristone and levonorgestrol: Mechanism of action. *Obstetrics & Gynecology, 100*(1), 65–71.

Martins, S. L., Curtis, K. M., & Glasier, A. F. (2006). Combined hormonal contraception and bone health: A systematic review. *Contraception, 73,* 445–469.

Mathias, S. D., Colwell, H. H., LoCoco, J. M., Karvois, D. L., Pritchard, M. L., & Friedman, A. J. (2006). ORTHO birth control satisfaction assessment tool: Assessing sensitivity to change and predictors of satisfaction. *Contraception, 74,* 303–308.

Mishell, D. R. (2002, August). The transdermal contraceptive system. *The Female Patient,* supplement, 14–25.

Nakajima, S. T., Archer, D. F., & Ellman, H. (2007). Efficacy and safety of a new 24-day Oral contraceptive regimen of norethindrone acetate 1 mg/ethinyl estradiol 20 ug (Loestrin24® Fe). *Contraception 75,* 16–22.

National Collaborating Centre for Womens and Childrens Health UK. (2005). *Long-acting reversible contraception: The effective and appropriate use of long-acting and reversible contraception.* London: RCOG Press.

Nelson, A. L. & Katz, T. (2007). Initiation and continuation rates seen in 2-year experience with same day injections of DMPA. *Contraception, 75,* 84–87.

Ngai, S. W., Fan, S., Li, S., Cheng, L., Ding, J. Jing, X., et al. (2004). A randomized trial to compare 24h versus 12h double dose regimen of levonorgestrel for emergency contraception. *Human Reproduction, 20,* 307–311.

Noveikova, N., Weisberg, E., Stanczyk, F. Z., Croxatto, H. B., & Fraser, I. S. (2007). Effectiveness of levonorgestrel emergency contraception given before or after ovulation—a pilot study. *Contraception, 75,* 112–118.

O'Connell, K., Davis, A. R., & Kerns, J. (2007). Oral contraceptives: Side effects and depression in adolescent girls. *Contraception, 75,* 299–304.

Petersen, R., Albright, J. B., Garrett, J. M., & Curtis, K. M. (2007). Acceptance and use of emergency contraception with standardized counseling intervention: Results of a randomized controlled trial. *Contraception, 75,* 119–125.

Rad, M., Kluft, C., Menard, J., Burggraaf, J., de Kam, M. L., Meijer, P., et al. (2006). Comparative effects of a contraceptive vaginal ring delivering a nonandrogenic progestin and continuous ethinyl estradiol and a combined oral contraceptive containing levonorgestrel on hemostasis variables. *American Journal of Obstetrics and Gynecology, 195,* 72–77.

Sabatini, R., & Cagiano, R. (2006). Comparison profiles of cycle control, side effects, and sexual satisfaction of three hormonal contraceptives. *Contraception, 74,* 220–223.

Sangi-Haghpeykar, H., Ali, N., Posner, S., & Poindexter, A. N. (2006). Disparities in contraceptive knowledge, attitude and use between Hispanic and non-Hispanic whites. *Contraception, 74,* 125–132.

Santelli, J., Lindberg, L. D., Finer, L. B., & Singh, S. (2007). Explaining recent declines in adolescent pregnancy in the United States: The contribution of abstinence and improved contraceptive use. *American Journal of Public Health, 97,* 150–156.

Saxena, S., Copas, A. J., Mercer, C., Johnson, A. M. Fenton, K., Eren, B., et al. (2006). Ethnic variations in sexual activity and contraceptive use: National cross-sectional survey. *Contraception, 74,* 224–233.

Schacter, H. E., Gee, R. E., & Long, J. A. (2007). Variation in availability of emergency contraception in pharmacies. *Contraception, 75,* 214–217.

Schafer, J. E., Osborne, L. M., Davis, A. R., & Westhoff, C. (2006). Acceptabilty and satisfaction using Quick Start with the contraceptive ring versus an oral contraceptive. *Contraception, 73,* 488–492.

Soon, J. A., Levine, M., Osmond, B. L., Ensom, M. H., & Fielding, D. W. (2005). Effects of making emergency contraception available without a physician's prescription: A population-based study. *Canadian Medical Association Journal, 172,* 878–883.

Wesson, J., Gmach, R., Gazi, R., Ashraf, A., Mendez, J. F., Olenja, J., et al. (2006). Provider views on the acceptability of an IUD checklist screening tool. *Contraception, 74,* 382–388.

Westoff, C., Jain, J. K., Milson, I., & Ray, A. (2007). Changes in weight with depot medroxyprogesterone acetate subcutaneous injection 104 mg/0.65 mL. *Contraception, 75,* 261–267.

Woods, J. L. Shew, M. L., Tu, W., Ofner, S., Ott, M. A., & Fortenberry, J. D. (2006). Patterns of oral contraceptive pill-taking and condom use among adolescent contraceptive pill users. *Journal of Adolescent Health, 39,* 381–387.

World Health Organization. (2004). *Medical eligibility criteria for contraceptive use.* 3rd ed. Geneva, Switzerland: World Health Organization.

Wysocki, S., & Moore, A. A. (2002). New developments in contraception: The first transdermal contraceptive system. *Womens Health Care, 1,* 9–23.

Zieman, M. (2002, August). Managing patients using the transdermal contraceptive system. *The Female Patient,* supplement, 26–32.

Zieman, M. (2002). Transdermal contraception. *The Female Patient, 27*(1), 17–18.

HIV/AIDS

Boehm, D. (2001). Women and HIV/AIDS: Act local/think global. *Journal of Obstetric, Gynecologic, and Neonatal Nursing, 30*(3), 342–350.

Cabral, R. J., Galavotti, C., Armstrong, K., Morrow, B., & Fogarty, L. (2001). Reproductive and contraceptive attitudes as predictors of condom use among women in an HIV prevention intervention. *Women & Health, 33*(3/4), 117–132.

Lauby, J. L., Semaan, S., O'Connell, A., Person, B., & Vogel, A. (2001). Factors related to self-efficacy for use of condoms and birth control among women at risk for HIV infection. *Women & Health, 34*(3), 71–91.

Morrison-Beedy, D. L., & Lewis, B. P. (2001). HIV prevention in single, urban women: Condom-use readiness. *Journal of Obstetric, Gynecologic, and Neonatal Nursing, 30*(2), 148–156.

INFERTILITY

Cheney, B. (2002). Helping couples concerned about infertility. *Womens Health Care, 1*(1), 21–23.

Hahn, S. J., & Craft-Roseberg, M. (2002). The disclosure decisions of parents who conceive children using donor eggs. *Journal of Obstetric, Gynecologic, & Neonatal Nursing, 31*(3), 283–293.

Swank, C. O., Christianson, C. A., Prows, C. A., West, E. B., & Warren, N. S. (2001). Effectiveness of a genetics self-instructional module for nurses involved in egg donor screening. *Journal of Obstetric, Gynecologic, and Neonatal Nursing, 30*(6), 617–625.

Tomlins, J. (2003). *The infertility handbook: A guide to making babies.* East Melbourne, Australia: Allen & Unwin.

INTERSTITIAL CYSTITIS

Bradley, C., & Singh, G. (2000). Interstitial cystitis: Evaluation and management. *The Female Patient, 25,* 83–88.

The Interstitial Cystitis Clinical Trials Group. (2005). A randomized controlled trial of intravesical bacillus Calmette-Guerin for treatment of refractory interstitial cystitis. *Journal of Urology, 17,* 1186–1891.

Moldwin, R. M. (2000). *Interstitial cystitis survival guide: Your guide to the latest treatment options and coping strategies.* Oakland, CA: New Harbinger Publications.

Myers, D. L., & Arya, L. A. (2000). Diagnosing interstitial cystitis in women. *Women's Health in Primary Care, 3,* 867–874.

Myers, D. L., & Arya, L. A. (2001). Treating interstitial cystitis in women. *Women's Health in Primary Care, 4,* 151–161.

Rabin, C., O'Leary, A., Neighbors, C., & Whitmore, K. (2001). Pain and depression experienced by women with interstitial cystitis. *Women & Health, 31*(4), 67–81.

MENOPAUSE, HORMONE THERAPY

Blake, J. (2006). Menopause: Evidence-based practice. *Best Practice & Research Clinical Obstetrics and Gynaecology, 20,* 799–839.

Brucker, M. C., & Youngkin, E. (2003). What's a woman to do? *AWHONN Lifelines, 6*(5), 408–417.

Cousins, S. O., & Edwards, K. (2002). Alice in menopauseland: The jabberwocky of a medicalized middle age. *Health Care for Women International, 23*(4), 325–343.

Ettinger, B., Barrett-Conor, E., Hoq, L., Vader, J., & Dubois, R. (2006). When is it appropriate to prescribe postmenopausal hormone therapy? *Menopause,13,* 404–410.

Finkel, M., Cohen, M., & Mahoney, H. (2001). Treatment options for the menopausal woman. *Nurse Practitioner, 26*(2), 5.

Fiorica, J. V. (Ed.). (2001). Postmenopausal hormone therapy and breast health: A review for clinicians. *Womens Health in Primary Care, 4*(supplement), 3–36.

Gass, M.L.S., Utian, W. H., Ettinger, B., Gallagher, J. C., Herrington, D. M., Lobo, R., et al. (2002). Report from the NAMS Advisory Panel on postmenopausal hormone therapy. Retrieved October 4, 2002 from http://www.nams.org.

Grady, D., Herrington, D., Bittner, V., Blumenthal, R., Davidson, M., Hlatky, M., et al. for the HERS Research Group. (2002). Cardiovascular disease outcomes during 6.8 years of hormone therapy. *Journal of the American Medical Association, 288*(1), 49–57.

Hanna, K. E. (2003). No fountain of youth: FDA & NHI review off-label use of hormones. *The Hastings Report, 33.*

HRT and SERMS: New guidelines for patient management. (2002, March). *The Female Patient, Supplement,* 1–38.

Joffe, H., Hall, J. E., Gruber, S., Sarmiento, I. A., Cohen, L.S., Yurgelun-Todd, D., et al. (2006). Estrogen therapy selectively enhances prefrontal cognitive processes: a randomized, double-blind, placebo-controlled study with functional magnetic resonance imaging in perimenopausal and recently postmenopausal women. *Menopause, 13,* 414–424.

Jun, M., Drieling, R., & Stafford, R. (2006). US women desire greater professional guidance on hormone and alternative therapies for menopause symptom management. *Menopause, 13,* 506–515.

Lange-Collett, J. (2002). Promoting health among perimenopausal women through diet and exercise. *Journal of the American Academy of Nurse Practitioners, 14,* 172–177.

Lyytinen, H., Pukkala, E., & Ylikorkala, O. (2006). Breast cancer risk in postmenopausal women using estrogen-only therapy. *Obstetrics and Gynecology, 108,* 2010–2019.

Magliano, D. J., Rogers, S. L., Abramson, M. J., & Tonkin, A. M. (2006). Hormone therapy and cardiovascular disease: A systematic review and meta-analysis. *British Journal of Obstetrics and Gynaecology, 113,* 5–14.

Mastroianni, L. D., & Segal, S. J. (2003). *Hormone use in menopause and male andropause: A choice for women and men.* Oxford, England: Oxford University Press.

Nelson, H. D., Vesco, K. K., Haney, E., Fu, R., Nedrow, A., Miller, J., et al. (2006). Non-hormonal therapies for menopausal hot flashes: Systematic review and meta-analysis. *Journal of the American Medical Association, 295,* 2057–2071.

Newton, K. M., Buist, D.S.M., Keenan, N. L., Anderson, L. A., & LaCroix, A. Z. (2002). Use of alternative therapies for menopause symptoms: Results of a population-based survey. *Obstetrics & Gynecology, 100,* 18–25.

North American Menopause Society. (2003). Role of progestogen in hormone therapy for postmenopausal women. *Menopause, 10,* 113–132.

Notelovitz, M., Funk, S., Nanavati, N., & Mazzeo, M. (2002). Estradiol absorption from vaginal tablets in postmenopausal women. *Obstetrics and Gynecology, 99*(4), 556–562.

Rodriguez, C., Patel, A. V., Calle, E. E., Jacob, E. J., & Thun, M. J. (2001). Estrogen replacement therapy and ovarian cancer mortality in a large prospective study of US women. *Journal of the American Medical Association, 285*(11), 1460–1465.

Sampselle, C. M., Harris, V., Harlow, S. D., & Sowers, M. (2002). Midlife development and menopause in African American and caucasian women. *Health Care for Women International, 23*(4), 351–363.

Sarrel, P. M., Kaunitz, A. M., Nachtigal, L. E., & Wysocki, S. (2002, December). Sexual dysfunction and the menopausal woman: Overcoming atrophic vaginitis. *Patient Care for the Nurse Practitioner,* Spec. ed., 4–19.

Segal, S. J. (2003). *Under the banyan tree. A population scientist's odyssey.* Oxford, England, Oxford University Press.

Sharp, H. T. (2006). Assessment of new technology in the treatment of idiopathic menorrhagia and uterine leiomyomata. *Obstetrics and Gynecology, 108,* 900–1003.

Speroff, L., Gallagher, J. C., Pinkerton, J. V., & Raisz, L. G. (2001, July). Menopause management: The impact of low-dose HRT. *Contemporary Ob/Gyn for the Nurse Practitioner* (suppl.), 4–26.

Stephens, C., & Ross, N. (2002). The relationship between hormone replacement therapy use and psychological symptoms: No effects found in a New Zealand sample. *Health Care for Women International, 23*(4), 408–414.

Wilonsky, S., & Wilkerson, J. T. (2002). *Heart disease in women.* New York: Churchill Livingstone.

MENSTRUAL CYCLE: ABNORMAL UTERINE BLEEDING, PMS, AMENORRHEA

Bosarge, P. M. (2003). Understanding and treating PMS/PMDD. *Nursing Management, 34*, (11-Supplement), 13.

Braverman, P. K. (2007). Premenstrual syndrome and premenstrual dysphoric disorder. *Journal of Pediatric and Adolescent Gynecology, 20*, 3–12.

Cohen, L., Miner, C., Brown, E., Freeman, E., Holbreich, U., Sundell, K., et al. (2002). Premenstrual daily fluoxetine for premenstrual dysphoric disorder: A placebo-controlled, clinical trial using computerized diaries. *Obstetrics & Gynecology, 100*, 435.

Cooper J. M., & Brady, R. M. (1999). Hysteroscopy in the management of abnormal uterine bleeding. *Obstetrics and Gynecology Clinics of North America, 26*(1), 217–236.

Dickerson, V. M. (2007, January). Premenstrual syndrome and premenstrual dysphoric disorder: Individualizing therapy. *The Female Patient, 32*, 38–46.

Jones, C. (2001). Premenstrual dysphoric disorder. *Advance for Nurse Practitioners, 9*(3), 87–90.

Labyak, S., Lava, S., Turek, F., & Zee, P. (2002). Effects of shiftwork on sleep and menstrual function in nurses. *Health Care for Women International, 23*, 703–714.

Speroff, L., & Fritz M. A. (2005). Dysfunctional uterine bleeding. In L. Speroff & M. A. Fritz, eds., *Clinical gynecologic endocrinology and infertility*, 7th ed. (pp. 548–571). Philadelphia: Lippincott Williams and Wilkins.

MENTAL HEALTH AND EMOTIONAL ISSUES

Antai-Otong, D. (2001). Dark days: Treating major depression. *Advance for Nurse Practitioners, 9*(3), 32–43.

Beck, C. T. (2001). Predictors of postpartum depression. *Nursing Research, 50*, 275–285.

Beck, C. T. (2002). Postpartum depression: A metasynthesis. *Qualitative Health Research, 12*, 453–472.

Beck, C. T. (2002). Revision of the postpartum depression predictors inventory. *Journal of Obstetric, Gynecologic, and Neonatal Nursing, 31*, 394–402.

Beck, C. T., & Gable, R. K. (2001). Comparative analysis of the performance of the postpartum depression screening scale with two other depression instruments. *Nursing Research, 50*, 242–250.

Beck, C. T., & Gable, R. K. (2001). Further validation of the postpartum depression screening scale. *Nursing Research, 50*, 155–164.

Corwin, E. J. (2002). Fatigue as a predictor of postpartum depression. *Journal of Obstetric, Gynecologic, and Neonatal Nursing, 31*(4), 436–443.

Dennis, C. L. (2005). Psychosocial and psychological interventions for prevention of postnatal depression: Systematic review. *British Medical Journal, 331*, 15.

Dietch, K. V., & Bunney, B. (2002). The silent disease: Diagnosing and treating depression in women. *AWHONN Lifelines, 6*(2), 140–145.

Edebohls, L., & Ecklund, C. (2002). Postpartum depression: Practical advice from two nurse practitioners. *Pediatric Nursing, 28*, 298–299.

Johnson, R. M. (2000). Diagnosis and managing seasonal affective disorders. *Nurse Practitioner, 25*(8), 56–62.

Norton, J. W. (2001). Personality disorders in the primary care setting. *Nurse Practitioner, 25*, 40–58.

Owen, C., Deslee, J., & Robbe, M.D.V. (2002). Barriers to cancer screening amongst women with mental health problems. *Health Care for Women International, 23*(6–7), 561–566.

Shell, R. C. (2001). Antidepressant prescribing practices of nurse practitioners. *Nurse Practitioner, 26*(7), 42–47.

Zamorshi, M. A. (2001). Anxiety disorders: Recognition and management in the ob/gyn setting. *Female Patient, 26,* 31–36.

OSTEOPOROSIS

Baron, J. A, Farahmand, B. Y, Weiderpass, E., Michaelsson, K., Alberts, A., Persson, I, et al. (2001). Cigarette smoking, alcohol consumption, and risk for hip fracture in women. *Archives of Internal Medicine, 161,* 983–988.

Consensus statement on osteoporosis: Prevention, diagnosis, and treatment. (2000). *Women's Health in Primary Care, 3*(9), 670–672.

Curry, L. C., & Hogstel, M. O. (2002). Osteoporosis. *American Journal of Nursing, 102*(1), 26–32.

Davidson, M., & DeSimone, M. E. (2002). Osteoporosis update. *Clinician Reviews, 12*(4), 76–82.

Ettinger, B. (2000). Sequential osteoporosis treatment for women with postmenopausal osteoporosis. *Menopausal Medicine, 8*(2), 1–4.

Gallagher, J. (2000). Diagnosing osteoporosis: The ABCs of Z and T scores. *The Female Patient, 25,* 66, 69.

Harris, S. T., Watts, N. B., Genant, H. K., McKeever, C. D., Hangartner, T., Keller, M., et al. (1999). Effects of risedronate treatment on vertebral and nonvertebral fractures in women with postmenopausal osteoporosis. *Journal of the American Medical Association, 282*(14), 1344–1352.

Holm, K., Dan, A., Wilbur, J., Suling, L., & Walker, J. (2002). A longitudinal study of bone density in midlife women. *Health Care for Women International, 23*(6–7), 678–691.

Lindsay, R., Gallagher, J. C., Kleerekoper, M., & Pickar, J. H. (2002). Effect of lower doses of conjugated equine estrogens with and without medroxyprogesterone acetate on bone in early postmenopausal women. *Journal of the American Medical Association, 287*(20), 2668–2676.

Lindsay, R., Silverman, S. L., Cooper, C., Hanley, D. A., Barton, I., Broy, S. B., et al. (2001). Risk of new vertebral fracture in the year following a fracture. *Journal of the American Medical Association, 285,* 320–323.

McClung, M. R., Geusens, P., Miller, P. D., Zippel, H., Bensen, W. G., Roux, C., et al. (2001). Effect of risedronate on the risk of hip fracture in elderly women. *New England Journal of Medicine, 344,* 333–340.

Miller, B., DeSouza, M., Slade, K., & Luciano, A. (2000). Sublingual administration of micronized estradiol and progesterone with and without micronized testosterone: Effect on biochemical markers of bond metabolism and bone mineral density. *Menopause, 7*(5), 318–326.

Stevenson, M., Lloyd Jones, M., De Nigris, E., Brewer, N., Davis, S., & Oakley, J. (2005). A systematic review and economic evaluation of alendronate, etidronate, risendronate, raloxifene and teriparatide for prevention and treatment of postmenopausal osteoporosis. *Health Technology Assessment, 9*(22), 1–160.

Torgerson, D. J., & Bell-Syer, S. E. M. (2001). Hormone replacement therapy and prevention of nonvertebral fractures. *Journal of the American Medical Association, 285,* 2891–2897.

POLYCYSTIC OVARY SYNDROME (PCOS)

Ahles, B. L. (2002). Toward a new approach: Primary and preventive care of the woman with polycystic ovarian syndrome. *Primary Care Update for OB/GYNS, 7*(6), 275–278.

Cheung, A. (2001). Ultrasound and menstrual history in predicting endometrial hyperplasia in polycystic ovary syndrome. *Obstetrics & Gynecology, 98,* 325.

Freeman, S. B. (2002). Polycystic ovary syndrome: Diagnosis and management. *Women's Health Care, 1*(4), 15–20.

Freeman, S. B. (2006). The metabolic syndrome: Revisited. *Womens Health Care, 5*(4), 52–74.

Hart, R., & Norman, R. (2006). Polycystic ovarian syndrome: prognosis and outcomes. *Best Practice & Research Clinical Obstetrics and Gynecology, 20,* 751–778.

King, J. (2006). Polycystic ovary syndrome. *Journal of Midwifery & Womens Health, 51,* 415–422.

Kovacs, G. T. (2000). *Polycystic ovary syndrome.* Cambridge, England: Cambridge University Press.

McCook, J. G., Reame, N. E., & Thatcher, S. S. (2005). Health-related quality of life issues in women with polycystic ovary syndrome. *Journal of Obstetrics, Gynecology, and Neonatal Nursing, 34,* 12–19.

Noller, D., & Paulk, D. (2006). Polycystic ovary syndrome. *Clinician Reviews, 16*(9), 32–42.

Sherif, K. (2006, February). Polycystic ovary syndrome in primary care. *The Female Patient, 31,* 25–29.

Stevens, S. (2005, November 14). Out of the dark polycystic ovary syndrome can early escape notice, but diagnosis and early treatment is important for women's long term health. Arlington Heights, IL: *Daily Herald.*

PRECONCEPTION CARE

CDC. (2006). Preconception health care: Recommendations from the CDC. *Clinician Reviews, 16*(7), 45–51.

Heath, C., & Acevedo, R. (2004, December). Preconception screening and counseling. *The Female Patient, 29,* 47–50.

Kirke, P. N., Mills, J. L., Molloy, A. M., Brody, L. C., OLeary, V. B., Daly, L., et al. (2004, May 21). Impact of the MRHFR C677T polymorphisim on risk of neural tube defects: Case-control study. *British Medical Journal* On-Line Version.

Moos, M-K. (2006). Preconception care. *AWHONN Lifelines, 10,* 332–334.

Moos, M-K. (2006). Preconception health: Where to from here? *Womens Health Issues, 16,* 156–158.

Seibel, M. M. (2006). The environment: Its risks to conception and pregnancy. *Sexuality, Reproduction & Menopause, 4*(1), 1–2.

Weisman, C. S., Hillemeier, M. M., Chase, G. A., Dyer, A., Baker, S. A., Feinberg, G., et al. (2006). Preconceptual health: Risks of adverse pregnancy outcomes by reproductive life stage in the central Pennsylvania womens health study (CePAWHS). *Womens Health Issues, 16,* 216–224.

SEXUALITY

Baxer, P. M. (2001). Midlife changes in sexual response. *ADVANCE for Nurse Practitioners, 9*(3), 67–69.

Berg, J. A. (2001). Dimensions of sexuality in the perimenopausal transition: A model for practice. *Journal of Obstetric, Gynecologic, and Neonatal Nursing, 30*(4), 421–428.

Ferguson, D. M., Steidle, C. P., Singh, G. S., Alexander, J. S., Weihmiller, M. K., & Crosby, M. G. (2003). Randomized, placebo-controlled double blind, crossover design trial of the efficacy and safety of Zestra for Women in women with and without female sexual arousal disorder. *Journal of Sex & Marital Therapy, 29*(s), 3–44.

Gott, M., & Hinchliff, S. (2003). How important is sex in later life? *Social Science & Medicine, 56*, 1617–1628.

McCaffrey, R., Barnett, S., & Thomas, D. J. (2001). Seeking satisfaction: Treating decreased libido in women. *AWHONN Lifelines, 5*(4), 30–35.

Wade, L. D., Kremer, E. C., & Brown, J. (2005). The incidental orgasm: The presence of clitoral knowledge and the absence of orgasm for women. *Women & Health, 42*, 117–138.

SEXUALLY TRANSMITTED DISEASES

Centers for Disease Control and Prevention. (2006, August 4). Sexually transmitted diseases treatment guidelines 2006. *Morbidity and Mortality Weekly Report, 55*, 1–94.

DiMaio, H. (2002). Chancroid infections in women. *Primary Care Update for OB/GYNS, 8*(6), 258–259.

Feroli, K. L., & Burstein, G. R. (2003). Adolescent sexually transmitted diseases. *MCN American Journal of Maternal-Child Nursing, 28*, 113–118.

Holzman, C., Leventhal, J. M., Qiu, H., Jones, N. M., Wang, J., and the BV study group. (2001). Factors linked to bacterial vaginosis in nonpregnant women. *American Journal of Public Health, 91*, 1664–1670.

Kelley, S. S., Borawski, E. A., Flocke, S. A., & Keen, K. J.(2003). The role of sequential and concurrent sexual relationships in the risk of sexually transmitted disease among adolescents. *Journal of Adolescent Health, 32*, 296–305.

Magnus, M., Schillinger, J. A, Fortenberry, J. D., Berman, S. M., & Kissinger, P. (2006). Partner age not associated with recurrent Chlamydia trachomatis infection, condom use or partner treatment and referral among adolescent women. *Journal of Adolescent Health, 39*, 396–403.

Manavi, K. (2006). A review on infection with Chlamydia trachomatis. *Best Practice & Research Clinical Obstetrics and Gynaecology, 20*, 941–951.

McClure, J. B., Scholes, D., Grothaus, L, Fishman, P., Reid, R., Lindenbaum, J., & Thompson, R. S. (2006). Chlamydia screening in at-risk adolescent females: An evaluation of screening practices and modifiable screening correlates. *Journal of Adolescent Health, 38*, 726–733.

Paskawicz, J. (2005). Latex allergy revisited: Clinicians, stay alert. *Clinician Reviews, 15*(11), 66–75.

Roddy, R. E., Zekeng, L., Ryan, K. A., Tamoufe, U., & Tweedy, K. G. (2002). Effect of nonoxynol-9 gel on urogenital gonorrhea and chlamydial infection. *Journal of the American Medical Association, 287*, 1117–1122.

Sheeder, J., Stevens-Simon, C., Lezotte, D., Glazner, J., & Scott, S. (2006). Cervicitis: To treat or not to treat? The role of patient preferences and decision analysis. *Journal of Adolescent Health, 39*, 887–892.

van Devanter, N., Gonzales, V., Merzel, C., Parikh, N. S., Celantano, D., & Greenberg, J. (2002). Effect of an STD/HIV behavioral intervention on womens use of the female condom. *American Journal of Public Health, 92*, 109–115.

SMOKING CESSATION

Bauman, K. E., Foshee, V. A., Ennett, S. T., Pemberton, M., Hicks, K. A., King, T. S., et al. (2001). The influence of a family program on adolescent tobacco and alcohol use. *American Journal of Public Health, 91*(4), 604–610.

Centers for Disease Control and Prevention. (1997). Perspectives in disease prevention and health promotion smoking-attributable mortality and years of potential life lost United States, 1984. *Morbidity and Mortality Weekly Report, 46,* 444–451.

Centers for Disease Control and Prevention. (1999). Cigarette smoking among adults–United States, 1997. *Morbidity and Mortality Weekly Report, 48,* 993–996.

Easton, A., Husten, C., Elon, L., Pederson, L., & Frank, E. (2001). Non-primary care physicians and smoking cessation counseling: Women physicians health study. *Women & Health, 34*(4), 15–29.

Faucher, M. A., & Carter, S. (2001). Why girls smoke: A proposed community-based prevention program. *Journal of Obstetric, Gynecologic, and Neonatal Nursing, 30,* 463–471.

Fiore, M. C., Bailey, W. C., Cohen, S. J., Dorfman, S. I., Goldstein, M. G., Gritz, E. R., et al. (2000). *Treating tobacco use and dependence: Clinical practice guideline.* Rockville, MD: US Department of Health and Human Services, Public Health Service.

Gaffney, K. F., Wichaikhum, O., & Dawson, E. M. (2002). Smoking among female college students: A time for change. *Journal of Obstetric, Gynecologic, and Neonatal Nursing, 31*(5), 502–507.

Gruskin, E. P., Hart, S., Gordon, N., & Ackerson, L. (2001). Patterns of cigarette smoking and alcohol use among lesbians and bisexual women enrolled in a large health maintenance organization. *American Journal of Public Health, 91,* 976–979.

MacDonald, M., & Wright, N. E. (2002). Cigarette smoking and the disenfranchisement of adolescent girls: A discourse of resistance? *Health Care for Women International, 23,* 281–305.

Roush, K. (2006). Nursing resources: Helping patients quit smoking: Information and resources are in abundance online. *American Journal of Nursing, 106*(7), 71–72.

The Surgeon Generals Report. (2001). Women and smoking. *Womens Health in Primary Care 4*(6), 399–400.

Thorndike, A. N., Biener, L., & Rigotti, N. A. (2002). Effect on smoking cessation of switching nicotine replacement therapy to over-the-counter status. *American Journal of Public Health, 92,* 437–442.

Urso, P. (2003). Match the best smoking cessation intervention to your patient. *The Nurse Practitioner: The American Journal of Primary Health Care, 28*(1-Supplement), 12–21.

U.S. Department of Health and Human Services. (1988). *The health consequences of Smoking: Nicotine addiction: A report of the Surgeon General.* Atlanta, GA: US Department of Health and Human Services, Public Health Service, Centers for Disease Control, Center for Chronic Disease Prevention and Health Promotion, Office of Smoking and Health. DHHS publication (PHS) (CDC) 88–8406.

U.S. Department of Health and Human Services. (1990). *The health benefits of smoking cessation: A report of the Surgeon General.* Rockville, MD: US Department of Health and Human Services, Public Health Service, Centers for Disease Control, Center for Chronic Disease Prevention and Health promotion, Office on Smoking and Health. DHHS publication (CDC) 90–8416.

URINARY TRACT INFECTIONS AND URINARY INCONTINENCE

Bachmann, G., & Witta, B. (2002). External occlusive devices for management of female urinary incontinence. *Journal of Womens Health, 11,* 793–800.

Bardsley, A. (2003). Urinary tract infections: prevention and treatment of a common problem. *Nurse Prescribing, 1*(3), 113–117.

Bent, S., Nallamothu, B. K., Simel, D. L., Fihn, S. D., & Saint, S. (2002). Does this woman have an acute uncomplicated urinary tract infection? *Journal of the American Medical Association, 287,* 2701–2710.

Burgio, K. L., Goode, P. S., Locher, J. L., Umlauf, M. G., Roth, D. L., Richter, H. E., et al. (2002). Behavioral training with and without biofeedback in the treatment of urge incontinence in older women. *Journal of the American Medical Association, 288,* 2293–2299.

Dougherty, M. C., Dwyer, J. W., Pendergast, J. F., Boyington, A. R., Tomlinson, B. U., Coward, R. T., et al. (2002). A randomized trial of behavioral management for continence with older rural women. *Research in Nursing and Health, 25,* 3–13.

Fihn, S. D. (2003). Acute uncomplicated urinary tract infection in women. *New England Journal of Medicine, 349,* 259–266.

Gibbs, C. F., Johnson, T. M., & Ouslander, J. G. (2007). Office management of geriatric urinary incontinence. *The American Journal of Medicine, 120,* 211–220.

Gray, M. L. (2004, May). Stress urinary incontinence: Myths, misconceptions, and other impediments to the diagnosis and treatment of stress urinary incontinence. *American Journal for Nurse Practitioners,* Supp., 15–22.

Holroyd-Leduc, J. M. (2004). Management of urinary incontinence in women. *Journal of the American Medical Association, 291,* 986–995.

Hooten, T. M. (2003). Optimizing treatment for acute uncomplicated cystitis. *Clinician Reviews, 13*(9), 109–119.

Katchman, E. A., Milo, G., Paul, M., Christiaens, T., Baerheim, A., & Leibovici, L. (2005). Three-day vs longer duration antibiotic treatment for cystitis in women: Systematic review and meta-analysis. *American Journal of Medicine, 118,* 1196–1207.

Kontiokari, T., Sundqvist, K., Nuutinen, M., Pokka, T., Koskela, M., & Uhari, M. (2001). Randomised trial of cranberry-lingonberry juice and lactobacillus GG drink for the prevention of urinary tract infections in women. *British Medical Journal, 322,* 1571–1573.

Manges, A. R., Johnson, J. R., Foxman, B., O'Bryan, T. T., Fullerton, K. E., & Riley, L. W. (2001). Widespread distribution of urinary tract infections caused by a multidrug-resistant escherichia coli clonal group. *New England Journal of Medicine, 345,* 1007–1013.

Martin, J. L., Williams, K. S., Abrams, K. R., Turner, D. A., Sutton, A. J., Chapple, C., et al. (2006). Systematic review and evaluation of methods of assessing urinary incontinence. *Health Technology Assessment, 10,* 1–132.

Newman, D. (2004, May). Therapeutic strategies for managing stress urinary incontinence in women. *American Journal for Nurse Practitioners,* (Supp)., 23–32.

Newman, D. (2006, March). Assessing the patient for OAB in primary care. *Clinical Advisor,* Supp., 9–14.

Newman, D., & Palmer, M.H. (2003). State of the science on urinary incontinence. *American Journal of Nursing,* Supp., 1–51.

Nickel, J. C. (2005, October). How to select the right drugs for UTIs. *The Clinical Advisor,* 62–66.

Palmer, M. H. (2004, May). Stress urinary incontinence: Revalence, etiology, and risk factors in women at 3 life stages. *American Journal for Nurse Practitioners,* Supp., 5–13.

Panzera, A. K. (2003). Overactive bladder: A practical guide for diagnosis and management. *Womens Health Care, 2*(11), 8–14.

Rode, M., & Rogers, R. G. (2007). The vaginal pessary: Practical treatment for pelvic organ prolapse and stress urinary incontinence. *The Female Patient, 32,* 15–21.

Roe, V. A. (2002). Antibacterials in women's health. *Womens Health Care, 1*(2), 7–19.

Sheeler, R. D. (2003, September). A contemporary approach to UTI therapy. *Patient Care for the Nurse Practitioner,* (special ed.), 1–6.

Sussman, D. O. (2006, March). OAB: A bothersome medical condition. *Clinical Advisor,* Supp., 3–8.

VAGINITIS/VAGINOSIS

Andrist, L. C. (2001). Vaginal health and infections. *Journal of Obstetric, Gynecologic, and Neonatal Nursing, 30*(3), 306–315.

Burkhart, C. G. (2006, November). A guide to recognizing and treating herpes. *The Clinical Advisor,* 26–33.

Elkins, B. L., Mayeaux, E. J., & Kodura, S. (2006, August). Bacterial vaginosis: Diagnosis and therapy. *The Female Patient, 31,* 41–46.

Geller, M. L. & Nelson, A. L. (2004). Diagnosis and treatment of recurrent and persistent vaginitis. *Womens Health Gynecology Edition, 4*(3), 137–146.

Geller, M. L, & Nelson, A. L. (2004). Infectious and noninfectious causes of recurrent and persistent vaginitis. *Womens Health Gynecology Edition, 4*(4), 171–178.

Holzman, C., Leventhal, J. M., Qiu, H., Jones, N. M., Wang, J., and the BV study group. (2001). Factors linked to bacterial vaginosis in nonpregnant women. *American Journal of Public Health, 91*(10), 1664–1670.

Huppert, J. S., Batteiger, B. E., Braslins, P., Feldman, J. A., Hobbs, M. M., Sankey, H. Z., et al. (2005). Use of an immunochromatographic assay for rapid detection of trichomonas vaginalis in vaginal specimens. *Journal of Clinical Microbiology, 43,* 684–687.

Klebaqnoff, M. A., Carey, C., Hauth, J. C., Hillier, S. L., Nugent, R. P., Thom, E. A., et al. (2001). Failure of metronidazole to prevent preterm delivery among pregnant women with asymptomatic trichomonas vaginalis infection. *New England Journal of Medicine, 345,* 487–493.

Lichtenstein, V. N., & Nansel, T. R. (2000). Womens douching practices and related attitudes: Findings from four focus groups. *Women & Health, 31*(2/3), 117–131.

Mashburn, J. (2006). Etiology, diagnosis, and management of vaginitis. *Journal of Midwifery & Womens Health, 51,* 423–430.

Ness, R. B., Hillier, S. L., Richter, H. E., Soper, D. E., Stamm, C., McGregor, J., et al. (2002). Douching in relation to bacterial vaginosis, lactobacilli, and facultative bacteria in the vagina. *Obstetrics & Gynecology, 100,* 765–772.

Raphaelidis, L., & Secor, M.C. (2006). Bacterial vaginosis: Diagnosis and treatment update. *Womens Health Care, 5*(3), 21–30.

Sobel, J. D., Ferris, D., Schwebke, J., Nyirjesy, P., Wiesenfeld, H. C., Peipert, J., et al. (2006). Suppressive antibacterial therapy with 0.75% metronidazole vaginal gel to prevent recurrent bacterial vaginosis. *American Journal of Obstetrics and Gynecology, 194,* 1283–1289.

VULVAR CONDITIONS

Arnold, L. D., Bachmann, G. A., Rosen, R., & Rhoads, G. G. (2007). Assessment of vulvodynia symptoms in a sample of US women: A prevalence survey with a nested case control study. *American Journal of Obstetrics & Gynecology, 196*, e1–e6.

Biofeedback Foundation of Europe. (1997). *Electromyography-Vulvovaginal pain disorders* (11th ed.) Brochure. Amersfoort, The Netherlands: Howard Glazer.

Dupree Jones, K., & Tyler Lehr, S. (1994). Vulvodynia: Diagnostic techniques and treatment modalities. *Nurse Practitioner, 19*(4), 34–46.

Fitzpatrick, C. C., DeLancey, J. O., Elkins, T. E., & McGuire, E. J. (1993). Vulvar vestibulitis and interstitial cystitis: A disorder of urogenital sinus derived epithelium. *Obstetrics & Gynecology, 81*, 860–862.

Foster, D. C. (2002). Vulvar disease. *Obstetrics & Gynecology, 100*, 145–163.

Giescke, J., Reed, B., Haefner, H., Giesecke, T., Clauw, D., & Gracely, R. (2004). Quantitative sensory testing in vulvodynia patients and increased peripheral pressure pain sensitivity. *Obstetrics and Gynecology, 104*, 126–133.

Goldstein, A. (2003, September 9). Vaginal pain and itching with no known cause? Retrieved June 22, 2004, from http://www.ourgyn.com/article.

Haefner, H., Khoshnevisan, M., Bachman, J., Flowe-Valencia, H., Green, C., & Reed, B. (2000). Use of the McGill Pain Questionnaire to compare women with vulvar pain, pelvic pain and headaches. *Journal of Reproductive Medicine, 45*, 665–671.

Harlow, B. L., & Stewart, E. G. (2003). A population based assessment of chronic unexplained vulvar pain: Have we underestimated the prevalence of vulvodynia? *Journal of the American Medical Women's Association, 58*, 82–88.

Holland, S. (2003, May). Dysesthetic vulvodynia. *Advance for Nurse Practitioners*, 42–46.

Jerzak, B. & Smith, S. K. (2006). Vulvodynia: Diagnosis and treatment of a chronic pain syndrome. *Women's Health Care, 5*(4), 29–50.

Klaperich, J. (2001, October). An Intimate problem. *Advance for Physician Assistants*, 42–47.

Lotery, H., McClure, N., & Galask, R. (2004). Vulvodynia. *Lancet, 363*, 1058–1060.

McCormack, W. M. (1990). Two urogenital sinus syndromes. Interstitial cystitis and focal vulvitis. *Journal of Reproductive Medicine, 35*, 860–862.

Reed, B. (2006). Vulvodynia: Diagnosis and management. *American Family Physician, 73*, 115–125.

Reed, B., Advincula, A., Fonde, K., Gorenflo, D., & Haefner, H. (2003). Sexual activities and attitudes of women with vulvar dysesthesia. *Obstetrics and Gynecology, 102*, 325–331.

Reed, B., Haefner, H., & Cantor, L. (2003). Vulvar dysesthesia (vulvodynia): A follow up study. *The Journal of Reproductive Medicine, 48*, 409–416.

Sadownik, L. (2000). Clinical profile of vulvodynia patients. *The Journal of Reproductive Medicine, 45*, 679–684.

Schmidt, S., Bauer, A., Grief, C., Merker, A., Elsner, P., & Strauss, B. (2001). Vulvar pain, psychological profiles and treatment responses. *The Journal of Reproductive Medicine, 46*, 377–384.

Stewart, D., Reicher, A., Gerulath, A., & Boydell, K. (1994). Vulvodynia and psychological distress. *Obstetrics and Gynecology, 84*, 587–590.

WEIGHT MAINTENANCE

Avonne, L. J., Blackburn, G. L, & Vash, P. D. (2001). Intervening in the obesity epidemic. *Patient Care for the Nurse Practitioner, 12*, 24.

Bray, G. (2002). Obesity: Is there effective treatment? *Consultant, 42*(8), 1014.

Daniels, J. (2006). Women's descriptions of a successful weight-loss experience: A qualitative study. *The American Journal for Nurse Practitioners, 10*(10), 67–74.

Davis, P., & Krauss, H. (2001). The impact of diet on chronic disease. *Patient Care for the Nurse Practitioner, 25–26, 29, 30.*

Fiegal, K. M., Carroll, M. D., Ogden, C. L., & Johnson, C. L. (2002). Prevalence and trends in obesity among US adults, 199–2000. *Journal of the American Medical Association, 288,* 1723–1727.

Gillman, M. W., Rifas-Shiman, S. L., Berkey, C. S., Frazier, A. L., Rockett, H.R.R., Field, A. E., et al. (2001). Risk of overweight among adolescents who were breastfed as infants. *Journal of the American Medical Association, 285*(19), 2461–2467.

Hogan, S. L. (2005). The effects of weight loss on calcium and bone. *Critical Care Nursing Quarterly, 28,* 269–275.

Hu, F. B., Li, T. Y., Colditz, G. A., Willett, W. C., & Manson, J. E. (2003). Television watching and other sedentary behaviors in relation to risk of obesity and type 2 diabetes mellitus in women. *Journal of the American Medical Association, 289,* 1785–1791.

Kane, A. K., Schatzkin, A., Graubard, B. I., & Schairer, C. (2000). A prospective study of diet quality and mortality in women. *Journal of the American Medical Association, 283*(16), 2109–2115.

National Institutes of Health. (2000). *The practice guide: Identification, evaluation, and treatment of overweight and obesity in adults.* Bethesda, MD: NIH.

Turner, J., Knosby, K., & Popkess-Vawter, S. (2002). Nurse practitioner and client partnerships in long-term holistic weight management. *American Journal of Nurse Practitioners, 6*(6), 9–18.

White, J. H. (2000). Improving outcomes for obesity. *The American Journal for Nurse Practitioners, 4*(10), 9–18.

WOMEN AND HEART DISEASE

Ali, N. S. (2002). Prediction of coronary heart disease preventive behaviors in women: A test of the health belief model. *Women & Health, 35*(1), 83–96.

Anderson, J. K., & Kessenich, C. R. (2001). Women and coronary heart disease. *Nurse Practitioner, 26*(8), 12–31.

Appel, S. J., Harrell, J. S., & Deng, S. (2002). Racial and socioeconomic differences in risk factors for cardiovascular disease among southern rural women. *Nursing Research, 51,* 140–147.

Arslanian-Engoren, C. (2002). Recognizing heart disease. *AWHONN Lifelines, 6*(2), 114–122.

Braun, L. T., & Rosensun, R. S. (2001). Assessing coronary heart disease risk and managing lipids. *Nurse Practitioner, 26*(12), 30–41.

Brown, B. G. & Crowley, J. (2005). Is there any hope for vitamin E? *Journal of the American Medical Association, 293,* 1387–1390.

Grady, D., Herrington, D., Bittner, V., Blumenthal, R., Davidson, M., Hlatky, M., et al. (2002). Cardiovascular disease outcomes during 6.8 years of hormone therapy. *Journal of the American Medical Association, 288,* 49–57.

HOPE and HOPE-TOO Trial Investigators. (2005). Effects of long-term vitamin E supplementation on cardiovascular events and cancer. *Journal of the American Medical Association, 293,* 1338–1347.

Jiang, W., & O'Connor, C. M. (2002). Depression and cardiac health in women: How close is the relationship? *Womens Health in Primary Care, 5*(6), 393–405.

Lee, I. M., Cook, N. R., Gaziano, M., Gordon, D., Ridker, P. M., Manson, J. E., et al. (2005). Vitamin E in the primary prevention of cardiovascular disease and cancer. *Journal of the American Medical Association, 294*, 56–65.

Manson, J. E., Greenland, P., LaCroix, A. Z., Stefanick, M. L., Mouton, C. P., Oberman, A. et al. (2002). Walking compared with vigorous exercise for the prevention of cardiovascular events in women. *New England Journal of Medicine, 347*, 716–725.

Meischke, H., Kuniyuki, A., Yasui, Y., Bowen, D. J., Andersen, R., & Urban, N. (2002). Information women receive about heart attacks and how it affects their knowledge, beliefs, and intentions to act in a cardiac emergency. *Health Care for Women International, 23*(2), 149–162.

Pai, J. K., Pischon, T., Ma, J., Manson, J. E., Hankinson, S. E., Joshipura, K., et al. (2004). Inflammatory markers and the risk of coronary heart disease in men and women. *New England Journal of Medicine, 351*, 2599–2610.

Pradham, A. D., Manson, J. E., Rossouw, J. E., Siscovick, D. S., Moulton, C. P., Rifai, N., et al. (2002). Inflammatory biomarkers, hormone replacement therapy, and incident coronary heart disease. *Journal of the American Medical Association, 288*, 980–987.

Quinlivan, E. P., McPartlin, J., McNulty, H., Ward, M., Strain, J. J., Weir, D. G., et al. (2002). Importance of both folic acid and vitamin B12 in reduction of risk of vascular disease. *Lancet, 359*, 227–228.

Regensteiner, J. G., & Gerhard-Herman, M. (2002). Aging and vascular disease in women. *Womens Health in Primary Care, 5*(4 suppl.), 1–40.

Rick-Edwards, J. W., Kleinman, K., Michels, K. B., Stampfer, M. J., Manson, J. E. Rexrode, K. M., et al. (2005). Longitudinal study of birth weight and adult body mass index in predicting risk of coronary heart disease and stroke in women. *British Medical Journal, 330*, 115.

Sampson, S. M., Lapid, M. I., Moore, K. M., Netzel, P. J., & Rummans, T. A. (2005). Depression in women with heart disease. *Womens Health in Primary Care, 8*, 476–489.

Sawtzky, J. V., & Naimark, B. J. (2005). Cardiovascular health promotion in aging women: Validating a population health approach. *Public Health Nursing, 22*, 379–388.

Sparks, E. A., & Frazier, L. Q. (2002). Heritable cardiovascular disease in women. *Journal of Obstetric, Gynecologic, and Neonatal Nursing, 31*, 217–228.

Wenger, N. K. (2002). How to keep her heart healthy. *Womens Health in Primary Care, 5*(7), 432–442.

Wenger, N. K. (2005). Why do women with acute coronary syndromes fare worse than men? *Womens Health Gynecology Edition, 5*(5), 273–274.

Wenger, N. K. (2005). Prevention of coronary heart disease in women: Challenges and opportunities. *Womens Health in Primary Care, 8*(3), 121–122.

Index